Faster Than Forty

Mark Gomes | Rick Miller

Faster Than Forty

Optimized Message, Inc.

Chicago

Optimized Message, Inc.
111 W Maple St.
Suite 1506
Chicago, IL 60610

ISBN 978-0-988-6266-0-7

DEDICATIONS

To Mom, for giving me life, guidance, and all you had to give. To my coaches, especially Dave, Mr. Hurley, and Mark. Your influence on my development as an athlete and individual were immeasurable. And to my beautiful girlfriend Jamie, who supported me through nearly three grueling years of training and remains by my side through seven years of eccentricities.

~ Mark Gomes

To my family (who have no idea what I do), and to my coaches, teammates, and competition, past and present (who have every idea).

~ Rick Miller

Table of Contents

Prologue

There is no official entry in my training log for February 5, 2009. That's ironic because of how important a day it turned out to be. It was the first day of an epic personal pilgrimage. It was the first day of nearly 1,000 consecutive days of training without a day off. Strung together in a long line, those days culminated in a single day – a few minutes, really – at a track outside of Cleveland, Ohio.

The precursor came in the fall of 2008.

A group of competitors from my college days began an e-mail thread proposing a ridiculous idea – training to compete at the 2011 USA Masters Track & Field Championships. This is the country's premier event for runners age 40 years or older. It's like the Senior PGA Championship in golf, except that most senior golfers gradually transition from the PGA to the senior tour with no discontinuity in competition. Many Masters runners haven't touched a track since their early 20s, and some haven't run a step in years before preparing for this event. This disconnect between golf and track exists because golf, by and large, is fun. Running oftentimes is not. I personally hadn't stepped on a track since 1996.

My last *real* race was in college in the spring of 1992. At Northeastern University, in Boston, I won a New England Championship, placed fifth at the IC4As (one of the largest collegiate track events on the Eastern seaboard), and set a school record in the 1,000-meter run – a record previously held by NCAA All-American and eventual USATF Cross Country Champion, Brad Schlapak.

In 1996, four years removed from college competition and the year after my old teammate Schlapak won the cross country nationals, it wasn't crazy to think that I could run again at a high level. I was only 25 years old. In 1996 I was wrong. After several months of somewhat dedicated training, my race times lagged those from my formative years at Stoughton High School. Exasperated, I sent my track spikes to what I supposed was their final resting place.

In 1996, my intent was to regain competitive parity with the nation's top athletes – athletes who would compete for a berth on the United States Olympic team. I was good, but maybe not that good. But 12 or 13 years later, my interest in a Masters comeback was piqued. I didn't feel much less athletic than I had been in 1996. I had dropped some bad habits, and some of the weight associated with them, and I was littering the field with the exhausted bodies of my Saturday flag football companions – a group of 20-somethings who once excelled on the high school gridiron. I still dominated beer-league hoops games. I thought it possible that my extended athleticism could prove advantageous against the nation's 40-year-old runners. Perhaps the idea wasn't so ridiculous after all. Nonetheless, the kneejerk enthusiasm elicited by the e-mail thread soon gave way to mid-life reality and the notion faded like many others.

A few months passed, then one of the guys resuscitated the Masters e-mail thread. Apparently, some guys had taken the ridiculous idea to heart. A few of them were getting serious. If I was going to throw my hat in the ring, it appeared time for me to get serious too. It was time to decide. Did I really have the capacity to get back in shape and race against the nation's top Masters?

I started jogging: two or three miles at a time, two or three times a week. When I went out for a 3.5-miler on February 5th, 2009, I had no idea it would mark the beginning of the longest training streak of my life. It also marked the beginning of a human laboratory experiment and a research effort much more comprehensive than any class project I ever completed at Northeastern – an effort that, in part, prompted this book.

Who should read this book and why?

➢ We hope any athlete approaching that ominous "Big 4-0" will learn from my experience – not just the training regimen, or the dietary changes, or the injury recovery and prevention techniques (yeah, Ace, at your age you're probably gonna get hurt), but also the psychological factors: the motives that spurred me to do it successfully and the side effects both good and bad.

➢ Even though this book is targeted toward athletes in their 30s and 40s, many high schoolers, collegians and post-collegians who are serious about running faster can benefit from the technical research. I can't tell you how many times – after field-testing a training technique or tweaking my diet – I wondered if my collegiate New England Championship *could* have been an NCAA championship. (Of course when my boys and I were tearing up the college track scene, we didn't give a rat's ass what the blathering old Masters guys were doing, so maybe I am the blathering old guy now.)

➢ Anyone who ran competitively in New England in the late 80s through the mid 90s should find this book highly entertaining. As we explored the psychological factors that motivated me to undertake this quest, we were forced to look at who we were as competitors "back in the day" – and most of these anecdotes took place far from a track or a road race. Runners seem to feel the need to turn everything up a notch – maybe more so than other athletes. This frequently leads to trouble and almost as frequently leads to comedy.

Lastly, here are a few tips about how to read this book... The book is organized chronologically, from that February day when I decided to chase a Masters title until the Masters Championships in 2011. Each chapter contains some common elements:

➢ A story – present day or ancient history – more often than not with a moral...
➢ A day-by-day account of my activity from my workout log
➢ Injury reports or other medical findings
➢ Dietary research or findings
➢ Race reports, records, and results
➢ Miscellaneous research, notes, and anecdotes

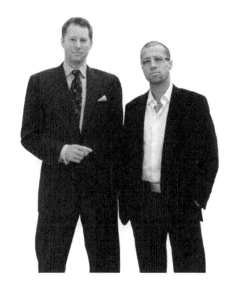

Here's one of many little-known facts you will learn about me in this book: I hate to read. Ironic, I know. But if you hate to read as well, you can skip to whichever element above is most important to you. Also, you can find links to original research sources, updated findings, and other cool stuff at our Web site:

www.fasterthanforty.com

Co-Authors Rick Miller and Mark Gomes, 2011

Neither my co-author nor I have a background in dietary science, exercise physiology, or medicine – however, we are both trained researchers and analysts. We present scientific findings contingent on two factors:

1. We've found enough credible sources to indicate the finding is true, and
2. I've applied the finding during my training in an unbiased manner that permits me to present results.

In the case of my applications, the findings pertain to how a particular tactic affected *me* during training. I may not be representative of how the same tactic would affect others, but rest assured I'm presenting what I learned as objectively and completely as possible. I would add that the science of running better is constantly evolving – in general and for me personally. As we explore new training techniques and technologies, the Faster Than Forty Web site will be the most current source for our findings.

In the case of sourced research, wherever possible we cite and provide links to the original studies or subject matter experts. If the URL to the Web page we cite is short, we provide it. If it is long and difficult to type, we provide the keyword string that will lead you directly to the page using the Google search engine.

Best of luck out there because there really is no finish line. Forty is nothing.

Mark Gomes

Chapter 1
Do Call it a Comeback!

Weeks 1-6

My situation is probably more universal than unique, but I find it a little uncanny – maybe even a little humbling – to think that most of what I am today stems from people I met because of my "first" running career. I manage a small investment research firm that provides analysts at Wall Street banks and hedge funds with the information they need to make smart investments. This is a blessing and a curse for my training regimen: In slow weeks I have an extremely flexible schedule conducive to heavy training; in busy weeks, like during earnings periods, I work ungodly hours and might find myself training at weird times of day.

Overall though, the blessings outweigh the curses – and I may not even have embarked on this career if it hadn't been for Tom Lahive, one of my teammates at Northeastern University. Tom recommended me for my first job "in the industry," and with his early guidance I honed my craft. I got a front-row seat to the Internet boom and bust at the turn of the century, leveraged that experience into more challenging positions, then ultimately left the corporate nest and ventured out on my own.

Running my own firm provides another blessing pertinent to rigorous training: geographic freedom. "Have Internet; will work," is my motto. Free to live anywhere, I convinced my girlfriend Jamie to spend the November-through-April months in warmer climates, paradise for most any athlete or beach-loving young lady. Much of my immediate family lives in Florida – which is where we spend most of our time now – but my journey to the 2011 USA Masters Outdoor Track Championships actually began as we were finishing up a stint in Cancun, Mexico.

The e-mail thread promoting a Masters campaign was still circulating among my old running buddies up in Boston, but although their challenge prompted my interest (and stirred some easy-to-stir competitiveness), it was a series of deeper thoughts that finally made me pull the trigger.

When I joined the Northeastern University track team in the fall of 1988, I had enough chips on my shoulder to stock Vegas for years; it's a wonder I could move my legs from all the weight. The resentment fueled me, and I burned that fuel efficiently: I won a New England Championship in the 1,000-meter run my first year (an unusual feat by a freshman), then set a school-record 2:24.5 over the same distance at the same meet a year later. But perhaps it was too much too soon. I beat the people I wanted to beat, put my name in the school's history books, and not long after, my attention span began to wane.

I encountered some of the same distractions every college athlete encounters – keg parties and girls – but ironically I was also distracted by school itself, by *life*. A business major, I took my studies to heart; I even launched a couple of businesses and started trading stocks from my off-campus apartment. Beating the market and making money became a more interesting game than running, and the frenzied pace catered to my self-diagnosed ADD. By my third year at Northeastern I was clearly going through the motions on the track. When my close friend and younger teammate Erik Nedeau came along and clipped my 1,000-meter record (first with a 2:22.5, then with an NCAA-leading 2:20.9), I didn't even have the urge to fight for it back...

...and it probably wouldn't have mattered.[1]

Mark Lech, the highly decorated track and cross country coach at Northeastern (now turning out sub-4:00 milers at the University of Maine) tried to find ways to motivate me, but no pep talk, no consulting session in his office, no subtle reminders that I was no longer the team prodigy inspired me. After four years of high school track and a few years of college, I was just bored with running around in circles.

It may have been a coach's last-ditch effort out of loyalty and love, or it may have been a cruel and unusual punishment – or a little of both – but when the outdoor track season started, Lech had a stroke of genius: run me in the steeplechase. It was three times as long as my specialty distance, and I'd have to jump large wooden hurdles and a water pit for six out of the seven-plus laps of the race. We had no one of note competing in the event. One of our cross country specialists ran it, but he could barely negotiate the water pit. One time he ditched so violently, we thought we'd have to call a lifeguard.

Coach Lech's gambit worked. The idea actually excited me – the barriers and water pit added an element of danger to an otherwise boring sport. I started practicing hurdle technique right away. I upped my mileage, regularly running from Northeastern's downtown campus to the athletic facilities in suburban Dedham (almost 10 miles), then I'd train over hurdles and the water pit until the bus was ready to bring everyone back to campus.

My first race was a win against Harvard in a time of 9:35, a pretty good showing for a first-time steeplechaser. The next time out I won again – against stiffer competition, in a faster time. I was motivated! If my progress continued apace and I could dip under 9:00, I'd have a legitimate shot at qualifying for the NCAA Championships. Lech enlisted the aid of a Northeastern University legend, All-America steeplechaser Bruce Bickford, to foster my unexpected success.[2] But Bruce was a fundamentally different animal than I was. Bruce was a distance runner by nature, who had enough athletic ability to hurdle the steeplechase's unforgiving barriers; I was an athlete that hurdled barriers by nature and happened to have built up enough endurance to cover the distance. His first change to my routine: land *in* the water pit with one foot for optimal efficiency. (My instinctive technique was to stay *dry*... I was easily jumping over the *entire* water pit and carrying about my business while the other runners were landing in it and running the better part of two miles with wet feet.)

My next race out was against Brown University. I attacked the first water pit with The Bicker's suggestion in mind, timing my landing to place one foot on the incline of the water pit. Everything went perfectly, except that when my lead foot landed on the incline, I sprained my ankle so severely it would be the last competitive race of my college career. I still finished the race in 9:15 – landing on NU's all-time steeplechase list in the process – but all things considered, my college career went out with a whimper.

Then college ended. Life moved on, and I spent my 20s and 30s chasing a career, not school records and NCAA qualifying times – and the former kept me busy enough not to think about the latter... for the most part. But regret is a complicated emotion. Depending on its cause, it can blur and fade over time or lay dormant below the surface, perfectly preserved.

When my Masters training streak started on February 5th 2009, I probably wasn't really conscious of my regrets from years past. I didn't speak about them with anyone – even my best friends and teammates (many of whom are still one and the same). When one of my college roommates, Dennis Shine, came to spend a week's vacation in Cancun with Jamie and I, it was clearly evident he wasn't missing competitive running or suffering the emotional strain of unfinished business. He could have reason to: He was a standout miler at Bishop Hendricken High School in

---

1 "Ned" went on to rewrite most of Northeastern's record books, compete in three Olympic Trials, and eventually win a bronze medal for the United States in the 1995 IAAF World Indoor Championships in Spain in the 1,500-meter run.

2 "The Bicker," as decades of Northeastern athletes affectionately call Bruce, was ranked #1 in the world at 10,000 meters and represented the U.S. in the 1988 Summer Olympics. He was an All-America steeplechaser at Northeastern in the late 70s.

Rhode Island, and when he joined the Northeastern team a few people thought he could be a four-minute guy, but the inevitable injuries that come with Division-I running kept him off the track enough to quell his motivation.[3] He hadn't appeared too regretful in the years after college, and isn't to this day. That could be Dennis' personality; he was the first guy on the team to take me under his wing and introduce me to aspects of life beyond the oval (namely wine, women and song), and he tends to live in the moment – but most of the other guys didn't appear to be missing anything either.

"Been runnin'?" is a mandatory question any time one of us picks up the phone to catch up with another.

"Eh, you know…" is the common reply, indicating the respondent is either living a life of complete sloth or at most logging the cursory three or four miles, three or four times a week. If one of the guys offhandedly mentions running a local 5K or admits he has strung together more than two weeks of a training streak, inboxes around the country light up with sarcastic e-mails.

But if I was leaning toward a comeback of any sort when I started my streak that February 5th, shuffling along the scenic Cancun running path with one of the old crew matching me step for step definitely pushed me over the edge. Literally and figuratively I was off to the races – with the next six weeks leading up to my first one in almost 12 years.

Training Log Week 1			
Day	Date	Notes	Mileage[4]
Thurs.	2/5/09	No entry	3.5
Fri.	2/6/09	4.8 miles at medium pace w/Dennis Shine, former Northeastern University miler.	4.8
Sat.	2/7/09	Dennis not exactly in "top form." This a.m. we did 2 miles and that was it for him. Additional afternoon 7 miles for me. Slow (55 min), but didn't feel like a crawl either. Could've gone further. Happy with it.	9.0
Sun.	2/8/09	Easy 5 miles with Dennis at 11a. It killed him. He crashed and slept until 4:30p. I ran 4 more miles on my own in the evening.	9.0
Mon.	2/9/09	No entry	4.5
Tues.	2/10/09	Dennis left today, but I feel like I'm building momentum. He was good for my morale, which is important because it's tough to get out every day and put in more and more miles. I realize despite 8+ years of running experience, I know little about how to train!	5.0
Weds.	2/11/09	OK… I've officially got a running streak going. Seven whole days. Yesterday felt rough, but ran a good 5 miles today -- 6:45 pace for the first 4 miles before hitting a wall.	5.0
Total		Averaged 7:43 per mile for the week	**40.8**

Injury Reports and Medical Findings

The scariest part of starting a training routine is "not knowing what you don't know." This especially pertains to injuries. I noticed problems with my calf muscles and the surrounding areas by Week 2, but was I truly injured, or were these the aches and pains associated with running seriously again after a long layoff? I had no idea.

---

3 In a fact little known to anyone – probably not even to Dennis Shine himself – his Bishop Hendricken 4 x 1,600m relay team still holds the Rhode Island state record (17:59.8), one of the oldest in the Rhode Island high school record books.

4 "Mileage" in one sense is extremely straightforward: the number of miles run on a given day. Some days, however, injury or workout strategy prevented me from running in the traditional sense. Mileage may include distance covered on an elliptical machine or converted distance from a stair workout or other activity. The "Miscellaneous" section of this chapter goes into more detail on our conversion processes. The "Notes" column in the log will clearly explain when I trained on a machine instead of traditional running.

Training Log Week 2

Day	Date	Notes	Mileage
Thurs.	2/12/09	5.5 miles. Took it easy for the first 3, but faster for the rest. Should've taken it easy for the whole run.	5.5
Fri.	2/13/09	4.8 miles very slow. Did some wind sprints, but for the most part didn't push it.	4.8
Sat.	2/14/09	3.5 miles at 6:40 pace. Felt some strains yesterday, so I planned to go slow... but I felt good, so I went with it (without pushing too hard). Fastest I've run since before this running streak started.	3.5
Sun.	2/15/09	Planned on 5 miles at 8:00 pace but felt real strong and picked it up every couple of miles. Ended up w/7.2 miles at 7:26, with the last mile under 6:30. Easily best run to date.	7.2
Mon.	2/16/09	Nice easy 5 miles as planned. Pace was almost exactly the same as yesterday but felt much slower. I think it's odd that I'm going to miss running the same course every day when we leave Cancun. I'm more concerned to lose the 500m markers on the running path. I can see them 15-25 sec ahead. They pull me toward them and I feed on imaginary cheers as I pass.	5.0
Tues.	2/17/09	A little further, a little faster. Felt basically the same as yesterday.	5.1
Weds.	2/18/09	Long day. 8 miles in 60 min. Was listening to a boring conference call on MP3, which made the extra miles even tougher to get through.	8.0
Total		Averaged 7:36 per mile for the week	**39.1**

Training Log Week 3

Day	Date	Notes	Mileage
Thurs.	2/19/09	Felt *great* today. 8.2 miles in less than 60 min (15 sec faster per mile than yesterday). Final mile around 6:40. Pushed the pace, but felt near effortless from start to finish.	8.2
Fri.	2/20/09	Felt slower, but somehow ran the same time. No matter. Miles are miles.	8.2
Sat.	2/21/09	8 miles in 56 min. Best effort yet. Stayed relaxed and slowly picked it up as I went.	8.0
Sun.	2/22/09	Easy day. Shuffled through a slow 8 miles. Thought I was at 8:00 pace, but turned out to be 8:14... Does it really matter?	8.0
Mon.	2/23/09	4.2 miles at 6:44 pace. Last day in Cancun.	4.2
Tues.	2/24/09	First run back in Boston. 40+ degrees, but felt like 20. Ran for 60 min and felt like about 7:30 pace (8 miles)... I'll measure it later.	8.0
Weds.	2/25/09	No numbers today... I just ran. Didn't know the time until I got back. Didn't measure the course until afterward. Turned out to be 6.8 miles at 7:05 pace. I prefer the numbers! Thank God for the weather: 52 degrees. No Cancun, but could have been worse.	6.8
Total		Averaged 7:20 per mile for the week	**51.4**

In Hindsight – *Early on, I prioritized my training like this: workouts at 70 percent importance, diet at 15 percent importance, and recovery at 15 percent importance. As such, my approach to injuries and recovery was "ice and ignore." I assumed the sore spots would eventually acclimate to the rigors of training – after all, they used to in college. Nothing was further from the truth. I now prioritize training, diet, and recovery each at 33 percent importance. To this day, my calves respond negatively to multiple sessions of heavy pounding, so I counter this with aggressive cross-training and professional physical therapy. And as you'll see, my approach to diet also changed significantly.*

Training Log Week 4			
Day	Date	Notes	Mileage
Thurs.	2/26/09	Ran 30 min out and 30 min back. Labored. Felt sluggish.	8.0
Fri.	2/27/09	Ate extra carbs last night and this morning (to help with the recent sluggishness) and ran on an elliptical machine to go easy on my calves, which have been a little sore since Week 1. The soreness hasn't been bad, but it has been a constant, albeit ignored, aspect of my training. I've been stretching, to no avail. I should start icing and consider a real pair of running shoes instead of my cross-trainers. Completed a hard 47 min on the elliptical, and a 13-min run home from the gym. 60 min total at a strong pace. Workout was easily an 8-mile equivalent. Very quick. More accomplished than yesterday.	8.0
Sat.	2/28/09	Slow and cold 8 miles. 65 min. Putting money in the bank one penny at a time today. Didn't worry about pace; just got it done. More worried about the soreness in my lower right leg. Definitely a weak spot, but hopefully it's just another body part getting used to the daily pounding.	8.0
Sun.	3/1/09	Another slow, cold day. Only 4+ miles in 33 min. Leg feels no better, but no worse either.	4.2
Mon.	3/2/09	Ran indoors today. *Much* prefer an indoor 11-lap track to going outside. My injuries felt better and I ran faster, longer. The gym worker told me it was a 10-lap track, but I figured it wasn't when I finished 5 miles at 5:50 pace... So, it was really 4.5 miles at 6:25 pace. Still pretty good. As soon as I got the laps-per-mile figured out, I ran another 2 miles at the same pace. I went back and did another 3.5 miles at 7:15 to make it an even 110 laps (10 miles) for the day. I was only a little fatigued afterward. Also, the injury feels fine.	10.0
Tues.	3/3/09	Another day of "alternative" training. Stayed in my apartment building and did repeat stairs... 33 floors, just under 4:00 per set. Based on my experience, each set is equal to about 2/3 of a mile (1,073 meters). I did 11 sets, which is something north of 7 miles. *Very* challenging, but easy on the injuries. Passed out right after dinner, then awoke in the middle of the night.	7.0
Weds.	3/4/09	Same workout as yesterday, but took it slower. Hoping to get on a track soon, but stairs are ok for now. I can feel the cardio effect, as well as the strain in my calves and thighs.	7.0
Total		Averaged 7:19 per mile for the week	52.2

Dietary Research and Findings

Diet is an important aspect of the training regimen that I initially overlooked for several reasons:

First, training at the collegiate level, no one on my team ever put much thought into diet; it was highly unusual to realize any real weight gain no matter what we ate. We operated on a calories-in/calories-out model with no concern for what the calories were made of or how they might affect performance, and certainly no one kept a log. If one of the guys had brought up the topic of diet, I can just imagine the remarks they'd have heard from the rest of the team. ("Aw, is Nancy having trouble fitting in her prom dress? If you're feeling self-conscious, increase your mileage, jackass.") If anything, we purposely flaunted our jacked-up metabolisms and our high caloric burn rates via all sorts of eating and drinking contests.

What a lot of us failed to realize, however, was that when college ended and we dialed back our training (or stopped altogether), we should have adjusted our diets accordingly. In our defense, because we were so fit for so long, few of us saw real weight gain in a short time frame – certainly not in a few months or even a couple of years after graduation. Fat is a slow, stealthy demon.

A second reason we paid little attention to diet: correlating diet to performance is very difficult. Did you just run your fastest 5K because you changed your carb-to-protein ratio, or was it because you increased your mileage several weeks back? Unless you're documenting everything in great detail and purposely keeping some training variables constant, it's hard to quantify diet's true effect. For a lot of athletes, even if they are casually thinking about diet, if they fall off the wagon for a few days or longer, their thought process is, "I'll up my training for the next few days to recoup." Then their diet discipline starts to falter.

Side Track: Eating for Sport

My first instance of competitive eating occurred at an off-campus dwelling dubbed "The Townhouse." The Townhouse was a three-floor apartment less than a mile from Northeastern University, within earshot of Fenway Park. For budgetary reasons, countless runners, pseudo-runners, and interesting third parties inhabited The Townhouse, including teammates, Dennis Shine and Tom Lahive.

One night after practice, I was preparing my dinners for the week. I was on a tight budget, and because of this I ate a lot of store-brand spaghetti – usually cooking it up by the boxful and rationing it over several days. This same night, on our front porch, Lahive was barbequing up a storm. He had double or triple the food budget I had, so his eating habits didn't much differ from the home cooking he was used to – and the depressing scent of charring steak filled The Townhouse. He stumbled into the kitchen, spatula still in hand, and eyed up my bulk batch of spaghetti. "Holy Moly!" his jester-like voice screeched, purposely trying to sound as sarcastically corny as possible. "You gonna eat all that?"

"Over the next few days, I am," I dryly replied, somehow knowing this wasn't going to be the end of the conversation.

"I dare you to eat it all right now."

"Now? If I eat this now, I won't have anything to eat for the rest of the week."

"If you pound that down, I'll feed you for the rest of the week," he challenged, waving a barbequed slab of meat in front of my face. For him, this was entertainment. For me, it was a chance to eat like home for a week. The bet was on:

➢ One full box, regular spaghetti
➢ One full jar, Prego spaghetti sauce
➢ One pound (precooked) ground beef
➢ 2 liters, store-brand fruit punch

I was not allowed to vomit at any point, and I had to finish the entire meal before the time was up.[5] I downed the first half in about 15 minutes. After that, I started pacing myself. Good thing I did. After 30 minutes I was pretty full and had to stand up to continue. I took smaller bites and smaller sips. With 20 minutes to go. I started sweating – literally and figuratively. The bites and sips got ever smaller with each passing minute. With 10 minutes left, there was still a half-pound of food and a half-pint of drink remaining. I looked down at my fork and had a flashback to Monty Python: *It's only wafer thin...* My stomach heaved in defiance. It was not easy, but I finished, and because The Townhouse offered plenty of witnesses, the concept of the eating contest gained a lot of notoriety. It was the first of many such competitions...

Third, most people like to eat! (I definitely fall into that category.) And many people consider eating one of the great rewards of heavy training. Just the thought of giving up one of life's simple pleasures while they put their body through more and more hell is too much to bear.

When I started my Masters training I felt I had a pretty good diet. I had matured out of my college/early-20s diet – which included a *lot* of presweetened cereal for breakfast, a *lot* of super-sized steak & Swiss or pastrami & Swiss grinders for lunch, and steak with pasta at least three times a week for dinner – and I moved on to more fish and chicken, with even some vegetables mixed in here and there. But even my "more mature" eating approach was not

---

5 Note: Total calorie count is roughly 3,600 (which in hindsight doesn't sound as bad as it felt, even though that's more than a full day's worth of fuel for the typical human – double for a female! By weight, including the drink, the meal was close to 9 lbs.)

enough to offset the performance plateaus I would encounter as my training progressed. In future chapters, the Dietary Research and Findings section will document very specific changes I made to my diet to best enhance my training.

I would argue these changes can benefit *all* runners, not just Masters.

Miscellaneous Research and Notes

Relative Effort: One challenge runners of all types face is measuring relative effort in reliable ways. In northern climates you likely must alternate between indoor training and outdoor training, depending on the weather. If you travel for work, you probably find yourself facing drastically different equipment from fitness center to fitness center as you bounce from hotel to hotel.

The biggest challenge in determining relativity occurs when you're forced to compare non-running activity to running activity. Doing a session on an elliptical machine or an exercise bike is obviously different than running on the roads or even a treadmill. And running on a treadmill is still different than running on the roads. The key *benefit* from a bike or elliptical is that you escape the pounding associated with the roads and treadmills. The key *drawback* is that you escape the pounding associated with the roads and treadmills – that pounding is strengthening muscles and tendons and preparing you for the rigors of racing. In the early stages of my training, I was focused on building my aerobic capacity, and I found the elliptical machine did a good job of that while coming the closest to mimicking a natural running gait without impact.

So how do you find relativity and a mileage "equivalent" between a machine and a run on the roads? Clearly it's not a direct correlation. Several variables affect your true level of effort (incline, resistance setting, machine lubrication level, etc.), so the first task is understanding what "effort" feels like.

If you're a novice runner, you may want to run a time trial to determine your starting level of fitness.[6] If you think you can do so without getting hurt, after a few days of easy running to get your legs under you, run a couple of miles at near-maximum effort on your local track (or hop in a 5K). Now you know what your race pace is (or 100-percent effort). After a few days of recovery and rest, try the same distance again, purposely running at what feels about 70- or 75-percent effort. Assess how you feel and check the pace. Practice running at this pace for a few days, then pick your machine of choice and try to duplicate the same level of effort over a similar period of exercise time. You may have to do this a couple of times because the machine will feel different at first – for bikes and ellipticals you're using different muscle groups, and even treadmills (with their moving belt) might require a try or two to effectively mimic outdoor running and the right level of effort. But now you should be able to make some comparisons...

 In Hindsight – *One piece of technology that helps solve the conversion conundrum is a heart rate monitor. I researched heart-rate training late in my Masters comeback, and this type of training proved useful on many levels – not just for comparing relative effort but for governing recovery between intervals and days between hard-workouts. Heart rate training requires a dedication to data and a level of patience many beginning runners can't stomach; hence why we provide the simple guidelines for comparative effort in this chapter. But my co-author and I have concluded that the heart rate monitor is essential for athletes that want to optimize their time investment in training. As more elite athletes adopt this tool, it will be an essential part of any training program.*

---

6 Former competitive runners probably won't need to do a time trial to assess their fitness levels. It only took me a few days of three-mile runs to figure out a comfortable training pace for distance runs when I began the streak.

Training Log Week 5

Day	Date	Notes	Mileage
Thurs.	3/5/09	Temp in the high 30s, so I got out in shorts, a t-shirt, and a long-sleeve. 8 miles, 1 hr. Still tired from the past couple days on the stairs, but it was good to be moving horizontally again. Stopped at Reggie Lewis Center to check memberships. The old NU equipment manager (Jack) works there. His daughter Lisa graduated a couple years after me and has 3 kids now, including an 11-year old daughter. Crazy!	8.0
Fri.	3/6/09	Ran the same 8-mile course as yesterday. Equal time. Equal sluggishness. Felt sluggish for the past few days. My diet, plus too many consecutive fatiguing workouts may be the culprit... so I ate and slept very well last night. If I'm still weak, I'll rest tomorrow with an easy "day off" 4-miler.	8.1
Sat.	3/7/09	Much better today. Ran a bit over a mile with Jamie (her first 1+ mile run ever). Very slow, but I was supporting her and trying to loosen up for my run. About 30 min later I did just under 7 miles at just under 7:00 pace. Still felt a little sluggish, but 7:00 is a lot better than 7:30, so no complaints.	8.1
Sun.	3/8/09	Great run. Went out not knowing if I'd go 6, 7, or 8 miles. Established a comfortable pace. By Mile 2 it was clear I'd go 8. Got to the Reggie Lewis Center 30 sec faster than usual (7:10 pace) and felt much better than usual. The 4-mile mark is the highest point of the run. As I started downhill I picked it up. By Mile 6 I had a chance to break 56:00 for the run, so I picked it up more. Crossed 8 miles at 55:51. Ended fast, but didn't tax myself. Rest and food seems to have broken me out of that sluggish funk.	8.1
Mon.	3/9/09	Thought I'd do a short run but ended up going 7.4 miles. Went out at an average pace and relaxed all the way back. 32 degrees but didn't feel that bad.	7.4
Tues.	3/10/09	Went out for a relaxed 8 mile *jog*. Checked my watch at the Reggie Lewis Center (3.7-mile mark) and realized I hadn't started it. Guessing it was about 27:00 at that point (7:18 pace), because I kept the same pace and did the last 4.3 miles in 31:06 (7:14 pace). Overall the run was faster than I thought I was going.	8.0
Weds.	3/11/09	Ran a *slow* 20-min warm-up with Jamie (at her request). 30 min later, I went out for a fairly hard 7 miles. Started 7:45 for the first mile and then went sub-7 the rest of the way. First 3.5 miles in 25:30 (7:17 pace). Final 3.5 miles in 23:49 (6:48 pace).	8.1
Total		Averaged 7:15 per mile for the week	**55.7**

Training Log Week 6

Day	Date	Notes	Mileage
Thurs.	3/12/09	Set out to take it easy today after yesterday's tougher run. Was doing the same 8-mile course at about 7:15 pace without much trouble, then my high-ankle/lower-calf started acting up after 5 miles. Around 6 miles, I decided to stop and stretch it out. Gingerly jogged straight home. Ice and anti-inflammatories tonight. Should've been more diligent about that over the last several nights. Gotta be more careful...	7.6
Fri.	3/13/09	Needed to rest the calf, so I did stairs today. It's been 2 wks since I've done less than 7-miles worth of effort, so this was an off day of sorts. For what it's worth, I cruised up the stairs faster than ever... a 14-sec/mile pace improvement (converted) vs. 2 wks ago.	5.0
Sat.	3/14/09	1-hr run in Uncasville, CT... all hills! Modest pace due to my leg injury. The Cambridge Boys[7] were unanimous in what they think the problem is. They suggested using a roller on the affected area.	8.0
Sun.	3/15/09	Back to the same old Boston 8-miler. Started slow to test the leg and picked it up as the run wore on. Went out in roughly 31:00 (7:45 pace) and came back in 27:00 (6:45 pace). Leg is still sore, but holding steady. Iced, did the roller thing, and stretched my hamstrings. Hopefully one of those activities will cure the injury.	8.0
Mon.	3/16/09	Did a hard 1 hr on an inclined elliptical machine today. Low impact on the body, but good work. Leg is feeling better.	8.5
Tues.	3/17/09	Monster day: 8 miles in 53:42 (6:43 pace). Bested last week's record by over 1 min. Out in 27:40 (6:55), back in 26:02 (6:31). No aches. No pains. Leg felt great. Felt a little sick after. Just like the old days...	8.0
Weds.	3/18/09	Virtual "day off." Ran 6 miles at 8:00 pace. Was a bit tired from yesterday, and I didn't want to risk injury. Did a lot of icing. Will probably also go easy tomorrow, to prepare for Sunday (first road race in years!)	6.0
Total		Averaged 7:10 per mile for the week	**51.1**

---

7 "The Cambridge Boys" was our nickname for the late 80s and early 90s standouts from Boston's Cambridge Rindge & Latin High School – many of whom competed against Northeastern University at the college level. Jamahl Prince (Boston College), Scott Cody (Providence College), Lance Campbell (Westfield State), Kenny Forde (Brandeis), Karim-Ben Saunders (Auburn) and Ramon Neves (Boston College) – all coached by Rindge & Latin's Frank McCarthy and Robert McGuire – were a few of the guys in this elite group.

If you can cover four miles in 30 minutes when running outdoors at 75-percent effort (7:30 pace) and 4.5 miles in 30 minutes when using the elliptical at the same effort (6:40 pace) – remember to use a consistent resistance setting on the machine – you now understand your relative pace from machine to road.

My co-author, Rick Miller, developed the following relativity metrics for bikes and treadmills while he was training for the Boston Marathon, when the bad New England weather and narrow, snow-covered roads forced him inside for roughly 30 percent of his training:

➢ Bike effort is equal to roughly 45 percent of road running effort; thus a 30-minute ride that yields 10 miles is equal to 4.5 miles on the roads.
➢ Treadmill effort versus road-running effort is close to 1:1 if you set the machine somewhere between a 0.5-percent to 1.0-percent grade, but in time-trial scenarios the treadmill still skews faster (up to 10 seconds faster per mile than what you might achieve on the roads).

Miller will tell you he ran like crap at Boston, but a 2:44 marathon with only four months of training – where one-third of that training was indoors – sounds pretty good to me.

Similarly, I've developed the following metric to estimate beach running (hard pack, not loose sand) versus road running:

➢ Road Time Equivalent = Beach Time minus 10 percent (e.g., a 7:20 mile – or 440 seconds – on sand is the rough equivalent of a 6:36 mile on paved road)

The only conversion rate I could not establish on a reliable basis was elliptical time to road time. Resistance settings and machine lubrication seem to vary too dramatically from brand to brand and even machine to machine when sticking with the same brand of equipment. I also found that the longer the elliptical session, the easier it was to hold pace because my muscles were spared the pounding they would take on the roads.

Nonetheless, here's another *very important* fact to keep in mind: All relativity metrics become moving targets over time. As your fitness improves, you'll be covering more ground with your 75-percent effort. Where you used to run 30 minutes at 75-percent effort and log 4.0 miles, soon you'll be running the same time and logging 4.5 miles. The corollary numbers on the machines will move as well and may even skew – especially if you spend an abnormal amount of time on one machine.[8] My opinion is, the numbers in your training log won't make you better; your actual effort will.

Final point for this chapter: Some of you may read the times and distances in my training log and be put off by them... "He ran four miles at 8:00 pace and he thinks that's an *easy* recovery day?" Or, "He ran a 5-mile road race at 6:00 pace and he thought that was *hard*?!?"

When I started this quest, a 75-percent-effort training run was about 7:30 pace – much, much slower than my typical training pace during my college days, but much, much faster than anything my girlfriend (a beginner) has ever run in her life. The times and distances in my log are relative; learn from my tactics and the progress of my fitness over time and apply my lessons accordingly based on who *you* are as a runner.

---

8 During an extended injury, Miller spent so much time on the bike that he could easily turn out 11 miles in 30 minutes at 75-80% effort – which at the 45% conversion rate would be 4.95 miles of running (6:02 per mile). His real running rate was actually much slower at that time, especially because the injury kept him off the roads for so long.

Chapter 2
Check One, Two; Bring it On…

Weeks 7-13

What prompts people to dedicate most (if not all) of their personal time to perfecting a sport? More specifically, what sparks a person to dedicate themselves to a seemingly thankless sport like running? In Chris Lear's fantastic book, *Running with the Buffaloes*, he quotes University of Colorado Cross Country coach Mark Wetmore thusly:

> "In football, you might get your bell rung, but you go in with the expectation that you might get hurt, and you hope to win and come out unscathed. As a distance runner, you know you're going to get your bell rung. Distance runners are experts at pain, discomfort, and fear. You're not coming away feeling good. It's a matter of how much pain you can deal with…"

This may be the truest comparison statement ever made between running and any of the so-called "glamour sports" – or even the comparison between competitive running and health-oriented jogging. Add to this truism a few more unpleasant facts:

➢ Most runners, even many pros, receive limited financial incentives or perks. If you're the 32nd-best wide receiver in the nation, you will make millions; if you're the 32nd-fastest 5,000-meter runner in the nation, you will make a smattering of low-level prize money from regional-level races and *maybe* an endorsement or two. You might never compete at Nationals.
➢ On college campuses all athletes enjoy some sexual appeal, but track guys – with their lanky builds and perpetually haunted facial expressions – still get far less play than their football or baseball counterparts. (Female runners, however, usually enjoy quite a bit of attention.)
➢ Even practices offer little joy. Where a soccer player might experience the intrinsic thrill of threading two defenders and scorching a goal off the far post during a scrimmage, a runner's enjoyment usually comes from negotiating a particularly challenging workout slightly faster or slightly less painfully than he did the week before.

So why do it?

Although neither author of this book is a trained psychologist, we've spent enough time hanging around a track or in the slop of a cross country course – and enough time hanging around other runners – to *begin* to understand. For some runners, the urge to compete through running is primal; it is a need to dominate and impose their will on those around them by forcing them to endure pain. Others have something to prove: the need to wave their medals from the podium and say, "I told you so." Maybe worse than either of those is the accumulated sense of immortality many runners acquire when they have elevated their fitness to near super-human proportions – a concept we'll explore later in this book.

In some cases, size, coordination, or other physical limitations drive people to run because no other sport is an option.[9] In yet other cases, they run for a sense of community and a general sense of fitness – but in real

---

9 We would argue that this happens far less frequently than non-runners would like to believe. Some of the guys on Northeastern University's track and cross country teams in the 80s and 90s could have played tennis or baseball or other sports. They just didn't.

competitors the latter motive is rare. It's a sinister finding, but all too true. Although non-runners often generalize the sect as a bunch of free-spirited health nuts seeking peace of mind, body and the purported runner's high, most competitive runners entered the sport as brutal sadomasochists, with health, fitness and a positive sense of accomplishment being fortuitous byproducts buried deep in a darker subtext. By 35 or 40 years old, health, fitness, and accomplishment may move toward the forefront of the list of motives, but for many of the characters in this book, they weren't what originally drew them to the sport as young athletes.

One frequently recounted story in Northeastern University track lore, depicting the vicious nature of the competition and the irreverence of the competitors, involved a distance runner named Matt (last name redacted to protect the guilty). In a tough 5,000-meter race on the track, Matt battled a runner from a rival college back and forth for all 12.5 laps. He prevailed in the final stretch, with both runners turning in close-to-personal-best times – something in the high 14-minute range. They hobbled to the infield grass, the other runner collapsing in a heap and vomiting violently. Matt staggered toward him, and anyone in the stands probably assumed he was offering some consolation. Matt's actual statement as he stood above his heaving opponent: "You're a fag."

As a child, I don't recall any particular athletic talent of note, and I wasn't shepherded toward any specific sport from a young age. I was the first of three children to my Cape Verdean parents, and the first in my family to be born in America. If you ask the women of Cape Verde, they'll tell you that Cape Verdean men are boisterous, headstrong, unfaithful and hard to satisfy. They'll also tell you that they are overzealous disciplinarians, partial to corporal punishment – U.S. translation: child abuse – and prone to alcoholism. (If you ask me, I'll tell you that the women of Cape Verde know their men.)

My father was most of these things, as was his father before him. To be fair, he wasn't a stumbling drunk – nor did he ever throw a clenched fist my way – but his brand of justice exhibited torturous creativity. I grew up in abject fear of missteps. "Good enough" never was, and great could always be much better. Obviously this didn't make for a fun childhood, and I volunteer these details only to provide some background about *my* motives to run competitively at higher and higher levels. One example:

During my senior year at Stoughton High School, I competed at the Massachusetts South Shore Principals Meet. This is a regional competition, one step below state-championship level. I won the 800-meter run in a school-record 1:55.1. I also earned bronze medals in the triple jump and 4 x 100-meter relay.[10] I arrived home, my neck encumbered with medals. They clinked and clanked noisily with each step I took toward the kitchen, where I usually could find my mother. I was halfway there when my father emerged from the bedroom. Our paths met, and I looked up at him in silence. Part of me hoped that one of my medals would speak out, "Hey! Check these out!" but the medals had gone silent, too.

"How'd you do?" he inquired.

To be honest, it wasn't out of character for him to ask. Still, I was a bit surprised... encouraged, even. My posture perked up, causing the medals to jangle a little.

"I won the half-mile and got third in the triple jump and 4 x 100!"

He inspected the medals, looked me in the eye, and said, "You'll do better next time." Then, he noted that my eyes were bloodshot and asked if I was taking drugs. Situations like these were murder on my self-esteem. However, they contributed to my hyperactive competitive drive, albeit in perverse and otherwise damaging ways. To his credit, I believe that my father gained a later-in-life understanding of these traits and their impact on his kids. Nonetheless, the effects of his rearing still echo through my core, and those of my siblings.

---

10 The oddity of this combination of events is not lost on me...

The chip on my shoulder that I carried from childhood wasn't the only factor that fueled my competitiveness in high school and college (future chapters will examine others) – and at age 40, many of my negative motivators have fallen away, although as I acknowledged in the prior chapter, not all have.

Whether you're training to be a standout Masters runner or you're just entering college, understanding your motives is important for one very tangible reason: pride, hate, desire, regret – these are powerful emotions that can drive you to ignore everything during your quest... including your risk of injury.

We have a saying: A great coach knows how to break you – *and* how to keep you from breaking yourself. I've been fortunate to have known a few great coaches in my career, and as I progressed beyond the first six weeks of my Masters training, it turned out I'd be calling on some of them.

As a kid back at Stoughton High School I found a role model that I still consult today: our winter and spring track coach, Dave Barbato. Coach Dave came across like a big brother or even one of the guys, but despite his peer-like presence, he was (and remains to this day) a hard-nosed, headstrong coach and individual. His toughness was superseded only by his principles, and he was a great runner in his own right. He set a Stoughton High School record in the two-mile run (9:34), which I believe still stands. He would accompany the high school team on runs and bring us to local road races – where he would routinely win by setting a near-reckless pace... and maintaining it. He impressed his tough training and racing style upon the entire team. Under Dave's tutelage, I broke several school records and won many titles. Most notably, my senior year when we traveled to Princeton, NJ, where I took first-place in the Eastern States Meet 1,000-yard run.

Dave augmented my competitive nature through example, not through a fear of discipline or verbal dismantling. Even as a 40-year-old, I still consult him, and in the next phase of my Masters training I did again – especially as I was about to begin racing.

Technical Tip – *Much effort is being devoted to the study of "athletic identity" and the transition from participation in sports at an elite level (usually intercollegiate or better) to a lifestyle that includes sports at recreational levels or less. In his senior thesis at St. Thomas University, Matt Kiss[11] reports that many collegiate and professional athletes are expected to possess strong athletic identities starting from early childhood until their retirement or termination from sport; this is identified as "identity foreclosure." Identity foreclosure restricts an athlete from developing a multidimensional self in the event he or she fails in athletics. For example, most student-athletes' strong athletic identities cause them to get so caught up in their commitment to their sports and studies that they miss out on valuable opportunities to diversity their personal identities. Consequently, this leaves many athletes unprepared for the work force and other life after the sport. This risk of substance abuse problems and even suicide attempts in this population was identified in a* Journal of Sport and Psychology *article in 2009.[12]*

In some of my teammates at Northeastern University – and truth be told, even for me – this identity crisis often didn't even wait until retirement. Anyone out for the season with a stress fracture or serious muscle pull would usually make his way to the campus bar more than a few nights per week to fill the time.

---

11 Matt Kiss is a training partner and character who appears much later in this book. At press time, he was completing his senior year at St. Thomas University and competing on the school's cross country team.

12 Journal of Sport & Exercise Psychology; Oct 2009, Vol. 31 Issue 5, p680

Day	Date	Notes	Mileage
Training Log Week 7			
Thurs.	3/19/09	Recovery days suck! Did an easy 8 miles (more than yesterday at a faster pace). The time implied I was going faster than I felt, but I was definitely sluggish. No matter... my injuries seem to be under control.	8.0
Fri.	3/20/09	Massage appointment in Cambridge to work on my calf muscles. Ran a 7.5 mile course home from there. Still felt a bit sluggish, but the cold and wind probably contributed to that. 6:51 pace was solid. Almost exactly what I wanted to accomplish today.	7.5
Sat.	3/21/09	Easy 5 miles. Came home slower than I went out. Waiting on the real spring to hit Boston.	5.1
Sun.	3/22/09	My first *real* race since the mid-90s. Ran the James Lamb 5-mile course in 30:34 (6:07 pace). Placed 8th overall. Only one or two older runners ran faster. Felt ok afterward, but my right soleus[13] is slightly strained and the left is moderately strained. They have proven incapable of handling any hard running. Hopefully, more icing and stretching will work. Maybe some weight training? The strains kept me from a warm-down. Overall, it was a good test.	6.0
Mon.	3/23/09	Don't know what to say about today. Went to the gym for alternative training to rest my soleus muscles. Managed 90+ min on a stationary bike at breakneck speed. I felt a little tired after 30 min, but I found a groove. It could have been any number of things: 1) I was motivated from yesterday's race. 2) I was drinking from one of those 180 Energy drinks every few min. 3) My MP3 player played a great song over and over ("Panic Switch" by Silversun Pickups). It may have been a combination of the three. Regardless this was *double* my output from Feb 27's alternative training. The bike read 34 miles (22.6 miles/hour). Warmed down with 2 miles on the elliptical (14+ min). Converted the output to miles using this formula: total workout time/average workout pace to date (7:18).	13.0
Tues.	3/24/09	Hard 61 min on elliptical machine. Lost 5lbs and my legs, calves and feet cramped for hours afterward. The machine read 10 miles, but it was not a straight conversion based on my settings. I estimate it's 8.5 miles of effort (7:11 pace). Been icing and stretching more each day. The solei are better, but still sore. Looking forward to hitting the roads, but rushing it would be stupid. This whole episode reminds me of Rocky IV. When I'm on the roads, I feel like Rocky. When I'm on the machines, I'm Ivan Drago.	8.5
Weds.	3/25/09	40 min hard on the elliptical in the early afternoon (5.6-mile equivalent). A few hrs later, I did 2.7 miles on the road. The solei don't feel ready for long runs, but I flew for those few miles (about 6:00 pace) with no ill after-effects. The high turnover of the previous few days did wonders. I need an easy day though... been going hard for 3 straight days. The run took me to Marathon Sports, where I bought two new pairs of shoes. They're supposedly tailored to my gait, weaknesses, etc.	8.3
Total		Averaged 7:10 per mile for the week	**56.3**

 In Hindsight – *Looking back on my first few weeks of training, a couple of important things stand out. First of all, I was clearly running with the wrong equipment. I can't be sure that better shoes would have prevented the onset of my calf-muscle issues, but they certainly wouldn't have hurt. Proving that two wrongs don't make a right, my lack of proper injury prevention and treatment certainly contributed to my calf injuries.*

On a positive note, without being aware of it, I did a decent job of incorporating easy days into my weekly routine. Also, though I should have started off with fewer miles in Week 1, my weekly progression was gradual. However, this wasn't the result of my wisdom; rather, it was the desire to run further and faster, offset by the impediment created by my soon-to-be-chronic calf strains.

---

13 The soleus is a powerful muscle in the back part of the lower leg (the calf). It runs from just below the knee to the heel, and is involved in standing and walking.

Training Log Week 8

Day	Date	Notes	Mileage
Thurs.	3/26/09	Not much fanfare for my 50th day of training. Felt good enough to hit the roads again (been shaking injuries pretty quickly). Planned on an easy 6 miles to test the solei. Started at 8:00 pace and felt a little rough. However, averaged 6:38 for the last 5 miles. Should have gone easier, but felt ok after. New shoes may have helped.	6.0
Fri.	3/27/09	Went out for what was supposed to be an easy 8 miles at 1p. Somehow finished in 54:27 (my second fastest time for the course). Wouldn't call it "easy" but wasn't pushing either. The last 7 miles were 6:38 pace, the same pace as the last 5 miles yesterday.	8.0
Sat.	3/28/09	Easy 1-hr run along the back trails at Foxwoods Casino. Haven't run through woods since NU track camp in the early 90s. Very enjoyable. Joined the Cambridge Boys later for craps.	8.1
Sun.	3/29/09	Hard to get motivated. Tired from last night at Foxwoods and the ride home. Plus, those trails left my legs sore in new places. Cold and rain didn't help either. Dragged myself into the gym for an easy 7.5 miles on the elliptical. Disappointed I didn't get any hard work done this weekend, but I guess a little rest isn't a bad thing.	7.5
Mon.	3/30/09	Challenging to get motivated again. The end of the fiscal quarter is a hectic time for my business. Plus, it was rainy and cold again. So, I ate a bunch of chocolate (high serotonin), sucked down some caffeine, did some stretching in the steam room to warm up, and then hit the roads. Ugh. The first 2 miles felt like someone put gum on the bottom of my shoes. Went through in 15:30. The next 2 miles felt better but were only marginally faster. Hit the halfway point in 30:30. There was a lot of wind... but still. Finally got going, completing the back half in 25:30 (6:23 pace), with the last mile likely under 6:00. I may have run negative splits for each of the 8 miles. Overall, it was a good lesson in "stick-to-it-iveness." The solei feel ok. Hopefully, that holds – they typically act up after any sub-6:30 action, but perhaps they have finally strengthened.	7.9
Tues.	3/31/09	Ran with the "Black & Tan" group:[14] 5.7 miles with the group at an easy pace. Afterward, I did some very light steeple drills then ran a brisk 3.4 miles with Chris Simpson. It felt pretty easy, probably because I was not running alone.	9.2
Weds.	4/1/09	Calf sore from yesterday's drills, so I used the elliptical. Hard 8 miles. Plan to increase to 60 total miles for next wk and perhaps 65 the wk after by implementing double sessions Mon/Weds/Fri. However, staying healthy is job #1. Stretching and icing seems to be paying off. Everything seems to be at 90% or better, including the solei.	8.0
Total		Averaged 7:09 per mile for the week	**55.2**

Injury Reports and Medical Findings

By Week 7 in my training cycle – notably after my first race – I developed an undetermined problem in my soleus muscle or my calf. It could have been a high-ankle sprain, for all I knew. What I learned was that any hard training resulted in next-day soreness along the outside of my leg, somewhere in the vicinity of my calf.

In hindsight – *My heavy pronation was the primary cause of my problem. It didn't help that I had/have a tendency to tense my calf muscles just prior to impact with the ground. I learned to stretch better and run less tensed. Specifically, there are stretches that hit the outside of the calf as well as the middle. The same goes for the interior. While stretching your calf, all you have to do to stretch the inside and outside of the calf is twist your hips and leg – first to one side and then the other. A full twist will result in a nice full stretch.*

As for my stride, I became very conscious of how I struck the ground. Now I do my best to stay completely loose when I land. This helps to prevent strains. It also helps me to run more efficiently – tensing one's muscles expends more energy than not tensing them! More importantly, my muscles are now working the way they should, instead of simply absorbing shock in a tensed position.

---

14 The "Black & Tan" guys are Masters runners, mostly Brandeis University alumni, who took their name from their favorite post-workout beverage. One, Chris Simpson, placed third in the 1,500 meters (4:08.5) at the USATF Indoor Masters Nationals in 2009.

Training Log Week 9			
Day	Date	Notes	Mileage
Thurs.	4/2/09	Went out for an easy 8 miles. Started very slow (over 8:00 for the first mile) but still finished in less than 56 min with very little effort. It was an enjoyable run.	8.0
Fri.	4/3/09	Double session today. Slow 4.6 miles at lunch with a former Brandeis runner, Terry Pricher.[15] The lunch run was only 8:00 pace. I was rushed in the afternoon, but I still managed a good stair workout (9 x 32 flights, 5.4 mile equivalent). All but the first set was under 4:00, with a couple under 3:45 – very strong for 32 flights. The stair workout should help strengthen my calves, hopefully helping eliminate my soleus issue.	10.0
Sat.	4/4/09	Struggled to complete 8 miles in less than 56 min. High wind and my MP3 player died with over 3 miles to go. I didn't realize this 8-miler made 18 miles in 23 hrs. Taking that into account, I feel pretty good about it. Injuries were quiet today. I learned that I was stretching my calves, but not my solei. I've rectified that situation and hopefully that will turn the tide in my injury battle.	8.0
Sun.	4/5/09	Great day. New shirt, new socks, new tights, and 58 degrees. Planned an easy 8 miles after the heavy workload Fri and Sat. Didn't work out that way. My legs wanted to go, so I let them. Went out in 28:30 (7:08 pace). Came back in 25:05 (6:16 pace). I ran almost as fast a couple wks ago, but felt sick afterward. This was easier. Just a brisk, controlled run. All injuries seem to have gone into remission. Couldn't ask for more.	8.1
Mon.	4/6/09	Triple session. A slow (7:45 pace) 4.6 miles with Terry Pricher, followed by a moderate (7:00 pace) 4 miles on the elliptical later in the day, capped off by a hard (6:40 pace) 4.2 on the inclined elliptical that night. The solei remain silent. My left knee and right Achilles are sore but just a little. All is good.	12.8
Tues.	4/7/09	Busy day. Ran 4.75 miles at near 7:00 pace before a Coyle & Cassidy High School track meet, where I helped out. Next, went to MIT with Doug Williams (ex-Brandeis University 400m runner). We ran an easy 3 miles, followed by some drills, followed by 4 x 400m at 78 sec each with 200m rest in between. Warmed down an easy 2 miles. Injuries not a problem. Gotta keep an eye on the knees, but the calves responded well to the intervals.	11.5
Weds.	4/8/09	Easy day. Ran 4.9 miles (8:20 pace) with Terry Pricher at 1p, followed by 4.6 miles at 7:14 pace with co-author Rick Miller and Gwil Jones – both Northeastern University track alums – at 6p. This wk was a pretty big increase in mileage, mainly because of double and triple sessions. Put lots of miles in the bank and gained the upper hand against any looming injuries.	9.5
Total		Averaged 7:12 per mile for the week	67.9

Dietary Research and Findings

Approaching three months into my training, I knew I needed to better understand the effects of nutrition. As my mileage and average pace increased, my weight continued to drop... so at first I just increased my food intake. One night I probably had *three* dinners at Bertucci's Italian Restaurant. Afterward I woke in the middle of the night, probably due to the carbo load, and struggled to get back to sleep. Not a good sign.

If I was going to eat more just so I could train more, I wanted it all to contribute to peak performance. Researching diet was a long process that continues to this day. Along the way, I flip-flopped between high-protein diets, high-carb diets, the 80-10-10 diet (80 percent carbs, 10 percent protein, and 10 percent fat), among others.

Food Tip – *Eating an apple immediately after working out provides much-needed carbs. It also makes a good pre-meal appetizer because its fibrous pulp helps you feel full sooner. That's not as important for younger guys, but for aspiring Masters, weight control can be an issue. My 5' 8" frame carried about 190 pounds a few short years ago. I subsequently dropped to 135 pounds, and I'm now holding steady at my target (150 pounds).*

---

[15] Terry can't go much faster due to recent knee and Achilles surgeries. But he'll ramp up quickly. In high school, he was among the best cross country runners in New York.

<u>**Nutrition Tracking:**</u> One reason many runners fail at, or simply forego, nutrition tracking is because it's difficult and tedious. The Web site FitDay.com offers a free service where you can enter the foods you eat and receive a total calorie count and nutritional assessment. (Coach Dave's wife, Sue, tipped me off to this great resource.)

I wanted a complete assessment of my nutritional deficiencies during a typical week. To do this, I made a list of *everything* I ate, including the quantities. This included weekdays, when I mainly stuck with skinless chicken, fish, fruits, vegetables, lentils, eggs, water, and protein shakes, *and* weekends, when I rewarded myself for a hard week of training and dieting by eating virtually anything I wanted (steak, wine, candy, soda, ice cream, etc).

I entered everything into the Web site. However, the site tracks intake by the day, so I divided my weekly consumption by seven for an average. (e.g., I don't eat beef during the week, but I was eating a combined 21 ounces of steak, hamburgers, etc. on the weekends. Thus, I entered 3 oz of beef as my daily amount on FitDay.)

It took awhile, but it was a worthwhile exercise. In addition to calculating caloric intake, the site also estimates caloric output based on your weight and activity level. If you maintain a steady weight, your caloric input and output should be identical. My input and output numbers were very close (about 3,200 calories per day).

In addition to calorie-counting, I wanted an understanding of my nutritional ratios. I read that a 4:1 ratio of carbs to protein was needed to properly process protein.[16] I expected my assessment to be about 70 percent carbs, 15 percent protein, and 15 percent fat, but I was surprised to see that my carb intake was lower than I expected. My ratio was 60 percent, 20 percent, and 20 percent. I used this baseline – and referred back to FitDay regularly – to make adjustments based on what I felt my training required, as you'll see in some of my log entries.

In addition to carbs/protein/fat ratios, FitDay assesses your intake of specific vitamins and minerals. I intentionally excluded my mega-vitamins from my entries, so I could see what I was getting from whole foods. I was well over 300 percent of RDA in most categories. I was only deficient in vitamin E at the time.

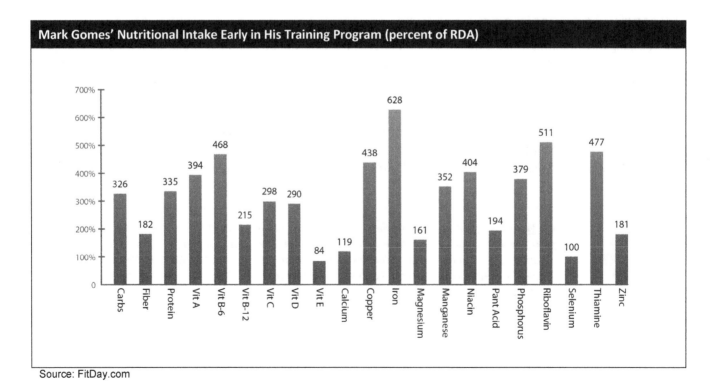

Mark Gomes' Nutritional Intake Early in His Training Program (percent of RDA)

Source: FitDay.com

---

16 Source: [Google: "UT Feature Story" + "John Ivy"]

Training Log Week 10			
Day	Date	Notes	Mileage
Thurs.	4/9/09	Labored through 8 miles. Tired from averaging 11 miles per day for the past 3 days. Managed to finish under 7:00 pace. Focused on staying loose and pushing through the fatigue. Solid day's work.	8.0
Fri.	4/10/09	Did a quick out-and-back 4 miler at noon (6:41 pace). Ran an easy 4.9 miles with Terry Pricher in the afternoon. Felt rough. May be feeling the effects of bumping the mileage up too much this week.	9.1
Sat.	4/11/09	Ran an unpleasant 5.8-miles (7:07 pace) after golfing 18 holes. It was 40 degrees and drizzly all day. Bad weather for 18 holes on 5 hrs sleep. Even worse for a run.	5.8
Sun.	4/12/09	Completely fatigued this morning. Didn't think I'd get anything productive done today. Did 3 fast sets of stairs (11:19) to start the day. That did little to wake my body up, so I headed to the gym for an elliptical workout. The first 30 min were sluggish. Finally, my legs woke up and I was off to the races. I worked for another 45 min and finished the day with the equivalent of 10+ miles (7:12 pace). Glad I didn't call it a day after the first 30 min. Great lesson in "don't give up." I'm on track for 60-65 miles for the week.	10.3
Mon.	4/13/09	Did 5.1 miles at 1p with Terry (7:55 pace). It was windy; I felt sluggish and had bowel problems for the last 2 miles. It wasn't a fun run. We ran up Storrow Drive to Mass Ave and back via Comm Ave. Planned on slogging through 6 miles in the late afternoon... but when I got out there, I actually felt good. Near-record splits for the first couple of miles, so I decided to do 8 miles instead. I kept powering up hills and hitting great splits. Capped it off with a 5:50 final mile to finish in a record 53:05 (6:38 pace). Very nice surprise. The right soleus is barking a little, but nothing disconcerting. I'll take it easy tomorrow because the Black & Tan guys will be working out at Harvard on Wednesday.	13.1
Tues.	4/14/09	Ran an easy 6 miles with Terry today, but that was all. Right soleus is acting up again... infuriating. Supposed to run 4.5 miles with Terry at lunch tomorrow and then workout with the Black & Tan at Harvard. I'll be icing the leg until then. I may have gotten ahead of myself last week. I've got 2+ years until the 2011 Masters Championships.	6.1
Weds.	4/15/09	Limped into the end of my wk with a crummy day of training, thanks to my sore right soleus. It can't seem to take a sub-6:00 mile. Had to forfeit the workout I had planned. Clearly have to leverage machines to let this thing heal. I need to stay injury-free as much as possible. Thankfully, I ran my fastest 8 miles this week. I also did some hurdle drills for the first time in 15+ years, so it was a good week, except for the soleus relapse.	6.9
Total		Averaged 7:23 per mile for the week	59.3

Race Reports, Records, and Results

2009 James Lamb Memorial 5-Miler: Stepping to the line for the James Lamb Memorial 5-Mile Race in Week 7 brought back a few thoughts and emotions. I'd only been training for a few weeks, so I didn't really feel the pressure to perform as I would have back in the day. However, I was anxious because my performance would serve as an important barometer for whether or not I still had something left that resembled talent.

The hardest part came when the gun went off. It had been so long since I had been tested, I wasn't sure I knew the proper pace at which to start. However, that aspect of racing is apparently something that becomes etched into a runner's permanent memory – in hindsight I feel that I went out just right. Every step along the way I grew more and more fatigued, but I ran at the right pace to finish the race completely spent without dying too soon.

The race itself was as hard as I remember five-milers being. After the first couple of miles it became a struggle, as it always had. True to past experiences, the fourth mile was an absolute bitch. Mile 5 was still the toughest, but I knew that the end of Mile 5 would bring an end to my suffering, so there was the psychological aid of seeing the light at the end of the tunnel. That's why I always treat the second to last mile like the last one... because the last one is all guts!

When it was all said and done, I was pretty pleased with my performance. The eighth-place overall finish and my time (30:34 for 5 miles) was definitely not bad for six weeks of training. The fact that only one or two guys that were

Training Log Week 11

Day	Date	Notes	Mileage
Thurs.	4/16/09	Sometimes I need to restrain myself. Former NU teammate Tom Lahive called to see if I was up for a lunch run. I tested my right calf and decided it could handle an easy 4.6 miles. To be safe, I wore a brace and wrapped the lower calf with an ACE bandage. We completed the course at 7:22 pace. Later, I headed to the gym and did a hard 47 min on the elliptical. The soleus appears to be OK, but the rest of me is gonna feel it.	11.8
Fri.	4/17/09	Suffered through a double-session. Did 4.9 miles with Terry. We stopped and walked for about 400m at the halfway point. Terry had a root canal two days ago and hasn't eaten much since, so it's heroic he even went out today. The walk was fine by me – I wasn't feeling so hot. Fighting a cold and still feeling yesterday. I did 4.6 miles at a decent clip in the afternoon, but that didn't feel great either.	9.5
Sat.	4/18/09	Long, low-impact day. 11 miles on the elliptical in 73:33, which is only 9 sec slower per mile than the frenetic 7.2-mile elliptical workout I did a couple days ago. Definitely one of my best workouts to date. It was as much a mental challenge as a physical one. I think this day will pay dividends. Injury-wise, my right knee is a little sore, but the calves feel great.	11.0
Sun.	4/19/09	Another day on the elliptical. 8.5 miles in 60:00. Not too hard, but not easy either. Solid effort after yesterday and another day of low-impact training for my calf. Back on the roads tomorrow.	8.5
Mon.	4/20/09	Tough day at work. By the time I put out my corporate fires, it was late, cold, wet, and I was pissed off... so I just hit the elliptical for a quick 6 miles. Glad I worked hard for the past several days, because I felt guilty afterward... but I was probably due for an easy day. The workout was a breeze.	6.0
Tues.	4/21/09	Jamie had her wisdom teeth pulled, so I didn't run until 8p. Decided warm temperature trumped rain and hit the roads. Good choice (sarcasm). Zoomed through 3 miles, but at 6 miles, my soleus tweaked again. I eased up for the next 400m and realized it was best to walk it in. Disappointing. Should've wrapped the thing. Glad I started the wk strong. My fastest 50 miles are already logged at sub-7:00 pace.	6.3
Weds.	4/22/09	Week 11 ended like Week 10... gimpy. 5.5 miles in the morning, then Harvard for the evening workout. My soleus wasn't worth risking, so I did 1 hr of hurdle drills with a few careful 200m (33, 31, and 29 sec) mixed in to simulate race conditions. I'll probably be sore; I feel like I did something worthwhile, especially since I'll likely be back on the elliptical.	8.0
Total		Averaged 6.57 per mile for the week	61.1

my age or older finished ahead of me also fueled my competitive fire. It was also the first time I've ever run faster than Coach Dave head-to-head. It only took me 38 years, and the fact that I feel good about it even though he's eight years older than I am shows you how funny the competitive mind is. Three of Dave's runners beat me, but no shame in that – they're all promising young athletes.

Overall, it was a very important day. I ran a decent race, which gave me the confidence to continue training toward the larger goals to come. I also won some loot for being the top "Sub-Master" (the 30-39 age category), which is never a bad thing.

Miscellaneous Research and Notes

Static and Dynamic Stretching: Very early in my comeback I recognized I would have to pay specific attention to stretching. In some ways age takes very little toll on your athletic ability; flexibility is not one of those ways. I learned quickly that flexibility was important not just for recovery but for reaching peak performance as well.

There are two basic types of stretching, static and dynamic. Most of us old dogs were taught the static way. Static stretches, like the common hamstring/hurdlers stretch, are good for lengthening muscle but they take away from that muscle's ability fire explosively; they decrease eccentric strength.

Dynamic stretching utilizes momentum to propel the muscle into an extended range of motion. It is stretching while moving, as opposed to stretching while standing/sitting still. Dynamic stretching prepares the body for physical exertion and sports performance. It increases range of movement and blood and oxygen flow to soft tissues prior to exertion. Important note: dynamic stretching does *not* exceed one's static stretching range of motion. (Using momentum to propel your limbs *beyond* their natural limits is called ballistic stretching and it regularly leads to injury. Evidence indicates ballistic stretching may even be counterproductive and cause a "stretch reflex," or muscular contraction – the exact opposite of your desired effect.)

The esteemed British coach Brian MacKenzie provides numerous examples of dynamic stretching exercises on his Web site.[17]

Training Streaks: I don't think I had ever logged as many training miles over a lengthy span as I did in my first 13 weeks of my comeback. I know I didn't run as many miles during my previous running streaks. If I had run more, it was during my freshman or sophomore cross country seasons at Northeastern University. The first week of the season was always around 90 miles (at cross country camp). I also remember running a *lot* of 10-mile runs... but the season was short, and the break between cross country season and indoor track decreases the chance that I ever put in 750+ training miles in 100 days.

It's possible that I came close during the summer after my freshman year at Northeastern, when I managed a sport card shop in Braintree, Mass. That summer, I lived at my grandmother's house in Dorchester, which was seven miles from the shop. I would bike to work (seven-mile bike ride = about three training miles) and run home at night, then, the next day, I would run to work and bike home. I ran my 10K PR that summer at a road race (31:08). Not bad for a middle-distance specialist.

The training streak I began at the onset of my comeback became a huge motivating force, which yielded benefits and detriments – as we will explore later in this book.

Elliptical Machine Settings: Through trial and error I was able to find a resistance level on the elliptical machine that approximated the corollary effort to running on roads; thus the mileage in my training log after Week 7 shows a 1:1 correlation between elliptical miles and true mileage. For me, on LifeFitness machines, Level 13 required the same effort as road running to reach the same distance. As noted in an earlier chapter, this setting became a moving target over time.

Training Log Week 12			
<u>Day</u>	<u>Date</u>	<u>Notes</u>	<u>Mileage</u>
Thurs.	4/23/09	Had a strong day on the elliptical. Best machine workout yet. Managed a 10-mile equivalent in about 66 min. The soleus is feeling better, but still sore. I'm gonna play it carefully. Don't want this to become chronic. That would be a waste of my progress to date.	10.0
Fri.	4/24/09	Another 10-mile equivalent elliptical, but an extra level (14) of resistance for the second half. I still completed the workout 1 min faster than yesterday. The times for longer runs seem a bit skewed, but it was very hard (physically and mentally). Another strong day.	10.0
Sat.	4/25/09	Started the day with a lot of stretching and a short warm-up run before doing a hard 3 miles on the elliptical. Around 6p, went out for 8 miles. Goal #1 was to go easy on my right soleus. I had it wrapped it up, ran easy, and took care with each step... and yet I hit very impressive splits with little effort. Powered through in 54:17 (6:47 per mile; 3rd fastest on that course to date).	11.1
Sun.	4/26/09	The right soleus got sore after I unwrapped it yesterday. I guess the wrap masked the fact that it was being taxed on the roads. I'm done taking chances. The left one hasn't made a peep since April 2, so I'm hopeful that the right one can be rehabbed without any time off. Doing more icing, massaging, stretching, and Ibuprofen popping. Needless to say, it was another day on the elliptical. Fairly easy 8 miles with a sub-6:00 final mile. If I keep doing an hour of work with some high turnover mixed in, I should keep getting stronger.	8.0
Mon.	4/27/09	Another day on the elliptical. It was really hard today. The boring Red Sox game didn't help. My body might be tired from increasing the resistance level a few days ago. (I've definitely been sore). It was tough psychological challenge for the last 4 miles, and I was completely spent afterward. That can't be a bad thing.	8.0
Tues.	4/28/09	8 miles on the elliptical again. Went much faster and felt much better than yesterday. In fact, that great 10 mile on April 24th was only a little faster (per mile), but with less resistance for the first half... so this was comparable. I wonder, what makes such a big difference from one day to the next? The soleus continues to improve, but I can tell it's still a problem.	8.0
Weds.	4/29/09	Hit the roads today. Ran an easy 5 miles with Terry Pricher at noon and then another easy 4 miles with him in the afternoon. Did some hurdle drills after. The soleus seems OK, but I'm gonna play it safe.	9.3
Total		Averaged 6.50 per mile for the week	**64.4**

---

17 www.brianmac.co.uk/dynamic.htm

Training Log Week 13			
Day	Date	Notes	Mileage
Thurs.	4/30/09	Did an easy 64 min with Terry. Long slow distance… Terry struggled but gutted it out. He seems determined to get in good condition before the upcoming Green Mountain Relay. Happy that my injuries haven't acted up for the past few days. Hopefully my attempt at rehab is sending them into permanent remission.	8.2
Fri.	5/1/09	Started the day with 5 miles with Terry at 1p (7:41 pace). Basic run. No injury concerns. Followed that up with a strong 8 miles on the elliptical around 7p.	13.1
Sat.	5/2/09	Ran a hilly 8.1 miles in Braintree/Weymouth that kicked my ass. Plus, I was holding back on the downhills to protect my calf injuries, so my time sucked. Definitely a tough workout though. I'm sure I needed some hills to compensate for all that time on the elliptical.	8.1
Sun.	5/3/09	Napped until 7p, so only had time for 5 miles (7:17 pace) on the elliptical. After that, I changed into some dry clothes and hit the road for another 4.6 miles (6:43 pace). My injuries are not bothering me.	9.6
Mon.	5/4/09	Another injury-free day. Did a 5/5 double, going easy at 1p with Terry and moderate at 7p on the elliptical. I don't feel like my body is fully recovering between workouts, so I've upped my protein intake and will take it easy for the next couple of days.	9.9
Tues.	5/5/09	Felt stronger today and more importantly, injury-free. Did 5 miles in the morning with Terry (7:22 pace) – his conditioning is returning rapidly. Later, we ran 4+ miles at a slower pace. Today marked the 3-month anniversary of my comeback. I may start doing some easy once-a-wk speed workouts.	9.7
Weds.	5/6/09	Basically a day off. 5.1 miles at 7:48 pace.	5.1
Total		Averaged 7.18 per mile for the week	**63.7**

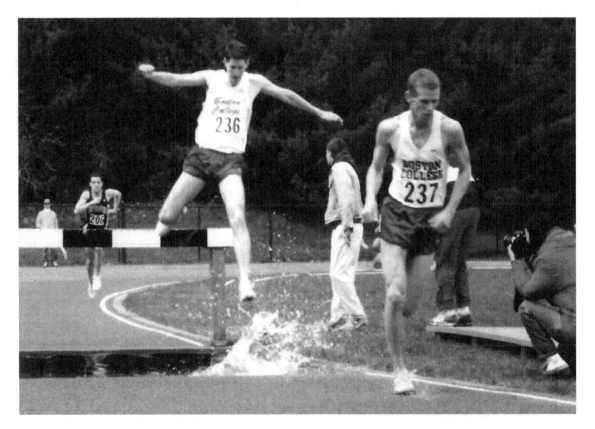

Mark Gomes (206) chases Boston College runners Mike Atwood (236) and Brian Culley (237) in the final steeplechase of his college career.

Chapter 3
Got Bear Hugs for My Brothers…

Weeks 14-20

If you Google-search the phrase "How fast does the average man run one mile," you'll receive about 250,000 results – of drastically varying relevance, of course. The largest "answer" Web sites, like Yahoo! Answers, Answers.com, and a few sports-oriented specialty sites indicate the average one-mile time for a typical American man is about 8:30. (None of these sites cites a legitimate study; the findings appear purely anecdotal based on comments from other site users.) Despite the lack of methodology and the fact that none of the responses consider that a large portion of American men can't even *finish* a full mile, 8:30 might pass the sniff test based on some data crunching we performed using recent race results.

Using data from 5K road races of varying size and prestige around the U.S., all completed in 2010, we found the average 5K time for a U.S. male was 26:48 – 8:38 per mile. Using several performance calculators, including the popular McMillan Running Calculator and our Faster Than Forty proprietary calculator, we estimate the man who runs a 26:48 5K would run 7:44 for the mile, all-out. (But keep in mind, these numbers are based on road race participants, which means these are men who already have a predilection to run, so 8:30 for the general public – which includes a lot of non-runners – may not be far off.)

Why does this matter? Aside from giving the male readers of this book a very, very general national benchmark to compare themselves with, it sets up the premise for this chapter: The competitive runner is barely the same species as the typical American man by a lot of measures, and he knows it.

This is both the source of the competitive runner's power and his greatest weakness. Young runners who – through talent and training – successfully advance their fitness toward national-caliber levels don't need to crunch numbers to know they're special. They hear it in their classmates' heavy breathing every time they climb the stairs to get to a second- or third-floor classroom. They see it (literally) when they watch America's legions of fat people walk through the mall. They feel it on Thanksgiving weekend when they've just coasted to a win at their local Turkey Trot while a large portion of the entrants are struggling to finish. They *believe* it after enough coaches/family members/teammates/etc. tell them they have a gift.

Because of the nature of these gifts – the speed, the strength, and maybe most importantly the high pain tolerance – it doesn't take long for competitive runners to feel more than special… they feel immortal. Not surprisingly, this leads to trouble on and off the track.

With the Northeastern University team in the early 1990s, this undercurrent of physical superiority was a constant. Although most of the track guys performed well in the classroom and mingled cordially with other students and athletes, behind the closed doors of the locker room they didn't hold many non-runners in high regard. Either you logged your miles and withstood the pain, or you did not. When one distance runner overheard a football player complaining about a 2.5-hour practice at the athletes' dining hall, he later wondered how that player would have felt if his practice was only slightly shorter and involved non-stop running – no breaks between plays, no stop-and-start drills. Whether it was true or not, the consensus in the track locker room was: no one trains harder, and pound-for-pound no one is tougher. (It probably didn't help matters that in the late 1980s and early 1990s the Mark Lech-coached track programs at Northeastern were at the top of their conference and regularly sending athletes to the NCAA Championships while most of the other sports at Northeastern were relatively weak.)

Off campus things were arguably worse. Despite mandatory early morning long runs on Sundays, the Northeastern runners had no aversion to Boston's watering holes on Saturday nights. Why would they? They could drink 10-15 beers and be ready to run a 13- or 14-miler by 8 a.m. on Sunday with nary an ill effect. The vicious cycle would occasionally transpire like this:

➢ A weight thrower on the team would get hired to bounce and work the door at a bar near Northeastern's campus or somewhere in the Lansdowne St. vicinity.
➢ The bulky weight throwers, who held a brotherly affection for their skinny runner teammates, would inform the runners which bars and which nights they'd be working.
➢ The runners would show up – usually on Saturday nights after meets, when everyone was still amped up – and proceed to drink heavily, behave loudly, and hit on women rampantly.
➢ The typical Boston bar patron, although often originally amused by the sight of six or seven walking skeletons guzzling beer and fearlessly flirting with his girlfriend, would eventually lose his patience and swing at someone. Then it was on...
➢ Weighing in at 135-145 pounds on average, the runners didn't pack devastating punches, but they were quick enough to land a shot or two and move – and when they had to, they could take their beatings and stay on their feet long enough for help to arrive. Eventually the weight thrower and his colleagues working the door would horse-collar the other patrons and toss them out.
➢ In the locker room on Monday, the weight guys would lecture the runners on what pains in the ass they were, and recommend they stay out of the bar for a while, but in a few weeks someone would start work at a new bar, or all would be forgotten at the old one, and the cycle would start all over again.

Being able to handle themselves in a fight was only half their arsenal. The other half, the most obvious half, was to simply outrun trouble. In the early 1990s, the south side of Northeastern's campus was bordered by a section of Roxbury that was still pretty rough. But living there was cheap, and the behemoth weight throwers – who feared no one – had no problem dealing with the sketchy neighborhood to be close to campus and the training facilities while paying a fraction of the rent on Gainsborough St. or Symphony Lane. They also had no problem with the occasional bat-shit crazy party.

One winter night, Rick Miller, Dino Dibiaso, and another distance runner, Matt, wandered out of a rager at a shot putter's place on Columbus Ave. It was late; it was cold, and there was hardly a soul around. As they crossed the road, a beat-up sedan that had been slow-cruising the street suddenly aimed and lurched toward them as they reached the median line. Miller and Dibiaso darted to the safety of the far sidewalk, but Matt took a step back, and like a bull fighter working his cape, casually flipped his half-full keg cup on the windshield of the car as it passed inches away. The plastic cup exploded, covering the windshield and hood of the car in beer, and the driver slammed on the brakes.

Matt looked at his teammates – who were not completely, but certainly a little bit, shocked – and simply said, "Run."

They sprinted toward campus via Camden St. because it was the shortest route but also because it dead-ended at a pedestrian bridge that crossed a set of train tracks that marked the south side of school.

"Nice call; they can't follow us," Dibiaso said as they reached the footbridge – just a second before the sedan popped up on the sidewalk behind them, its driver- and passenger-side doors already open. The three men who jumped out were large, thuggish, and not in a let's-talk-this-out sort of mood.

"I'd keep running," Matt advised sardonically, and the three harriers went up and over the footbridge with the occupants of the sedan sprinting after them. Crossing the bridge, the race was closer than any of the runners would like to have admitted, but by the time they reached Huntington Ave., 200 yards away, they had built a 40- or 50-yard lead. The only thing that surprised them was that their pursuers kept coming. They ducked into the doorway of Maxwell Jumps, the closest thing Northeastern had to a campus bar. The manager and the doormen recognized the runners – regular visitors, to say the least – and knew right away something was wrong; they hustled them inside and stopped the pursuers at the door.

After taking a minute to catch his breath, Dibiaso looked at Matt and asked, "Matt, what the f---? Why the hell did you do that?"

Matt's answer: "Because someone had to show them that aiming their car at us was bullshit... And because I *could*." At no point in the process did Matt think: a) I might get caught by some very bad dudes, or b) even if they do catch me, I'm the one that might get hurt.

In the day-to-day rigors of training, the same attitude held. The team would regularly train through minor injuries, like shin splints, and occasionally more serious ones, like stress fractures.

Later in life, it's more difficult – and makes even less sense – to try and "train through." The body heals at a slower pace, prolonging your discomfort, and as you favor your original injury (with conscious or sub-conscious changes to your gait) the likelihood that you injure something else increases. Having an alternate training plan is essential to maintaining your fitness when you do get hurt and providing the psychological escape hatch to get off the roads.

As I learned in the next phase of my Masters training, it's still hard to admit you need to back off – but recognizing that you do and yielding to the realization can make the difference between some minor amendments to your regimen and some serious lost time.

Training Log Week 14

Day	Date	Notes	Mileage
Thurs.	5/7/09	Average pace and "fastest 50 miles" were both much slower last week. Probably ought to dial back the mileage and allow my body to recoup. However, today I did an extra long warm-up before hitting the roads for a hard 8 miles. I went through each of my first 5 splits in record time (sub-33:00 at 5 miles). After that, it got rough. Mile 6 was close to 7:00, as was Mile 7. To top it off, my left calf (not the soleus, thank God) was getting sore... so I shut it down, walked a bit, and jogged home as a warm-down. I had a protein-heavy dinner tonight, and I'll keep pushing the protein for the next several days and see what that does.	8.2
Fri.	5/8/09	Planned on a nice slow 5 miles, but I suffered a mild strain of my left calf (*not* the soleus) just after the 1-mile mark... and I was only going 8:20 pace! It's now pretty obvious that I've worn my body down. I shuffled back to the gym and did an easy 4 miles on the elliptical.	6.0
Sat.	5/9/09	Did an easy 4 miles on the elliptical, followed by some light rowing and lifting. Switched my diet from being carb-heavy to being protein-heavy. My injury setback might be exactly what I needed to break out of a sub-optimal routine and start training a little smarter. I plan to use the elliptical until the calves are mostly healed and then train smarter on the roads (and with my diet).	4.0
Sun.	5/10/09	Did 6 easy miles on the elliptical. I'm treating this as a "wk off." Diet-wise, I'm cutting back on calories because *not* regularly going 8 miles hard will certainly cause me to gain weight, and I'm still focusing on high-protein foods (salmon, eggs, lentils, etc.). The extra protein is making me a bit more tired, but not training as hard offsets that. I will experiment with coordinating my diet and training regimen going forward.	6.0
Mon.	5/11/09	*More* elliptical work. I did 8 easy miles (61:47). Easy on my calves, easy on my body. I only planned on doing 6 miles, but I'm pent up: 9:15 won the NCAA New England Championships steeplechase. In college I ran 9:15 in only three attempts at that distance.	8.0
Tues.	5/12/09	Getting old sucks. The tendon is still too tweaked to risk road work. Need to reconfigure my workout schedule to incorporate cross-training and rest... Considering the past 3 months, it makes sense to give my calves a proper chance to heal. Did an easy 5 miles on the elliptical today. The training streak keeps me motivated, so I'm gonna keep it going.	5.0
Weds.	5/13/09	Did a very slow 4.3 miles (8:30 pace), half on the roads & half on Harvard's track. The leg was still tender on the run. The Black & Tan guys did the back end of a ladder (1,000m, 800m, 400m, 200m). I did 30-45 min of hurdle drills. Not as important as speed work, but probably the best use of my time and capability. Memories of jumping the whole water pit back in college always get me fired up.	4.3
Total		Averaged 7:38 per mile for the week	41.5

Injury Reports and Medical Findings

Kinesio Tape: The calf injury from Week 14 ultimately caused me to investigate Kinesio Tape. Kinesio Tape is a medical product similar to traditional athletic tape; the Kinesio Tape pulls the upper layers of skin, creating more space between the dermis and the muscle. This space houses various nerve receptors that send specific information to the brain. When the space between the epidermis and the muscle is compressed, such as during an injury, these nerve receptors are compressed and send information to the brain regarding continuous touch, light touch, cold, pain, pressure, and heat. This information causes the brain to send out certain signals to the body on how to react to particular stimuli. Kinesio Tape alters the information that these receptors send to the brain and causes a less reactive response in the body, allowing the body to work in a more normal manner and removing some of the roadblocks that normally slow down the healing process.[18]

Ex-teammate Tom Lahive claimed Kinesio Tape helped him through a triathlon without injury, but at first it didn't do anything for me. I later learned that the effectiveness of Kinesio Tape is strongly correlated to the skill of the therapist who applies it. There is a specific method for applying this tape, and it differs from the method trainers and therapists have used in the past to apply standard athletic tape. It took me a while to find a therapist who did it right, but once I did, Kinesio Tape proved very useful in mitigating my injuries.

Training Log Week 15			
Day	Date	Notes	Mileage
Thurs.	5/14/09	Weighed in at 149lbs. That's low, considering the low mileage I've been putting in lately. I felt strong as I walked toward the gym. I hit the elliptical for a hard 5 miles and tore it up. Started strong and picked it up at the 2.5-mile mark. Stayed relaxed and broke the last 2.5 miles into bite-sized chunks. It got tough with a mile to go, but I only needed to get to the 4.5-mile mark. The last 800m is just a kick.... My final time was 31:15 (6:15 pace), very fast.	5.0
Fri.	5/15/09	Ran a very easy 5+ with Terry today. He's still sore from his half-marathon last weekend and I'm still being cautious with my injuries. Today was my 100th straight day of training, which ties my lifetime record. Over this span I've gone 766.1 miles averaged at 7:16 per mile.	5.1
Sat.	5/16/09	Another easy day of 5+ miles. I was in Maine for my cousin's bachelor party. Last night was a late and ruckus affair. Got to bed at 4a but somehow managed to wake up before most of the other guys and take a leisurely jog around town. Halfway through, my calf tightened up a bit so I stopped to walk it off. My diet was not exemplary, but I took in as much pasta as I could before the booze and junk food went down. I'm sure I'll gain a couple lbs this weekend, but I'll work it off easily by next week.	5.7
Sun.	5/17/09	Another 4a night, another 5-miler in Maine. Today was pretty effortless. A little hilly, but not much challenge at a slow pace. No injury trouble, which is encouraging. May be ready for a light speed workout soon. My diet was pretty much identical to yesterday. (I tried to sandbag the booze this weekend. No hangover. No impact on my run. It's all good.)	5.6
Mon.	5/18/09	Sticking to the plan of caution, did a slow 4 miles on the elliptical. For cardio, it was almost like doing nothing at all. I felt better afterward than I did beforehand. Diet-wise, it was a transition day. After the bachelor party weekend, I ate leftover junk food along with my normal diet. I weighed in at 154lbs at the gym (versus my target training weight of 150lbs), so I plan to get back to the diet tomorrow.	4.0
Tues.	5/19/09	Couldn't take another easy day. Ran pretty hard for 5.1 miles and the time showed it. After going through Mile 1 in 7:00, I ripped the next 5K in 19:11 (6:11 pace). Cruised in with a 6:37 mile, which gave me 32:48 for the entire 5.1 (6:25 pace). It felt good to drop the hammer after the past 11 days. More importantly, my body felt 100%. I'll be icing the calves though. Back to my normal diet, so I should be back to 150lbs in no time.	5.1
Weds.	5/20/09	Terry Pricher and I hit the Charles River for 4.8 miles. Felt like our typical recovery run, but the pace was 7:28, which is faster than most of our runs together. He's clearly getting in shape. Meanwhile, I was a little tight for the first 800m (not surprising after yesterday), but my injuries were 99% silent. Feel ready to kick the mileage back up. Today closed out the second wk of my recovery. My totals were disappointing, but clearly necessary.	4.8
Total		Averaged 7:42 per mile for the week	35.2

---

18 Source: [Google: medicinenet.com + what is Kinesio Research and Findingstape]

Dietary Research and Findings

Diet and Recovery: I started researching muscular regeneration and glycogen replenishment techniques when I realized my recovery times weren't what they used to be. One study found that combining heavy carb-intake, with heavy caffeine loading is the optimal way to regenerate muscle tissue in the hours after a hard workout. Another study found that simple carbs (fruits, milk, and even sugar) are best *immediately after* a workout. Carbo-loading – when you pound carbs while cutting back on your training – maximizes glycogen reserves. [19]

I adjusted my diet although the regimen didn't leave much room for eating things I like. I increased my carbohydrate intake, focusing on whole wheat pasta, wheat germ, and fruits and vegetables. I added a banana-blueberry protein smoothie to my diet – which tasted great, unlike some of the other drinks I tried. The protein shakes added a lot of calories, so staying at my target weight of 150 pounds was a challenge, even with consistent training... but it was a worthwhile sacrifice.

Training Log Week 16

Day	Date	Notes	Mileage
Thurs.	5/21/09	In Dublin, OH to visit Jamie's family. Planned on 6-7 miles. Unfortunately, my calf tightened up at the 4-mile mark. I walked it off and jogged back home. After dinner I went out for a moderately hard bike ride: 30 min+, a 4.6 mile equivalent. The calf isn't 100%, though it felt good over the past couple days. Have to do more cross-training to let it heal.	8.9
Fri.	5/22/09	Went to the Columbus Zoo with Jamie's family. Later did 45 min (moderate) on the elliptical (6+ mile equivalent), plus some light lifting: modified curls that mimic the running motion because I don't get that on the elliptical. I don't use the elliptical's arms; they seem more suited for cross country skiers. With the curls, I do high reps/low weight at a quick speed, then switch to more weight at a slower speed. The injuries are still a factor. I'm sure they'll feel better soon, but I need to avoid hard pounding until they get checked out. As for diet, it's Memorial Day weekend. I plan to eat! (I'll make it up next week.)	6.2
Sat.	5/23/09	11:30a, started with a tough bike ride (10.5 hilly miles in 33:20, with a short warm-down). Definitely felt "the burn" in my thighs, plus the cardio effect. Hit the elliptical around 10p for 30 min of recovery. Felt great during and after. The injuries feel better, but still gotta get them checked out when I get home. I need a more logical training schedule. Easy days, setting up hard days, and lots of LSD. I've done a good job of getting in shape, but it has been haphazard.	8.7
Sun.	5/24/09	75 min on the elliptical. I pushed the final 15 min, but otherwise it was laidback and a solid 9.5-mile equivalent. Also did a fair amount of stretching, walking and using The Stick for massage.[20] I had a good breakfast before the workout, confident it wouldn't hurt my performance. If anything, it helped. Ate a lot of food at the family cookout.	9.5
Mon.	5/25/09	Yesterday's gluttony paid off. The plan was to do as much elliptical LSD as possible today. Blew through 1 hr without a problem, so I started thinking that 12 miles was possible. After 90 min I still felt strong, so I kept going. Around 110 min I was starting to feel tired, but not bad. At 2 hrs I called it. I saw no reason to go more than 15 miles. Immediately after, I ate an apple and did some 10lb running curls. Then, I hit the hot tub to relax and stretch. After that, I had a little coffee, an apple, a cookie, a shower, and gave myself a long stick massage. Think I could do more 2-hr days if I had enough things to keep me entertained.	15.0
Tues.	5/26/09	Did nearly 8 miles in a 60-min elliptical session. Only a little sore after yesterday's long run. I also scheduled an appointment for my calves. The doc I picked is the head-honcho at Harvard Pilgrim's downtown branch. Yesterday's 15-miler drew a reprimand from Coach Dave. He believes that my training schedule is erratic. He's absolutely right. A training schedule needs to make sense.	7.8
Weds.	5/27/09	8 miles elliptical, moderate pace (6:49). Soon, I'll be running speed workouts on Wednesdays, but for now I'm not even on the roads. Doctor's appointment tomorrow.	8.0
Total		Averaged 7:33 per mile for the week	**64.0**

---

19 www.exrx.net/Nutrition/Glycogen.html

20 www.thestick.com

Below are some key points from this calculated dietary shift:

Key Dietary Points

- ➢ Maintain a high-carb diet to keep glycogen levels high
- ➢ Maintain a high-protein diet to inhibit muscular breakdown and spur muscular recovery/regeneration
- ➢ Eat a snack pre-workout (30-90 min): low-GI food… small banana smoothie and a little pasta
- ➢ Eat a snack immediately post-workout (5-10 min after): high GI food… rice, potato, bread – with caffeine
- ➢ Drink post-workout (5-10 min after): Endurox or whey & banana smoothie with Gatorade
- ➢ Eat a meal post-workout: Fish, Pasta, Milk, Fruits (Smoothie w/dinner)
- ➢ Eat a post-dinner/pre-sleep snack: protein drink
- ➢ Add Omega 3 & Omega 6 foods/supplements
- ➢ Add Daily multi-vitamin(s)

Training Log Week 17			
Day	Date	Notes	Mileage
Thurs.	5/28/09	9 miles elliptical, as scheduled. Lesser resistance, but I compensated by keeping a quick pace. Saw the doc today. Apparently, the problem is in the top of my Achilles tendon, which feeds into my soleus. Starting physical therapy on Tuesday. No pain right now, but I need to minimize the road miles for several wks. Any road miles should be flat and at an easy pace.	9.0
Fri.	5/29/09	Strong 9 miles on the elliptical. Feeling pretty good after 2 easier wks, but still need to get those injuries taken care of. I have to find the maximum level of training my body can endure without triggering recurring injuries. It's funny payback for not running long mileage when I was younger and near-impervious to injury!	8.2
Sat.	5/30/09	Party day planned. Jamie and I hosted an "Earthfest" concert gathering at our place, which started promptly at noon. No Saturday sleep-in. Had to get up early enough to get a quick 4+ miles on the elliptical before the guests arrived. The legs feel good, but I may have some shin splits creeping in.	4.7
Sun.	5/31/09	Nice, easy 65 min on the elliptical (7:32 pace). Effortless. The tendons didn't make a peep and nor did the shin splits, though it's still sore to the touch.	8.6
Mon.	6/1/09	Typical 5-miler with Terry. These have become effortless for me, which may validate my new (smarter) training philosophy. We always have a good dialog going, but being in better shape may help the time pass. After the first 800m, everything felt good. I miss those hard 8-mile runs past NU, but they'll be back. First physical therapy appointment tomorrow.	5.1
Tues.	6/2/09	Did 8 miles on the elliptical at an accelerating pace. Each 2-mile split faster than the last, culminating in a hard 800m to finish the workout. Felt nearly effortless. Saw a physical therapist for the first time since 1992. She confirmed that I was training improperly. I need to dynamically stretch before workouts and statically stretch afterward. She green-lighted me for controlled running activity. Hard days need to be followed by easier days, road days to be followed by cross-training days, and strength training every other day. For strength training she advised PLANKS.	8.0
Weds.	6/3/09	With the medical ok, I hit the track for a light speed workout. I felt good. I did a light 800m at sub-6:00 pace, followed by a 67-sec 400m, 29-sec for 200m, and 1:52 for 600m before feeling a tweak in my calf again. I immediately stopped (as opposed to running through it or hopping on the elliptical).	4.5
Total		Averaged 7:01 per mile for the week	49.0

In Hindsight – *Later in my training log, you'll see that muscular recovery becomes problematic again. I was working hard, but my body wasn't able to recover fast enough. I found lots of recovery tips, especially around diet, but also a lot of confusing and conflicting data. I concluded there may not be a perfect answer. However, there's a pretty clear consensus that a low-GI (glycemic index)[21] snack is good before workouts to provide a slow, steady source of energy. A high-GI food is good post-workout for quick energy/recovery – as is a combination of water, carbs, protein, electrolytes, and amino acids.*

I decided to try the pre-workout low-GI/post-workout high-GI thing and combine that with Endurox as my post-workout drink. Endurox contains a combination of the aforementioned proteins/electrolytes/amino acids. On hard days, I started utilizing Accelerade for pre- and intra-workout fuel. Based on research, it seemed to be an improvement over what I had been doing.

Food Tip – *I read that cooking salmon at high temperatures can convert the Omega-3 fatty acids (good fat) into bad fat.[22] Preparation should be done in foil at lower temperatures, and any defrosting should be done in the refrigerator.*

Do not eat too much asparagus in one sitting. Asparagus is high in fiber, and a large dose can cause unexpected gastrointestinal distress.

Training Log Week 18

Day	Date	Notes	Mileage
Thurs.	6/4/09	The calves are a little tight, but not too bad. After yesterday's bust, I needed a hard workout, so I went nearly all-out on the elliptical. Turned in my fastest 8 miles ever (6:10 pace) and felt pretty good. May take it easy for the next 10 days. The Bay State Games Trials are June 16th at Harvard. I don't want to be hurt because the BSG Finals will be one of few chances to run the steeplechase this year.	8.0
Fri.	6/5/09	Easy 6 miles on the elliptical. An inauspicious 4-month training anniversary, but it's Friday night. Off to dinner!	6.0
Sat.	6/6/09	Did 7 miles along the Charles River with Jamie riding the bike. Good change of pace to keep from getting bored. I kept the pace easy to protect the tendons, but felt kinda tired. It may have been residual fatigue from Weds. and Thurs. Regardless, the calves felt fine and that's all that matters.	7.0
Sun.	6/7/09	Felt fatigued, so I took it easy. 47 min of moderate work (biked along the Charles with an elliptical recovery run). 6.3 "equivalent" miles. I want to be healthy and fresh for the Bay State Games Trials, especially if I need to run fast to make the Finals. If I need rest in the next few days, I'll take it. Recovery is my bottleneck. I'm willing and able to work hard, but my body doesn't seem to recover fast enough.	6.3
Mon.	6/8/09	Felt much better today, so I did a little catching up. Did 5+ miles with Terry at noon at normal pace. Effortless. In the evening, I worked on the elliptical for an easy 7 miles. Again, effortless. No complaints.	12.2
Tues.	6/9/09	Typical lunch run with Terry, plus a little extra on my own.	6.0
Weds.	6/10/09	More mileage than planned, but most of it was very slow and easy. 5-mile lunch run with Terry, but intentionally slow (7:51 pace). Later, I hit Harvard to run with Brian Burba,[23] whom I hadn't seen in 13 years, and the Black & Tan guys: 4.8-mile jog to Harvard (7:55 pace), plus a 2.2-mile warm-up with the group (7:47 pace), then Brian surprised us all by doing 8 x 400m at 80 sec w/400m rest. I handled the pace well. By the final 400m I was pent up, so I took Brian through 200m in 37.5 sec and then did the last 200m in a smooth 30 sec. After, we did an 800m jog and a 10-min walk to warm down.	16.5
Total		Averaged 7:28 per mile for the week	61.9

---

21 The glycemic index, or GI, is a measure of the effects of carbohydrates on blood sugar levels. Carbohydrates that break down quickly during digestion and release glucose rapidly into the bloodstream have a high GI; carbohydrates that break down slowly, releasing glucose more gradually into the bloodstream, have a low GI.

22 Source: www.paleohacks.com

23 Brian Burba is a former co-worker and was a standout Massachusetts high school runner. He finished third in the 1988 Eastern Massachusetts Championships' one-mile run and went on to run at Brown University until back surgery sidelined him.

Training Log Week 19

Day	Date	Notes	Mileage
Thurs.	6/11/09	Easy recovery day. Took a stretching/yoga class, followed by a leisurely 4 miles (8:00 pace) on the elliptical.	4.0
Fri.	6/12/09	Did a 5.2-mile double today. The first 5.2 was with Terry at noon. 7:40 pace and it felt effortless. The second 5.2 was on my own. Thought the pace was only slightly faster, but the final time was 36:38 (7:07 pace). It felt almost as effortless as the first run... a nice surprise. Running some decent times again, with good form, without getting hurt...	10.3
Sat.	6/13/09	Ran an effortless, but deliberate 6 miles. Though I never felt like I was pushing it, I ran mostly negative splits (how the Kenyans train). Mile times were roughly 7:40, 6:45, 6:35, 6:38, 6:32, 6:21, so I went 32:51 for the last 5 miles (6:36 pace). The final mile was consciously brisk, but still easy.	6.0
Sun.	6/14/09	With Bay State Games trials in two days, I wanted to do something vigorous. My race will be at 5p, so I started my workout at 5p. After 20 min stretching in the steam room, I did a 60-min Fartlek workout on the elliptical. Worked in 4 x 800m pickups at sub-6:00 pace. I did 1 mile at training pace in between. The 800m reps were in 2:53, 2:47, 2:45, and 2:35. It was fairly effortless.	8.0
Mon.	6/15/09	Pre-race 4-miler on the elliptical. Short and slow. I feel ready for whatever tomorrow brings. I slept extra long last night, so my sleep and speed-work schedules are both optimal for what I need tomorrow. Will continue carbo-loading (eating almost nothing but pasta and banana-blueberry shakes) and get 7-8 hrs sleep tonight. Not too little; not too much.	4.0
Tues.	6/16/09	Won the Bay State Games Trials 5K (which was also the steeplechase qualifier) by 30 sec with little effort (17:17; 5:34 per mile). I could've run a lot faster, so I'm happy. According to my performance prediction calculator, I should be able to run under 10:40 for the steeplechase, 25 sec short of the average winning time at Masters Nationals. After I got home, I hit the gym to loosen up and did a 4-mile recovery on the elliptical.	9.0
Weds.	6/17/09	Ran a "Kenyan 9-miler" (all negative splits) on the elliptical. Started slower than 8:00 pace and finished faster than 6:00. The Sox put on a nice show against the Marlins, which helped the time pass.	9.0
Total		Averaged 7:18 per mile for the week	**50.3**

Training Log Week 20

Day	Date	Notes	Mileage
Thurs.	6/18/09	Nice easy 8 miles with Terry. 66 min (8:15 pace).	8.0
Fri.	6/19/09	"Kenyan" 8 miles on the elliptical. 55:50 (6:59 pace).	8.0
Sat.	6/20/09	Hard 7 miles on the roads plus a 1-mile warm down. Didn't plan on running hard, but the pace came easily for the first 6 miles, including a sub-19:00 5K mixed in. I could've run my best 8, but I didn't want to turn a training run into a road race.	8.0
Sun.	6/21/09	Just a quick, easy 4.6 miles on the elliptical for me. Meanwhile, the Brandeis boys ran a 200-mile relay race (the Green Mountain Relay), which took them just over 24 hrs.	4.6
Mon.	6/22/09	Did a nice, long pre-workout "stick" and stretching session in the steam room. 74 min on the elliptical. Started out easy, then picked it up for 3 or 4 miles, then took it easy for the last 1.5 miles. Finished the day with some light weight lifting.	10.0
Tues.	6/23/09	The miles were easy, but the day was hard. Did the regular 5+ at noon with Terry. At 6:30p, I took a 1-hr yoga/Pilates class. That's always good for leg strength, as well as core, which kills me. I breezed through the leg strength work but was dying during the abs. From what I understand, weaker areas of the body can tire during a race and drag on performance by expending energy reserves. My abs are clearly a weak area, so I'll keep at it. After the class, I dragged myself onto the elliptical for 8 miles. All in all, I put in close to 3 hrs of training -- it showed in my post-workout weight: 143lbs, the lightest I've been in 21 yrs.	13.2
Weds.	6/24/09	Terry and I went out for a lunchtime run, but went little further today. He's still hurting from his 20-mile contribution at the Green Mountain Relay, but he felt it was time to start boosting our mileage up, so we added 2.2 miles to our 5.15-mile loop. We took it easy (8:30 pace).	7.4
Total		Averaged 7:32 per mile for the week	**59.1**

Race Reports, Records, and Results

2009 Bay State Games Trials: At Bay States Games Trials, the steeplechase qualifier is a 5,000-meter run (combined with the 5,000-meter trial itself). Apparently back in the day, not many facilities had steeplechase equipment, so they opted for this unusual trial format. I did not prefer this system, but I didn't get a choice... As the race got underway, I tucked in behind two Tufts University runners who led us through a pedestrian first mile in 5:40. Another runner took the lead at that point, but I opted to stay behind the Tufts teammates. They were creating a nice draft for me, cutting the headwind on the backstretch of the Harvard track.

One of the Tufts guys faded at the 2,500-meter mark. I stayed with the other. The next 1,700 meters were tougher for me, but not exceedingly so. Not being familiar with the 5,000-meter distance, I simply didn't know how I should feel... I got over it by relaxing, putting my head down, and just tuning out.

The second Tufts runner fell apart at 4,500 meters. I took over second place but pretended to be tired so the leader (only 20 meters ahead and frequently looking over his shoulder) wouldn't think of me as a threat. I didn't know how good he was, but I was willing to bet I could out-sprint him.

With 350 meters to go, I started to sneak up on him. There were no spectators on the back straight, so no one warned him of my movement. I quieted my footsteps and slid into the second lane so he couldn't see my shadow, which was being cast slightly forward and toward the infield. With 200 meters to go, I pulled up to his shoulder. As he turned his head to see what was going on, I took off... quickly. He didn't even appear to give chase. I was gone before he could react. I closed the final 200 meters in about 31 seconds.

As it turns out, the sprint was unnecessary. The guy I passed was DQ'd because he had jumped into the race at the 200-meter mark. Shades of Rosie Ruiz! Officially, I won the race by 30 seconds (17:17.2 – 5:34.5 per mile).

I could have run a lot faster, so I was really happy with the race and time. According to my calculations, my performance was better than 10:40 for the steeplechase – pretty good, considering I had been training for only four months (and had two more years to train).

Miscellaneous Research and Notes

A substantial amount of evidence suggested I should have been running more of my miles at an easier pace. I was potentially burning myself out and risking injury by trying to do 50 miles each week under 7:00-per-mile pace. It's not like I wasn't warned... Coach Dave had been strongly recommending that I take a day off periodically. Unfortunately, I knew myself well enough to know that breaking my training streak could give me an excuse to get lazy. As a compromise with Coach Dave, I focused on dialing back the intensity and having one day each week allocated to a slow, short recovery run. Along with the reprimand, he provided some insight into a more structured training schedule:

> *"Have a plan and abide by it. If you plan to run 60-70 miles in a week stick to it. If 60-70 miles includes a 17- to 20-mile day, good. If it doesn't, then don't do it. It is careless and potentially harmful. Try to evenly spread out your training over a seven-day schedule but include a long day at the beginning of the week after a race and then taper down before a race. If no race is involved, then a long run is advised at the beginning of the week because it is necessary, [plus] you get it out of the way early in the week when you are fresh. Friday or Saturday should be shorter because fatigue is heavy at the end. Plus a rest day or short day helps rejuvenate the legs."*

Because I was not racing seriously early in my comeback, I created a 60-mile-per week schedule. I wanted mileage at 70-plus per week, but my body couldn't handle it.

I settled on the following:

- ➢ Sunday – Race or 8 miles
- ➢ Monday – Easy 12 miles
- ➢ Tuesday – 10 miles
- ➢ Wednesday – Speed work or 8 miles
- ➢ Thursday – 9 miles
- ➢ Friday – Moderate 8 miles
- ➢ Saturday – Easy 5 miles

The Oregon Training Style: I watched a DVD on the training techniques employed at the legendary University of Oregon. Oregon spawned superstars like Alberto Salazar and, of course, Steve Prefontaine. It's also the birthplace of Nike, co-founded by Coach Bill Bowerman. During his 24 years at Oregon, Coach Bowerman produced 31 Olympic athletes, 51 All-Americans, 12 American record-holders, 24 NCAA champions, and 16 sub-4:00 milers, all while winning four NCAA team titles.

The DVD confirmed many things I suspected and revealed some things I didn't know. It wasn't a major departure from the philosophies of my high school and college coaches, but it presented the material in a big-picture way. (My problem in high school and college was that I never sought to understand the big picture.)

The main takeaways from Oregon's training tactics are as follows:

- ➢ Toe-runners shouldn't run as many miles as heel-to-toe runners; they have a greater risk of injury. They make up for it with more effective interval training. The DVD compared Rudy Chapa (a high school 10K record holder) and Alberto Salazar. Chapa was a toe-striker and was only assigned 40-50 miles a week – a shockingly low total to me. Salazar was a heel-striker and assigned 60-70 miles a week – which still seemed low to me, but not shockingly so. Interestingly, Terry Pricher told me that Salazar's time as a dominant runner came to an end after he significantly upped his mileage. He went from being a globally top-ranked runner to not even being the top American. Flatter performances led him to increase his mileage even more – the exact opposite of the right thing to do – but I can see how he would think that more training was needed to improve his performance.

- ➢ Interval training is the most effective way to achieve peak performance. Base training is critical to *maintaining* peak performance, but intervals are how you peak. Oregon's interval schedule starts with longer intervals at pace that is relatively comfortable for the runner. As the weeks progress, they slowly decrease the distance of the average interval (not necessarily by eliminating long intervals, but by introducing shorter intervals). Simultaneously they increase the pace per interval. As a runner's major race approaches, the interval pace matches the runner's goal time, thus simulating the goal-pace.

- ➢ 5K runners start with repeat mile intervals but eventually incorporate 200-meter intervals. A late-season workout might be 3 x 1 mile at close to goal-pace, plus 8 x 300 meters at goal-pace. 1,500-meter runners start the season with repeat 1,000/1,200-meter intervals. Similar to traditional intervals, they also do "repetitions" later in the season, where the runner does all-out or near all-out intervals, but get a *full* recovery period in between.

- ➢ Hill work is used for strengthening, and the program employs tempo runs (distance runs at hard, but specified pace), Fartlek training (distance runs with periods of faster-pace running mixed in). Oregon also leverages circuit training, where the runner does some sort of easy interval with exercises like calisthenics and planks mixed in. All of these workouts are considered hard days.

All other days are very easy to recover and prepare for the next hard workout.

Chapter 4
Questions of Science; Science and Progress…

Weeks 21-27

The following story is a must-read for everyone who wants to run faster – which I assume is most of you. The number of 1990s New England track nerds reading this book purely for the nostalgia and the thrill of seeing their names in print is pretty small.

In weeks 9-12 of my training – after a 13-year layoff – I ran a little more than 250 miles, averaging 9 miles a day at slightly slower than 7:00 mile pace. Even though I have a decent running resume, this was aggressive so early into my training program. In my excitement and rekindled love for the sport, I was running hard almost every day and doing a lot of double sessions. When my Soleus and Achilles injuries started flaring up (starting in Week 7 and really becoming problematic in Week 10), I moved to my backup training plan, the elliptical machine, but I didn't alter my effort levels or change anything else about my routine. I just got off the roads and waited for everything to heal.

That was *not* the right way to train, but I didn't know it then. Needless to say, my body broke down, as is well chronicled in my running log's late-April and early-May entries. There's a reason I'm reiterating this here. We talked a little about the "tough guy" attitude of my college team in Chapter 3, but anyone can fall victim to the "neurosis of not training." Running is one of the few sports where most of your success is predicated on micromanaging your body's every sensation. Whether you're trying to qualify for NCAAs or you're training just to finish your first marathon, if you're not hurting – or you're not hurting *too* bad – your natural impulse is to push a little harder, squeeze in a few more miles.

In the midst of that crazy April, I logged my best training run since college: 53:05 for 8 miles (6:38 pace), which was even more exciting because it happened only a few hours after a lunchtime 5-miler with my running buddy Terry. Remember, I wasn't a big distance trainer, even in college, so logging a 13-mile day was kind of a big deal. Coincidentally, this run happened on April 13th. It wasn't a Friday, but that would've been fitting, because that day and that run marked the beginning of my breakdown.

It took a couple more weeks and a streak-threatening injury (which happened on a very slow, uneventful run – not a barn-burner) for me to rethink my training regimen. After adhering to the "train-hard" school of running my entire life, I finally gave in and began adhering to "train-smart" philosophies. Since then, I stayed healthier and ran a decent race at the Bay State Games Trials. Despite this, I wasn't completely sold on the "train-smart" school of running. The reasons were two-fold:

1. The word "effortless" started appearing regularly in my training log after the breakdown, but I found it hard to believe that an athlete could improve without effort. The second reason was a related issue, but it bothered me much more than the first.

2. Since that fateful eight-mile training run in April until I came to this realization, my training streak more than doubled. Although I made a significant effort to train "smart" not "hard," I went 74 straight days without a clear sign that the school of smart training had given me one iota of improvement. Psychologically, this was a tough pill to swallow, especially because the train-hard methodology provided me with new signs of improvement almost every week.

But nearly five months into my comeback, that all changed.

On Saturday, June 27th 2009 (see Week 21), I set out to run eight miles. I didn't have a pace in mind and didn't expect much, *and* I had a greasy burger and fries for lunch – because even with my Draconian diet, I indulged on the weekends. That being said, it was late in the day, so I wanted to get the run done and get my Saturday night started (so I could do some more indulging...)

I started out at a deliberate, but reasonable pace on one of my regular routes, which got me to the Boston Commons in 6:45. Pretty quick for the first mile of that course. In fact, I don't remember ever running it much quicker previously. My two-mile split was a notable (for me) 13:15. I didn't feel great, but I was definitely settling into the pace. By the three-mile mark, I was totally warmed up and in cruise control. My split was 19:40.

At that point, I realized that I had a shot at equaling my April 13 time... and I wanted to do it out of pure competitiveness. But more importantly, I wanted it as first-hand validation that training smart was *at least* as effective as training hard.

That being said, I didn't want to risk injury, so I focused on proper form. I concentrated on relaxing my hands, as the legendary Olympic champion Emil Zatopek used to advise. I concentrated on relaxing my legs, especially my quads, as my Northeastern University teammate Chris Bianchi used to do (looking almost sleepy as he ran his sub-14:30 5Ks). I focused on efficient strides because I tend to over-stride, which costs momentum and creates a higher risk of injury.

The fourth mile of the course is the toughest, but I still managed a smooth 6:30. I hit the halfway point at 26:10 – a record, if memory serves me correctly. From there, I had four downhill miles and 26:55 left on the clock in which to do them.

Mile 5 was predictably quick. It's straight downhill, so going fast wasn't an issue – but overusing my quads or injuring my calves was. I held my form, which cost me a few seconds, but it was the smart thing to do. I clocked a 5:20 fifth mile for 31:30 total time, just a minute slower than the all-out 5-mile road race I ran in Taunton a few months prior. Not bad for a training run.

Staying smooth during Mile 6 took more concentration. This run was not "effortless." Also, I started to think about a run I completed on the same route the Saturday before. I had a good pace going through Mile 6 then, but I could only muster 7:00 for the seventh mile. The smart thing to do then was to call it a day, and I did – even though it further augmented my doubt in "training smart." I didn't know if the current run was going to be any different, but there was only one way to find out.

I turned my attention to *not* running 7:00 for Mile 7 while keeping the bigger picture in mind: This is a training run, not a race. Stay smooth; train smart.

I crushed a 5:55 for the seventh mile. I passed Mile 7 in 43:30, leaving me with 9:30 to equal my fastest 8 mile training run since I was a 21-year-old collegian. And I felt fine. I wasn't thinking 9:30; I was thinking 6:30. A 6:29 final mile would get me below 50 minutes for the run... so I focused on holding strong, and hold strong I did. Final mile: 5:50. Final time: 49:20 (6:10 per mile average).

If I remember right, 6:10 for 8 miles was not a leisurely jog even during my college days. I was tired, but not exhausted. It was hard and fast but also a smart, controlled run. Not a race, but a good tempo run. Most importantly, everything seemed to be in working order. I felt great and nothing was tight or hurting, even hours later. Training smart worked!

That run completely changed my attitude toward training. It made me think about my goals and my chances of winning the Masters Nationals in 2011. I felt my odds of breaking 10:00 in the steeplechase had just gotten a lot better. In the whimsical recesses of my mind, I had to wonder if Hal Higdon's 34-year-old Masters Steeplechase record (9:18) could fall to a guy who didn't believe in training smart until he was 38 years old.

The moral of this story: It can be psychologically harder to train smart than to train hard. *Not* cranking out a challenging pace for the third day in a row or *not* tacking on two or three more miles even though you feel good – because you think over-investing now will put you that much farther ahead come race day – can be harder to let go than forcing yourself through your planned workout when your body is clearly telling you to stop. And training smarter may take a few extra weeks or even a few months to show results. But training smart *will* pay off. If you've planned enough time between the beginning of your training and your target race (and you better have; there's no sense planning to run a race you can't train properly for), training smart will get you to the line ready to perform and with a much greater chance of being healthy.

So how do you train smart? The remaining entries in my log and the research in this book will give you the blueprint to do just that.

Training Log Week 21

Day	Date	Notes	Mileage
Thurs.	6/25/09	Hit the elliptical *before* yoga/Pilates because when I did the class before the elliptical it really hurt. The class was no easier but more importantly, my elliptical was 10 min faster than before. This is clearly the proper order of operations. The ab work was brutal, but I'm improving. Strength, flexibility and core are important for the steeplechase and the class focuses on those. It's a great complement to my mileage.	8.0
Fri.	6/26/09	Dino Dibiaso[24] joined Terry and I for the lunch run. Dino was a top cross country and track runner at NU. After a long post-college layoff, he started running again. His training mainly consists of running 10 miles per day. Dino was a hybrid hard trainer/smart trainer in college but moved into the smart-training camp as he got older. He has stayed healthy and is running half-marathons near 1:20, so I would count him as evidence that smart training works.	9.5
Sat.	6/27/09	Ran the 8-mile course and after starting out slow, absolutely crushed it! Final time – 49:20! Best training since college, and I felt relaxed and in control the entire way. Proof that being smarter with my training is working.	8.0
Sun.	6/28/09	Ran 4.6 miles near my friend John Cassarini's house. My third straight day on the road. I haven't done this since mid-May. It was also my third day without knee braces. I don't remember the last time that happened. Calves are a little tight (clearly from yesterday's work) and knees are a bit sore, but nothing major.	4.7
Mon.	6/29/09	Relaxed 9.3 miles on the elliptical. I wanted to go 10-12 miles, but ran out of time; the gym closes at 9p. John Lester and the Red Sox kept me entertained, shutting out the Orioles.	9.3
Tues.	6/30/09	Long day. Terry and I went for an "easy" 5 miles after work, but it didn't feel easy. It was a long wk and I was a bit tired. After our run I dragged my butt to the gym for 4 miles on the elliptical and a 1-hr yoga/Pilates class. The class killed me. There was a heavy focus on abs (my biggest weakness). After 45 min I was toast.	9.2
Weds.	7/1/09	Solid 10 miles of work on the elliptical (7:07 pace). I planned to work over steeples, but thunderstorms forced me to delay that. The Bay State Finals are next Saturday, so I'll be taking it a little easier over the next 10 days.	10.0
Total		Averaged 7:07 per mile for the week	**58.7**

---

24 Dino Dibiaso recorded a 4:11 mile and 14:35 5K while running for Northeastern University, and he still ranks as one of the fastest 3,000-meter runners in school history (8:17.8). As a Master, he has run 3:00:18 for the marathon.

Training Log Week 22			
Day	Date	Notes	Mileage
Thurs.	7/2/09	Doubled up today with 5 rainy miles with Terry at lunch and 7.5 dry miles on the elliptical in the evening, followed by a long set of runners' curls. Terry ran great. We went sub-7:20 pace, which is quicker than usual. I felt great during both workouts, like the day I ran my breakout 8 miles. That day I had a burger for lunch, and last night I had Indian beef. I wonder if I need more red meat in my diet.	12.5
Fri.	7/3/09	Terry and I did 8 miles, running the course that goes by the Reggie Lewis Center. We agreed to take it easy, so we stayed at a steady 8:00 pace throughout. Terry doubled yesterday with a 60-min bike ride, and he doesn't like the heat. I finished off with a 3:30 closing 800m which actually tired me out a little.	8.0
Sat.	7/4/09	Jamie and I slept in and attended a family cookout, so I did a quick 8 miles on the elliptical.	8.0
Sun.	7/5/09	I had the idea to walk 9 holes of golf at Newton Commonwealth Golf Course with Jamie and then run the 7.5 miles home. The idea worked out fine. The run was mostly downhill, which contributed to a sub-7:00 pace.	7.5
Mon.	7/6/09	Nice easy 8 miles on the elliptical.	8.0
Tues.	7/7/09	My first steeplechase is Saturday, and I am overdue to practice steeples. I strapped on a backpack and ran to Harvard (4 miles) as a warm-up. Loosened up and did some drills. I eased into some pit jumps, initially just jumping onto the steeple, then eventually jumping in the water. I planned on landing on one foot, but defensively landed on two. (Maybe a good idea for injury prevention.) Next, I did some 400m and 200m intervals with one hurdle plus the steeple pit. During the fourth interval, I felt something in my Achilles again. The Achilles has to be 100% if I'm going to do steeple workouts going forward. In the meantime, I hope it holds up for the race. On a positive note, I got over the hurdles and through the water pit without much trouble. My form is weak, but that's ok at this stage.	6.0
Weds.	7/8/09	Maybe it's the weather or the re-tweaking of my Achilles, but I am a little depressed. The realization of how taxing the steeplechase will be on my 38-year-old legs is a little hard to take. I should have known, but I didn't think about it. With the race coming on Saturday, I did 6 miles on the elliptical. Felt strong. Tomorrow, I'll be back on the elliptical, with some speed mixed in.	6.1
Total		Averaged 7:22 per mile for the week	56.1

Injury Reports and Medical Findings

Flat Feet: After multiple visits in the spring/summer of 2009, it became clear that my physical therapist was *alleviating* my Achilles problem rather than *eliminating* it. I suspected that my flat feet might have had something to do with the injury. Sure enough, much research suggested that flat feet were the culprit. The foot's arch is designed to absorb the shock of foot strikes. People with flat feet or "pes planus" don't have that shock absorber, which increases their odds of developing overuse injuries like Achilles tendonitis or plantar fasciitis.

Basically, when I run, I'm taking on a lot more punishment than someone with strong arches. It's not an issue at shorter distances and slower pace, but during a hard 8-miler it could be the runner's equivalent of playing football without pads.

According to Running Shoes Guru:[25]

> *A flat foot is the most visible sign of over-pronation, meaning that your arch collapses during the impact on the ground. As a consequence, your ankle twists inward and your knees overcompensate.*

> *Flat feet are a particular concern for runners [because] during the running gait the arch is supposed to support, on average, 3 times their body weight.*

Across various research sources, I found Achilles tendonitis was a frequent consequence of having flat feet. One thing that really hit home was that over-pronation worsens with more mileage (more foot-strikes) and a quicker pace (which results in a more forceful foot strike).

---

25 www.runningshoesguru.com; [Google: running shoes guru + "flat feet"]

Training Log Week 23

Day	Date	Notes	Mileage
Thurs.	7/9/09	Hit the elliptical for a Fartlek workout after a "non-diet" lunch of spaghetti and meatballs. 2-mile warm-up, then 5 x 1 min at sub-5:00 mile pace; 2 min rest in between; 2-mile warm-down. The rest was unnecessarily long, but I wanted turnover, not anaerobic work. Later, I had an ice cream sandwich, a bag of popcorn, and a Sprite at the movies. Not my typical training food, but I've run well 36 hrs after red meat and junk food, so this is an experiment.	6.0
Fri.	7/10/09	Got lots of rest last night, as is customary two nights before a race. I did a quick and easy 4 miles on the elliptical, followed by light stretching in the steam room. Hit the pasta hard all day and bought some 3/16" needle spikes in the afternoon – hopefully the right tools for the job. One more big pasta meal tonight before my first steeplechase since 1991.	4.0
Sat.	7/11/09	Seeded 6th going into the Bay State Games, but my real concern was running under 10:40. My calf/Achilles injury from steeple practice Tuesday loomed as a serious threat to my goal. I feared it wouldn't hold for the full race. The injury definitely slowed me down. Finished 4th in 10:34. (See Race Reports below for details.)	7.0
Sun.	7/12/09	Despite overcoming my injury and hitting my goal time I wasn't fulfilled by yesterday's race. I abandoned the easy recovery run and did an elliptical Fartlek workout: 2-mile warm-up, then 6 x 800m Fartlek with 800m recovery (at sub-7:00 pace). I planned the reps at just under 3:00 each, but with each rep, I decided to go faster. The 6th one was around 2:30. After the reps I kept going through 10 miles in 65:00. Still not satisfied, I did 2 more miles in 11:30. Finished in 1:16:30 -- my most vigorous elliptical workout to date. Did running curls and stretched. This was *not* an example of "training smart" and afterward I hoped I didn't do anything foolish.	12.0
Mon.	7/13/09	Did 8 miles on the elliptical at 6:50 pace.	8.0
Tues.	7/14/09	Started with 5 miles on the elliptical in 34:28 (6:54 pace). Jumped right off the machine and into yoga/Pilates. Typical ball-buster, but I noticed progress. I've struggled to keep up on the ab exercises, but today I came close. I was wiped out, but I got back on the elliptical for another 5 miles. Need to take it easy tomorrow.	8.0
Weds.	7/15/09	Did 9 brisk miles on the elliptical (6:43 per mile). Planned on doing 8 miles, but when I got there I still felt good, so I tacked on the extra mile. I'm quite happy with my weekly mileage but more importantly, the pace isn't nearly as taxing as it used to be. I hadn't averaged 7:00 pace since my breakdown a couple months back, so I've reached the same intensity level via "training smart."	8.0
Total		Averaged 7:00 per mile for the week	56.0

Newton Running[26] says:

> *Studies of elite runners, those who run barefoot, and anyone running at 6-minute mile pace or faster run on their forefoot.*

So, it was probably not coincidental that my Achilles problem didn't flare up during slower runs. I probably could have run 70 miles a week at 8:00 pace with no problem… but I couldn't do 55 miles at sub 7:00 pace. This actually encouraged me. If my flat feet were the problem, the right shoes (or orthotics) could solve it.

Post-Workout Routine: One of the biggest drawbacks to training in your 30s and 40s is not the workouts themselves – they feel the same as they did in your teens and 20s (albeit maybe a little slower) – it's the post-workout process to stay healthy. On days when I pounded the roads, a full post-training routine could take over an hour. It started with Advil (usually one; sometimes two) and an Endurox shake, then some quick stretching. Next, I tried to ice everything from my knees to just above the ankles. I occasionally iced my quadriceps, especially if they were sore for several days in a row.

Once I had the ice bags on, I'd use ACE bandages to affix rolled up socks to the balls of my feet to help keep my calves/Achilles in a stretched position. This was something I decided to try on my own. Many of the middle-aged comeback runners I knew suffered from calf/Achilles injuries. I theorized these injuries might stem from years in the workplace, wearing dress shoes with prominent heels. Larger-heeled shoes shorten the calf and Achilles over time, which leads to pull-type injuries when people resume a serious training regimen. Most running-shoe stores sell knee-high compression socks that come with straps to point your feet upward, thus achieving the same effect as my

---

26 http://www.newtonrunning.com

rolled-up socks. However, I found the compression socks to be a hassle to put on, and they didn't do a great job of pointing my feet up – they merely tugged my toes up. My rolled-up socks seemed to really help.

After I'd ice, I'd take a hot shower to thaw out and stretch some more. By that time, the Endurox had gotten into my system, so I'd prepare a banana/blueberry protein smoothie and work myself over with "The Stick." Finally, I'd re-affix the rolled up socks to my feet and put on my calf compression sleeves. Then it would be time to relax, watch TV, and eat dinner (all in bed).

It was a lot of stuff and I'm not sure how much of it was absolutely necessary, but I think most of it helped and none of it hurt. Considering the importance of staying healthy, I felt it was better to be safe (and even silly) than sorry.

Dietary Research and Findings

Diet and Recovery (Cont.): Research studies indicate that the synthesis of glycogen between training sessions occurs most rapidly if carbohydrates are consumed immediately after exercise. Delaying carbohydrate ingestion for just two hours after a workout significantly reduces the rate at which muscle glycogen is resynthesized and stored. Research suggests you should consume 0.7 grams of simple carbohydrates (preferably glucose) per pound of body weight within 30 minutes after a run – and again every two hours for four to six hours to maximize the rate of glycogen synthesis (which equals about 60 ounces of Gatorade or 28 ounces of chocolate milk for a 150-pound runner). If you don't get it all back right away, it's not the end of the world because glycogen will be resynthesized during the 24 hours between workouts – but for optimal effectiveness, sugar-up sooner.[27]

Despite the many highly advertised commercial sports drinks, any drink that contains a large amount of glucose is great for recovery. For example, research published in the *International Journal of Sport Nutrition and Exercise Metabolism* in 2006 showed that chocolate milk is just as good, or better, than other recovery drinks after exhausting exercise. Some studies have found that consuming carbohydrates and protein together speeds muscle glycogen storage, but other studies have not found this to be the case. The total amount of calories consumed seems to be more important for recovery than the carbohydrate-protein mix.[28]

I established a pattern of strong training on Saturdays. I suspected that had something to do with my Friday-night and Saturday-morning nourishment, when I strayed from my weekday diet. Noted physiologist Jason Karp offered some corroboration for my suspicions and a train-low, race-high philosophy:

> *While immediate post-workout carbohydrate ingestion is the best strategy for optimal performance, it may not be the best strategy for runners specifically preparing for the marathon, a race which requires the largest glycogen storage capacity possible, a very efficient capacity to make new glucose, and a very effective system of fat use. Molecular evidence suggests that the opposite strategy – holding out on the muscles by delaying the consumption of carbohydrates – may be even more beneficial. By "starving" the muscles of carbohydrates, they are forced to use fat more effectively and even more glycogen may be synthesized when carbohydrates are finally introduced.*

> *Low muscle glycogen content has been shown to enhance the transcription of genes involved in protein synthesis. Think of this strategy as creating a threat to the muscles' survival: When you threaten the survival of muscles by depriving them of their preferred fuel, a strong signal is sent to make more of that fuel to combat the threat and to use other sources of fuel more effectively. The downside to training in a low-glycogen state, however, is that it's hard to maintain a high intensity [because] such high-intensity running is dependent on carbohydrates for fuel. A lot more research needs to be done in this area, but if you're going to try training with low muscle glycogen, make sure you consume lots of carbs before your marathon, so you "train low, race high."[29]*

---

27 www.runningtimes.com; [Google: "running times" Karp + physiology]

28 ibid

29 ibid

Training Log Week 24

Day	Date	Notes	Mileage
Thurs.	7/16/09	Tuesdays and Thursdays have become my "hard work" days because these are yoga/Pilates days. I finished my running before class, starting with a fast 5-mile elliptical at 2p (6:18 pace). At 5p, I went with Terry for our standard 5.2 miler (7:46 pace), my first road run since injuring my calf July 7th. Felt fine. Yoga/Pilates started at 6:30 and was tough as usual. I'm definitely sensing improvement across the board – especially with the abs. Later, I strayed from my diet and went out for steak and lobster. Considering the quality of my post-steak workouts, I'm not going to shy away from an occasional porterhouse.	10.2
Fri.	7/17/09	It's Friday night. Last weekend revolved around the Bay State Games Finals, so I'm ready for a weekend of fun. Did 8 miles on the elliptical (6:58 pace) and some light stretching.	8.0
Sat.	7/18/09	Hopped on the elliptical early and did a moderate 10K (6:48 pace). Later, out with friends in my neighborhood, I sprinted a short distance to grab something I left in my apartment… and tweaked my Achilles again. This has become such a regular occurrence that it barely upsets me. I have to get back to an intense rehab routine. No races or speed work until it's 110%.	6.2
Sun.	7/19/09	Went boating with some friends. By the time we got home the gym was closed, so I hit the roads for an easy 7 miles (7:57 pace). The Achilles was noticeable throughout and worsened in the last few miles. Back on the Achilles recovery plan tomorrow. I know I can get it to 100% healthy, but can I keep it there?	7.0
Mon.	7/20/09	On the elliptical, I can work pretty much as hard as I want without Achilles pain. This is good because I can still pack in cardio work. The range of motion doesn't fully replicate running, but it's good enough. Did an 8-mile Fartlek workout, focused purely on turnover: 2-mile warm-up then 200m pickups every 800m for 4 miles. That's a lot of rest, but I was focused on speed, completing each 200m in 30 sec or less. The elliptical isn't really built for that kind of speed, but it went well nonetheless. Afterward, I did running curls and spent the night rehabbing (ice, cross-friction massage, compression sleeve, and light stretching).	8.0
Tues.	7/21/09	Physical therapy appointment at Harvard Vanguard. My regular PT referred me there for Kinesio taping. Therapist gave my leg a thorough exam and recommended only elliptical or swimming for the next 4 wks. She provided me with new exercises and taped me up. Logged a standard 8-mile elliptical, followed by yoga/Pilates.	8.0
Weds.	7/22/09	Quick 8 miles on the elliptical today. The Achilles is almost pain-free again, but I will follow the PT's orders.	8.0
Total		Averaged 7:02 per mile for the week	**55.4**

Training Log Week 25

Day	Date	Notes	Mileage
Thurs.	7/23/09	Good session today. Brisk 8-mile elliptical (6:33 pace), then yoga/Pilates. Starting to breeze through this easily… even the abs. I have to wonder if last night's dinner had something to do with it. Jamie and I went to Parish Café, where I ate a steak sandwich and most of her meatball sandwich, plus ice cream, apple pie, and an ice cream sandwich for desert. The junk food probably didn't do anything, but the red meat about a day prior has equated to stronger performances.	8.0
Fri.	7/24/09	Hamstrings are pretty sore from yesterday's yoga/Pilates. The class involved more leg-explosion exercises than usual, but I didn't think that would leave me sore. I'm happy. Hard to shake the "no pain, no gain" philosophy. Still had a good session on the elliptical: 8 miles in 51:46 (6:28 pace). Followed that with drills and physical therapy exercises.	8.0
Sat.	7/25/09	The road is better prep for racing, but injuries make elliptical work a necessity. It's good to find that machine work is nearly as valid as road work. That said, I set a new training record on the elliptical: 8 miles in 46:55 (5:52 pace), my first sub-6:00 training session since college. As was the case in previous records, I went out quickly and focused on relaxing during the final 3 miles.	8.0
Sun.	7/26/09	After yesterday's workout, I took it easy: 8.2 miles in 1:00:45 (7:25 pace) on the elliptical.	8.2
Mon.	7/27/09	Long day. Did a lunch run with Terry to see how the Achilles would handle an easy 5 miler (7:38 pace). It wasn't too bad but wasn't great, so I stopped 0.4 miles shy of the finish. In hindsight, this was not a good example of "training smart." We walked a warm down. Later I hopped on the elliptical for a quick 5.75 miles (6:32 pace). Everything felt fine.	10.5
Tues.	7/28/09	Typical Tuesday: elliptical, followed by yoga/Pilates.	8.0
Weds.	7/29/09	Did a brisk 8 miles (6:43 pace) elliptical. Training streak now at 175 days. However, I feel great, although I'm lucky nothing's breaking down after deviating from my "train smart" philosophy a few times recently.	8.0
Total		Averaged 6:43 per mile for the week	**58.7**

My event of choice was not the marathon, but I liked the theory nonetheless. I suspected that red meat deprivation during the week enhanced my body's absorption of its nourishing properties when I did eat it (almost exclusively on Fridays). I also tended to eat *more* food on Friday night and Saturday morning. As a result, I probably went into my Saturday workouts – which usually occurred at dusk – with more types of, and a higher quantity of, training fuels than I did at any other point in the week. Being able to achieve peak performance is clearly a function of timing – timing of rest, timing of interval workouts, etc. – and I believe nutrition is one more thing to time properly for optimal performance.

Race Reports, Records, and Results

<u>2009 Bay State Games Finals</u>: I was seeded sixth going into the 2009 Bay State Games Finals in Massachusetts, a meet that attracted mostly 18-to-24-year-old high schoolers and collegians trying to get some work in over summer break. *My* concern was finishing the steeplechase under 10:40. One problem: I injured my calf hurdling steeples in practice the week before, and that loomed as a serious threat to my goal. Even as I warmed up, it wasn't feeling great at all. I knew there was a real chance it wouldn't hold up for the entire race. Nonetheless, this was my only chance to run a steeplechase that year, so the show had to go on.

Early in the race, I settled into fifth place. The calf injury definitely impacted my form and slowed me down. The race-day heat also played a role. I was breathing hard most of the race, as were several of my competitors. (After the race many of them said they ran disappointing times). At the second-to-last water pit, I made a move and took over fourth place. I had an advantage at the water pit all day and never actually landed in the water. A bit on my old athleticism was still there! On the last lap I made another move but the guy in third place responded with a surge of his own. I tried to sprint, but my calf wasn't up to the task, so I let him go.

I finished in fourth with a time of 10:34.

It was about 76 degrees at race-time, at least 10 degrees warmer than the day of the Bay State Games Trials. All things considered, it was a good step toward my ultimate goal. Between the heat and the injury, I probably lost 10 seconds or more. Still, I ran to within 19 seconds of the time needed to win the Masters Nationals. And I had two more years to improve.

Beyond seeing the progress from all my hard work, I also learned a couple of things:

1. I should have started training over hurdles several weeks sooner. Waiting until two weeks before the race was cutting it too close and was exacerbated by some rain that eliminated a few hurdle days.
2. I needed interval training. I had a great base, but running repeated 80-second 400-meter splits over hurdles and water is something that requires interval work if you want to do it well.

Final note: My number for the race was #40. It might have been an omen, but I was thinking, "I'm not 40 yet!"

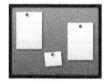 **<u>Bulletin Board Material</u>** – *I learned that my time at the Bay State Games Finals was the second-fastest in America in the 35-to-39-year-old division in 2009. It was the sixth-fastest among Americans over 30 years old, and sixth-fastest among 35-39 year-old Americans going back to 2003. I was five seconds shy of hitting the USATF's All-American standard for my age group. Not bad for five month's worth of work.*

As for 2009's fastest 35-39 age group time in America, that honor went to Ivan Ivanov. He blew away my performance, and everyone else's, running 9:56.4 at the USATF Masters Championships in Oshkosh, WI (with a similar temperature as the Bay State Games; probably a few degrees warmer). I couldn't find any other racing results for Ivanov but learned that he's a Bulgarian-born runner who won the NCAA Division II Steeplechase Championship in 1996. His 8:57 still stands as the fastest time ever run on his home track (University of Nebraska Kearney).

The 40+ division had an even better runner in Bart Wasiolek of Connecticut. He ran a 9:44 Steeplechase in April 2009 for a #1 age-group ranking. The year prior, he ran 4:34 for one mile. Also of note, a runner named David Smith (43 years old) ran four events over the course of four days at the USATF Masters Nationals. He ran 16:00.09 in the 5,000 meters on Thursday (seventh fastest in the nation in 2009), 10:25.01 for the steeplechase on Friday (fourth fastest), 34:00.51 in the 10,000 meters on Saturday (second fastest), and 4:19.95 for 1,500 meters on Sunday (tenth fastest) – a very impressive feat of stamina.

Training Log Week 26

Day	Date	Notes	Mileage
Thurs.	7/30/09	Typical Thursday: elliptical, followed by Yoga/Pilates. Nothing exciting to report.	8.0
Fri.	7/31/09	Had a PT appointment with Angela Mergel at Harvard Vanguard. She gave me electro stimulation for the Achilles, followed by a sports massage on my calf. My lateral gastroc (outer calf) is very tight, so that was an area of focus. Not a pleasant massage! After, I did some light stretching. Had another strong day on the elliptical: 49:35 for 8 miles (6:12 pace). Wasn't hard, and I recovered quickly. I had a feeling it would be a strong day because last night I went outside my diet. Need to see if this works for speed work and races.	8.0
Sat.	8/1/09	New training record. I hosted a pre-party for a Boston city-hall concert, so I had to get my run done early… and fast! I beat last week's record by 8 sec, covering 8 elliptical miles in 46:46 (5:51 pace). Not road work, but a solid accomplishment. I've been bettering my times on the same machine on the same setting, so it still feels like progress.	8.0
Sun.	8/2/09	8 miles on the elliptical in 52:19 (6:32 pace).	8.0
Mon.	8/3/09	8 miles on the elliptical in 51:28 (6:26 pace).	8.0
Tues.	8/4/09	Training streak is officially 6 months… and I'm officially caught in a grind. Nothing much to say. Today, 8 miles on the elliptical in 52:59 (6:37 pace), followed by yoga/Pilates class. In a couple more wks, I can try testing my Achilles out on the roads again.	8.0
Weds.	8/5/09	Another strong elliptical workout (8 miles in 49:24 – 6:10 pace). Arguably my best wk of work to date.	8.0
Total		Averaged 6:22 per mile for the week	**56.0**

Training Log Week 27

Day	Date	Notes	Mileage
Thurs.	8/6/09	Terry joined me on the elliptical. Nice to have some company. Hard workout by mistake though. I set the resistance at Level 14 (vs. 13). Thus, I started tiring at 5 miles and struggled. Terry wasn't done yet, so I dropped the resistance level and plodded through another 1.2 miles. Terry's pace on Level 13 was actually a bit slower than his road pace, which validates the times I've been logging. Yoga/Pilates followed.	9.2
Fri.	8/7/09	Easy day. Did 8 miles elliptical in 54:45 (6:51 pace). Afterward, I golfed with Dennis Coraccio in New Hampshire. He's 57 and still plays basketball with my old work colleagues.	8.0
Sat.	8/8/09	Breezed through 8 miles on the elliptical in 54 min (6:45 pace). I kept going and finished 11 miles in 1:14:00 (6:44 pace).	11.0
Sun.	8/9/09	Hard 8 miles on the elliptical: 48:28 (6:03 pace).	8.0
Mon.	8/10/09	73 min elliptical, for an easy 10 miles (7:18 pace).	10.0
Tues.	8/11/09	Easy 8 miles on the elliptical in 55:42 (6:58 pace).	8.0
Weds.	8/12/09	Cranked out 8 miles on the elliptical in 46:52 (5:51 pace).	8.0
Total		Averaged 6:38 per mile for the week	**62.2**

Miscellaneous Research and Notes

Faster Than Forty Performance Prediction Calculator: A good way for older athletes to measure their performances is to compare them to the world or American records for their age group. For example, my steeplechase time at the Bay State Games Finals was 13.6 percent shy of Hal Higdon's Masters steeplechase record (9:18.6). Four weeks prior to that, my road 5K was 21.0 percent short of Brian Pope's Masters 5,000-meter record (14:17.4) and 10 weeks prior to *that*, my five-mile time was 28.5 percent slower than Steve Spence's 23:47 standard. By this measure, I could compare apples to oranges and conclude that each race I had run showed significant improvement over the previous race (more so than I originally thought, in fact).

To determine their present-day potential, I believe Masters athletes can compare their *old* personal records (PRs) to the corresponding records and estimate what they might run later in life. For example, in high school, I fell 8.1 percent short of the national high school 800-meter record. In college, I came within 4 percent of the NCAA 1,000-meter record (2:24.5 vs. 2:18.7). From these findings, I concluded that I realistically had the ability to run within a similar range of the current Masters records.

I entered all of my high school, college, and sub-Masters PRs into a spreadsheet and compared them with the corresponding high school, college, and Masters records (the American records in each case).

From that exercise, it was clear that my 1,000-yard and 1,000-meter times (high school and college, respectively) were closer to national records than any other event. The further the distance was from 1,000 meters, the further I came from the corresponding record. I dubbed this is my "Event Bell Curve" (or EBC for short).

Drilling deeper, I entered my best times for each year in high school. As I suspected, my EBC was similar in each year. In other words, my times as a high school freshman were predictive of where I would see the greatest success in my running career – the 1,000-yard or 1,000-meter runs. In those events, I set my high school record, won the high school Eastern States Championship, won a New England Championships title at Northeastern University, and set a Northeastern University record that was previously held by NCAA All-American, Brad Schlapak.

Getting back to the point, calculating an EBC during my freshman year of high school would have helped determine my optimal event. Instead, I ran the two-mile that year, an event in which I never did anything of consequence. Luckily, I had a smart coach who quickly figured out where I belonged and put me in the 1,000-yard run. I think calculating an EBC is something everyone should do at least once.

Once turned out to be enough for me. The 1,000-yard and 1,000-meter runs remained my optimal events throughout my high school, college, and post-college career. My personal experience alone is not a valid data set, but similar data I have collected from other athletes implies we are all born with a physical pre-disposition to one perfect event... and if that's the case, everyone should find theirs sooner, not later!

One last thing – in high school, I came within 5 percent of the national high school 1,000-yard record. In college, I came to within 4 percent of the NCAA record, despite having lost focus in my junior and senior years. (My PR was set as a sophomore.) That made me think I had the potential to get within 3 percent (or less) of a Masters record. As my sub-Masters race distances grew shorter (going from 5 miles to 5,000 meters to the 3,000-meter steeplechase), my times came closer to the established Masters records in each event.

This made me rethink my overall Masters strategy... Perhaps I would be wise to focus on the 800-meter run for optimal performance (and keep the steeplechase as a fun diversion). One big question loomed: Would my Achilles withstand the more intense foot-striking of the 800-meter run?

Faster Than Forty

Rank	Time	Runner	Country	Date	DOB	Age
\multicolumn{7}{}						

Rank	Time	Runner	Country	Date	DOB	Age
1	1:48.8i	Johnny Gray	USA	3/2/2001	6/19/1960	40
2	1:50.3	Jim Sorensen	USA	6/30/2007	5/10/1967	40
3	1:50.7	Colm J. Rothery	IRL	9/5/2000	1/28/1960	40
4	1:51.3	Peter Browne	GBR	8/19/1991	2/3/1949	42
5	1:51.5	Ronald Mercelina	NED	9/24/1986	4/18/1946	40
6	1:51.6	Robert Mc Cubbin	AUS	3/13/2004	3/8/1963	41
7	1:52.4	Carlos Cabral	POR	6/1/1994	6/20/1952	41
8	1:52.6	Tony Young	USA	4/12/2003	4/12/1962	41
9	1:52.5	Ken Popejoy	USA	5/31/1991	12/9/1950	40
10	1:52.7	Darrell Maynard	GBR	8/24/2002	8/21/1961	41
11	1:52.8	Babacar Niang	FRA	6/29/1999	9/9/1958	40
12	1:53.2	Anselm Le Bourne	USA	7/23/2000	4/20/1959	41
13	1:53.5	Ron Bell	GBR	7/14/1987	10/1/1946	40
14	1:53.7	Saladin Allah	USA	7/9/2001	1/1/1960	41
15	1:53.7	Alain Flamee	BEL	6/2/2002	3/10/1961	41
16	1:53.9	Kip Janvrin	USA	4/25/2007	7/8/1965	41
17	1:54.1	Dave Taylor	GBR	9/6/2006	1/9/1964	42
18	1:54.2	Maximillian Freund	GER	8/9/2008	8/23/1967	40
19	1:54.5	John Hinton	USA	4/15/2006	5/1/1962	43
20	1:54.5	Klaus Mainka	GER	7/16/1977	3/12/1936	41

All-Time Rankings: Men's Masters 800 Meters (as of Feb. 1, 2010; i = indoors)

Source: www.mastersathletics.net

Chapter 5
Here We Are Now, Entertain Us

Weeks 28-40

The setting was Northeastern University, circa 1989, on a particularly boring weekday morning. Given the psychological makeup of the competitive runner, boredom equaled trouble.

I strolled across campus to the track locker room in Cabot Gym just to see if anything was going on. It was pretty quiet there – just a few guys coming in from early runs or getting ready for workouts. Ken Kaczinski was in the latter group. Kaczinski wasn't actually on the team at the time. He was an upperclassman who had exhausted his eligibility (a common happening at Northeastern, which had five-year curriculum). Still, he was always a welcome presence in the locker room and a good source of veteran insight.[30]

On that particular day, he was a good source of something else…

"What's up, Gomes?" he greeted me.

"Nada. What's up, Kaz?"

"Nada. Going for a run. You in?"

"Nah. I've got the day off. What else is going on?"

"Selling my car. Want it?"

"Dunno. What'cha got?"

"1980 Corolla. You can have it for 25 bucks."

(That's right, he said $25.)

Sadly, even at that price, that was a lot of money for me. At the time, my monthly budget was $300… for *everything*. I was sharing a basement room in an off-campus townhouse for $143 per month. I set aside $100 per month for food and $40 for utilities. This left roughly $17 per month for entertainment. I did a quick analysis:

On the upside, despite the initial sacrifice, a car had the potential for a lot more than 1.5 months' worth of entertainment. On the downside, I knew this car had to come with some problems. There was no mention of a title, no mention of a registration – and I knew that Kaczinski (like many of Northeastern's crazy runners) had no problems interfacing with the various drifters, street people, and other near-do-wells that inhabited Roxbury and approached Northeastern students with all sorts of offers for low-cost contraband. But Kaczinski was always good to me, so I was pretty sure the car would have four tires and a steering wheel. For $25, I figured that was all it needed.

"Deal." I fished into my pockets and handed him the money.

He handed me the keys. "Here you go. It's parked out in front of Maxwell Jumps."

---

30 Kaczinski's 9:04 steeplechase best still ranks on the Northeastern University all-time list.

"Thanks Kaz!" I sprinted out of the locker room toward Maxwell's, the campus bar. My boring weekday morning just received a jolt of excitement… Time for a joyride! I skidded to a halt in front of Maxwell's and my new set of wheels – which wasn't hard to identify, as it was *clearly* the only $25 automobile on the block.

The car was a dull, indecipherable color. The tint looked like spray paint or maybe even house paint. I didn't take a close look. I was too busy fumbling with the key to unlock the door. Finally, I got into the car and took a look at my surroundings. Steering wheel? Check. Instrument panel? Check. Stick shift? Check… er, wait a minute. The stick shift was made out of copper. Actually, it was a copper pipe. A removable copper pipe. I didn't care though; I quickly rationalized that the removable pipe was a form of anti-theft device. The car had a steering wheel and four tires, and it was obviously driveable or Ken couldn't have navigated it to park on busy Huntington Avenue. That was all I needed.

I put the key in the ignition and was happy to hear the engine turn over. A minute later I was driving down the streets of Boston enjoying my new $25 whip. I took it for a ride around the block and through the Fenway district. As I was looping around the park past the museum, I came to a red light and stopped. Much to my dismay, I was promptly rear-ended by another vehicle.

I got out of my car, and the driver behind me got out of hers. She clearly looked frazzled. There was blood on her hands and a little bit on her face – but it didn't look like she received the injuries from our very minor fender-bender. It looked like she had killed someone. I wanted nothing to do with that.

I asked myself a quick question. Which was of more benefit: recouping damages to a $25 car that I probably legally did not own, or getting the hell away from whatever was going on with this woman? I asked her if she was okay, hoping to quickly send her on her way. In a trembling little voice she said, "Yes."

I told her she could go, and she didn't hesitate to react. She got back in her car, pulled around my hoopty and was gone. As for me, I drove the car back to campus as fast as I could. I parked it in the same spot where I found it and ran back to the locker room.

Kaczinski was gone, but my roommate Tom Lahive was at his locker getting ready for a run.

"Hey, Lahive," I said.

"What's up, Gomser?"

"Wanna buy a car?"

"How much?"

"Fifty bucks."

"Sold!" (Lahive needed a much shorter cost-benefit analysis than I had needed.) He gave me the $50, and I gave him the keys.

Lahive was crazy. He was liable to do anything, anytime, anywhere, for any reason. I actually felt bad for that car – but I had just turned a 100-percent profit in less than an hour, a fact that I knew would infuriate Lahive when he learned it later, so I didn't feel *too* bad. Any concerns I had for the hoopty were soon validated though. Later that night, Lahive grabbed Damon, another Northeastern track guy, and went for a ride. They cruised around the city and eventually found themselves driving around the Fens – the same park district where I was rear-ended earlier.

Tooling around in an illegal ride wasn't exciting enough for Lahive, though. To spice things up he decided to take the car off road and drop it straight in the swampy pond in the middle of the park. He threw the transmission in neutral, and the car coasted toward the muck. Looking at Damon in the passenger seat, he calmly said, "Get out."

The car was picking up steam as it rolled downhill toward the water.

"What?" Damon asked incredulously.

"I said, get out!" Any friend of Lahive was no stranger to insanity, so Damon jumped quickly from the moving vehicle. Lahive jumped as well, just seconds before the car careened into the pond, but much to his dismay, it didn't sink... at least not as fast as he had hoped. The windows were up, which may have slowed its descent, so Lahive rolled up his pants legs, wrapped his hand and arm with his shirt, waded into the shallow mire, and smashed the driver-side window. Water started rushing in, much to Lahive's delight.

Damon, now fully emotionally invested in the destruction, raised his leg and karate-kicked through the passenger-side window. Unfortunately for him, a large shard of glass opened up a nasty gash the full length of his lower leg. When it was all said and done, the car sunk, Lahive was happy, and Damon's track season was over. It was not the strangest thing to have happened...

Technical Tip – *The biological/physiological effects of driving and destroying a stolen car don't vary much from the biological/physiological effects a runner feels as he lines up for a big race. The bigger the stakes, the bigger the body's chemical reaction. Score-oriented sports may provide a one-two punch. The first punch is the fear. Stepping to the track with a championship at stake, with fans and family watching and teammates depending on you, causes a certain degree of fear... and fear produces a triumvirate of chemical goodies: endorphins, dopamine, and norepinephrine.[31] The endorphins mitigate pain while the dopamine and norepinephrine act as performance enhancers. The second punch is the reward. If you <u>win</u> the race, the resulting boost of additional dopamine makes you crave more. The greater the release, the greater the addiction-like symptoms. This cycle can repeat with greater magnitude until the athlete stops winning – but the effects of a loss can be devastating. The brain can cut the dopamine supply in less than two seconds, and euphoria can change to depression.[32] This may explain the bad behavior in many athletes; when the chemical connection is cut, they need to replace it fast... on or off the track or playing field.*

Training Log Week 28

Day	Date	Notes	Mileage
Thurs.	8/13/09	5.2 miles on the roads with Ryan O'Connell[33] and Steve Carnevale, two of Coach Dave's guys from Coyle & Cassidy High School. My quads were sore before I finished. I may have to combine elliptical work with quad strengthening exercises to be ready for the roads.	5.2
Fri.	8/14/09	Quads sore from yesterday, so I only ran 4 miles, albeit at a brisk pace (6:28).	4.0
Sat.	8/15/09	Started my workout with a barefoot mile on the treadmill in 8:00. A lot of research indicates barefoot running will strength muscles in the feet and assist with Achilles issues. After that, I hit the elliptical for an all-out 7-miler. I finished that in 39:55 (5:42 pace) -- very fast, hard workout.	8.0
Sun.	8/16/09	Easy 9 miles at 6:59 pace. The last mile was my 1,500th since my comeback started.	9.0
Mon.	8/17/09	Pretty easy 8 miles at 6:44 pace. Nothing exciting.	8.0
Tues.	8/18/09	Last wk I missed my yoga/Pilates classes. I got back to the full program today, starting with 8 miles on the elliptical at 6:38 pace, then class – with an emphasis on leg strength and stretching, which I like. Class ended with a heavy dose of abs, which was tough. I felt sick/exhausted after, but the improvements are noticeable.	8.0
Weds.	8/19/09	Terry joined me for a 1-hr session on the elliptical. He's definitely getting in shape... hung with me for 6 miles, at which point I started picking it up. I got through 8 miles in 54:30, which left the door open to complete an extra mile before the hour was up. I busted out a 5:23 to complete 9 miles in 59:53. A good workout considering yesterday's butt kicking. (My hamstrings were sore and tired all day.)	9.0
Total		Averaged 6:39 per mile for the week	51.2

---

31 Source: [Google: psychology today + adrenaline + dopamine]

32 Source: [Google: money.cnn.com + dopamine]

33 Ryan O'Connell ultimately garnered a third-place finish in the Mass. State Meet for Coach Dave and went on to run for Springfield College, where he qualified for the NCAA D-III nationals multiple times. His PRs as of this writing were 1:56 for 800 meters and 3:51 for 1,500 meters.

Training Log Week 29

Day	Date	Notes	Mileage
Thurs.	8/20/09	Tough day. Started with 4.7 miles with Terry, but I had a sour stomach, so it wasn't so easy. I felt better at night, so I hit the elliptical for an easy 7 miles (6:51 pace) and then went to yoga/Pilates. Thankfully, the instructor, Ali, went easy on us. Lots of stretching, which was a welcome rest after Tuesday's workout.	11.7
Fri.	8/21/09	Started with 6.75 miles on the bike (equivalent to 3 miles at 7:30 pace) then jumped on the elliptical for 5 miles at 6:41 pace. Altered my diet to focus on protein. Although carbs help optimize my workouts, protein may be more important for maintaining my body. I'll focus on protein most of the time and save carbs for pre-workout meals (lunch) and days before I plan on doing extra hard workouts or races.	8.0
Sat.	8/22/09	A basic day of training, but not a *normal* day. Did 8 miles at 6:49 pace in the a.m. to get it done before our annual Newport Polo Tailgate Party. As is tradition, I wore a cow costume to entertain the kids. This involves much running around, including the traditional lap around the grounds – when I chase the players/horses around the field as they high-five the crowd. It's 400-800m at a brisk pace. I was pretty tired afterward!	8.0
Sun.	8/23/09	John Oliveira, Dennis Shine, Rick Miller, and I went for a short run in Newport, RI. Dennis and Johnny O did 3 miles. Miller and I went 4 miles, but I did an add-on just to make sure. Totaled 4.2 miles at 7:21 pace. Today was my 200th straight day of training. This doubles my old record. I've "run" 1,560 miles at an average of 7:11 per mile – 56 min of cardio per day and an equivalent of 7.8 miles.	4.2
Mon.	8/24/09	1:30p run with Terry and Miller in Boston. Covered 5.1 miles in 38:22 (7:31 pace). We all felt *awful*. A weekend of partying will do that when you're old. My afternoon elliptical wasn't much better until the end. First mile was 9:00! The second was in 8:00. I didn't hit my stride until the final 3 miles. I got back to my normal eating/drinking routine and almost felt human by bedtime.	13.1
Tues.	8/25/09	8 miles on the elliptical at 7:07 pace... *slow*. I felt off again today and couldn't make it through Ali's yoga/Pilates class. Gonna take it easy tomorrow. May need even more easy days. I'm hoping it's just residual effects of the weekend's festivities and my switch to a more protein-oriented diet.	8.0
Weds.	8/26/09	Standard 5.2 miles with Terry at 7:25 pace. Felt good for the first time in days, could have gone faster.	5.2
Total		Averaged 7:06 per mile for the week	**58.1**

Training Log Week 30

Day	Date	Notes	Mileage
Thurs.	8/27/09	The easy day did me some good. Did 8 miles on the elliptical at 6:10 pace. Last week's diet shift to protein may have had an impact on my performance, but I'm feeling stronger now. My Achilles also feels better, so maybe the protein is helping my legs get stronger and healthier. I've gained a few pounds, but I can live with the trade-off, if it enables my Achilles to get to 100%.	8.0
Fri.	8/28/09	Another strong day. 8 miles on the elliptical, 1 sec faster than yesterday.	8.0
Sat.	8/29/09	Planned on taking it easy but felt strong and banged out my 3rd straight elliptical of 8 miles under 50 min (49:58; 6:15 pace). I'll definitely take it easy tomorrow.	8.0
Sun.	8/30/09	Felt strong again but slowed the pace to 6:39 (versus 6:10-6:15 over the past 3 days) to incorporate some rest. Felt effortless and I added an extra mile, completing 9 miles in just under 1 hr. My shift to more protein seems to have worked, but my weight continues to rise. I was 154lbs after my workout, 6lbs more than usual. My target weight is 150lbs, but I'm going to increase it to 153lbs (my college racing weight). Hopefully, that will strike the right balance between health and efficiency.	9.0
Mon.	8/31/09	Brisk 8-mile elliptical (6:05 pace) after yesterday's "recovery run."	8.0
Tues.	9/1/09	Typical Tuesday elliptical work and yoga/Pilates. Only finished 7 miles before class. That may have helped in the class because I felt pretty strong.	7.0
Weds.	9/2/09	Easy 8 miles at 6:52 pace. Finished the wk with 56 elliptical miles at 6:23 pace - my best wk in almost a month. I'm adjusting well to the protein-oriented diet. I can load up on carbs before important workouts, but protein seems critical to muscular development and recovery, which is more important at my age.	8.0
Total		Averaged 6:23 per mile for the week	**56.0**

Training Log Week 31			
Day	Date	Notes	Mileage
Thurs.	9/3/09	Took it easy today; 6 miles on the elliptical at 6:29 pace. I may hit the roads tomorrow and test the Achilles.	6.0
Fri.	9/4/09	After a long hiatus from road running, I tried a tempo run. I was a little too excited and went out too fast for my fitness level. After 3.5 miles at 6:20 pace, I had to stop for a min. After that, I modified the workout to fit the theme. I averaged 6:17 per mile for 8 miles but made a couple more stops, making the run more of an interval workout (essentially 2-mile repeats at 12:34, with 1 min or so in between). Most importantly, the Achilles felt great. We'll see if that holds.	8.0
Sat.	9/5/09	The Achilles felt fine, but I stuck to the elliptical today. Easy 8 miles at 6:48 pace. I'll probably stay on the machine for the next few days. I'm heading to Chicago on Thursday and will probably be on the roads every day during the trip.	8.0
Sun.	9/6/09	Another 8-mile day on the elliptical, as planned. I dropped the pace to 6:17 and will likely go easy tomorrow.	8.0
Mon.	9/7/09	Did an easy 8 miles on the elliptical (6:41 pace). Spoke to Terry and planned a stair workout tomorrow. Been a while since I did a real workout…	8.0
Tues.	9/8/09	Did 5 sets of stairs (32 floors each). Terry did well: 3:45 to 4:00 per set. Under 4:00 is solid. My times were encouraging -- 3:45, 3:30, 3:15, 3:12, and 2:52. The last 3 sets were all PRs. The last one was agony. We capped the workout with a 4-mile warm down (a pedestrian, but painful, 8:24 per mile). Good strength work.	7.0
Weds.	9/9/09	Terry and I did our normal 5.2 miles at 7:20a. I felt sluggish before the run, but that changed when I started moving. Light-footed throughout. I spent the rest of the day barefoot doing toe-curling exercises, which are supposed to alleviate the side-effects of having flat feet (most notably, Achilles tendonitis). According to a passage in *Born to Run*, Alan Webb started as a mediocre runner. He had flat feet and size-12 shoes. As the story goes, he worked on strengthening his feet and arch, which changed his shoe size to 9/10. The rest is history. If foot exercises produce one-tenth of Webb's results, I'll be happy. If it just makes my Achilles problem go away, I'll be ecstatic.	5.2
Total		Averaged 6:41 per mile for the week	**50.2**

Injury Reports and Medical Findings

Injury Diagnosis: Another universal challenge related to competitive running – but of particular importance to athletes in their 30s or 40s (or beyond) – is diagnosing injuries and choosing the right way to deal with them. We've created an "injury hierarchy," as follows:

➢ Level 1 Injury – Daily aches and pains associated with training, alleviated by DIY home treatments or preventative measures (e.g., icing, ibuprofen, targeted stretching, preventative wraps, etc.)
➢ Level 2 Injury – Something worse than daily aches and pains, and something you can't treat yourself, but the treatment is non-medical in nature (e.g., massage therapy, Kinesio tape, etc.)
➢ Level 3 Injury – A legitimate training-related health problem (e.g., a stress fracture, muscle pull/tear, etc.) that requires medical treatment and/or physical therapy

In college, competitive athletes usually have regular access to school doctors and the team's training staff. Once you're on your own, the time (and sometimes money) you need to visit a doctor makes Level 3 injury maintenance a challenge – so you need to make an educated guess as to whether your problem requires routine DIY maintenance, something requiring professional assistance, or something requiring medical assistance.

After trying things on my own, then consulting doctors and physical therapists, then finally trying massage, I learned that my calf/Achilles/soleus problem was a Level 2 injury. The massage therapy sessions were uncomfortable, even painful at times; however, I sensed that the areas the therapist worked on felt a lot looser than they did when I first went to see her. She also believed that the fluke strain I felt in my calf dashing back to my apartment in Week 24 was likely from overworking it with The Stick. The tightest areas remained the outsides of my calves, probably due to my over-pronation.

Day	Date	Notes	Mileage
Training Log Week 32			
Thurs.	9/10/09	Couldn't sleep last night. Had a fantasy football draft that ended at 12:30a. After that, I had to pack for my morning flight to Chicago, so I finally got to bed around 3:30a, but I didn't really sleep. Got to Rick Miller's place in Chicago by late-morning, but our schedule allowed only a 2-hr nap before our run. Miller and I ran 6 miles along the lake (6:57 pace). Very humid out, but the run was easy. I'm sure my lack of sleep will catch up to me tomorrow. We're going out on the town tonight, so I don't see this ending well!	5.9
Fri.	9/11/09	After a long night of partying, I had nothing left in the tank. Went out for my bare minimum (30 min or 4 miles). Just followed Clark St. for 15 min, turned around and came back. Mercifully, the traffic forced me to stop several times. I cramped up a lot and felt completely out of shape. I'll check Map My Run later to determine the distance. Despite today's horror show, I'm having fun with the boys.	4.7
Sat.	9/12/09	It's been so long since the old team has partied together that we're all out of "partying shape." Nobody was willing to come running with me, so I ventured out for the same route as yesterday. Ran the still-unknown distance 30 sec faster (29:30) because I wanted to get back and take a nap. One more night with the boys.	4.7
Sun.	9/13/09	Last night felt like the last lap of a championship mile... but with booze instead of track spikes. Today we dragged ourselves to Northeastern University alumnus Jeff Baker's place for the NFL season openers. During halftime of the late games I decided to get the run over with, so I could get out for the Bears/Packers Sunday night matchup. I completed the Clark St. course in a slow 31:13. The real surprise: when I went to Map My Run to check the mileage it was 4.65 miles (6:30 per mile on average this weekend).	4.7
Mon.	9/14/09	Ran with Miller and Chicago's "Fleet Feet" Running Club. 7 miles with the group at 6:57 pace, plus about 0.75 miles to and from the event. I felt great and wanted to go faster, but I had no idea where we were. Probably all the better – this was my 6th straight day on the roads. I noticed a slight twinge in my Achilles. If the tendon hasn't healed, I may be in big trouble. I'll take it easy then test the leg on the track in a few wks.	8.6
Tues.	9/15/09	Busy day work-wise, which was disruptive to today's training. Did 2 miles at 6:35 pace on the elliptical, but my clients kept interrupting. By the time I got free, it was past 11p, so I hit the roads for 4 miles (6:55 pace).	6.0
Weds.	9/16/09	Terry and I felt good on our 5-mile loop, so we kept going and did 7 miles at 7:09 pace. My weekly mileage was well below average, but this was the first wk of running on roads every day since May.	7.0
Total		Averaged 6:49 per mile for the week	**41.5**

On the topic of massage, esteemed coach Tom Cotner[34] recommends that vigorous massage take place as far before or after a hard workout as possible. He believes that a deep tissue massage can be as tough on the muscles as a hard workout, so timing is important.

As a precautionary measure for the calf/Achilles, I started wrapping my right ankle with an ACE bandage and taping it with my foot pointing down a bit. I first tried this in a drill/track workout in Week 39. I hoped that restricting the motion of my ankle would limit the pressure I exerted on my lower leg. It worked like a charm. I got through the workout without serious (or even moderate) pain. Better yet, I woke up the next day with no discomfort at all. I believe that the combination of massage therapy, precautionary wrapping, and a few weeks of "smart training" finally enabled me to work through these injuries get back to 100 percent.

Dietary Research and Findings

Diet, pH, and Lactic Acid: In an effort to improve race performance, I researched the physiology of lactic acid. According to research posted by the Canadian Athletics Coaching Centre (among other places), fatigue during long sprints and middle-distance racing, say 400 meters to 1,500 meters, results from limitations imposed by anaerobic metabolism. Although anaerobic metabolism can generate energy at a very high rate, it results in metabolic acidosis from the production of lactic acid, which is closely correlated to fatigue. At physiological pH, the produced lactic acid during intense exercise is almost completely dissociated into lactate (La-) and hydrogen ions (H+). It is the increased

---

34 Dr. Tom Cotner is a renowned distance coach for Seattle's Club Northwest and coached the Masters champions David Cannon and Tony Young.

Training Log Week 33			
Day	Date	Notes	Mileage
Thurs.	9/17/09	Easy 4 miles on the elliptical (6:30 pace). I've been going pretty hard for 33 wks without a day off, so a few easy days may be more helpful than not. After my workout, I drove to NYC in advance of some business meetings on Friday.	4.0
Fri.	9/18/09	Got home from NYC at 6:15p. Jamie had a girl's night out and I had a poker game, so we had to leave almost as soon as I got home. Went out for a quick 4.7 miles (30:00) at my cousin's before our poker game.	4.7
Sat.	9/19/09	The elliptical machines at the gym were all taken, forcing me onto a stationary bike. This was actually good because I've meant to do more quadriceps-related work. I believe the elliptical favors hamstrings over quads when compared with road running. I made the most of the bike, hammering 10 miles in 27:17 (just under 22 mph). Counting it a 4.2-mile equivalent.	4.2
Sun.	9/20/09	7 miles on the elliptical (strong and effortless) at 6:46 per mile. My recent rest appears to be doing me some good. It may be time to start upping the mileage again.	7.0
Mon.	9/21/09	I may do a speed workout this week, so I stuck to the elliptical to keep the Achilles rested. That didn't mean an easy day though. I tore through 8 miles in 47:42 (5:58 pace). The last 2 miles required a lot of mental toughness; a good day of physical and mental training.	8.0
Tues.	9/22/09	Brutal 24 hrs! At noon Terry and I did the same stair workout as 2 wks ago (5 x 32 flights). We both improved markedly. I went 3:11, 3:07, 3:01, 3:08, and 3:10 (15:37 total) vs. 3:45, 3:30, 3:15, 3:12, and 2:52 last time (16:34 total). Almost puked after the 4th one. Later, we joined the Brandeis boys for an easy run and drills: 2.6 miles followed by 50m drills (butt-kicks, high-knees, hamstring snap-downs, frogs, strides, and pushups). Finished with an easy 1.5 miles. (Almost 20 miles in less than 24 hrs counting yesterday's elliptical.)	11.5
Weds.	9/23/09	Terry and I were pretty sore and tired today. Did a very easy noontime recovery run. We crawled through a social 5.1 miles in 41:54 (8:13 pace). I think we earned the easy day!	5.1
Total		Averaged 6:46 per mile for the week	44.5

hydrogen ion production that causes a drop in intramuscular pH – also known as acidosis – which is what really causes an athlete to fatigue and slow at the end of intense exercise. The lactate itself does not cause this.

Reportedly, you can mitigate acidosis by introducing a buffer to absorb the excess hydrogen ions. Buffers include sodium bicarbonate (a.k.a. baking soda), beta alanine, and cal-mag (calcium-magnesium) or related supplements. Baking soda (*not* baking powder) supposedly has the most immediate impact. You can take it one to two hours before a race. As an alkaline, baking soda raises the pH level in the blood and muscles, thus extending the amount of time a runner can go all-out before acidosis sets in.

In tests, baking soda has been known to knock several seconds off runners' 800-meter times. However, baking soda will result in an upset stomach or similar adverse effects (think explosive diarrhea) in approximately 50 percent of people who try it. As a result, you should test baking soda at an unimportant race or training session to see how you will react, before using it in championship situations.

Many top coaches aspire to perfect "bicarbonate loading" as a secret weapon for their athletes. The ideal dose seems to be 300 milligrams of sodium bicarbonate per kilogram of body weight. That's a little more than one teaspoon per 35 pounds, mixed with a little less than half a liter of water, taken over a 90-minute span, starting two hours before race time. This manner of dosing is intended to minimize the gastrointestinal side effects... or at least delay them until after the race.

Beta alanine seems to be the best long-term solution to offset the acidosis related to lactic acid production because it stimulates the body's natural ability to generate the buffer. The downside is that it takes at least two weeks for beta alanine supplementation to have any effect. Also, the longer-term side effects of taking beta alanine are not known. As such, using beta alanine for cycles exceeding 12 weeks is *not* recommended.

Training Log Week 34

Day	Date	Notes	Mileage
Thurs.	9/24/09	More sore today than yesterday. Haven't been this sore in a long time… and couldn't be happier. Hit the elliptical for 8 miles at 6:22 pace – solid day of work.	8.0
Fri.	9/25/09	Did a standard 5.2 miles with Terry today. I worked hard yesterday, so I was ok with our pedestrian 7:47 pace.	5.2
Sat.	9/26/09	Had a golf tournament in Maine, so training would have to wait until later. By the time I got home, Jamie and I had to leave for dinner with the Dolans (Tim and Jami). The Dolans live on a golf course, normally great for running. However, we got there after nightfall and coyotes live up and down the course! Luckily, Tim has an elliptical, so I snuck in a quick 30 min before dinner. Not the best day of training, but they can't all be great.	4.0
Sun.	9/27/09	After a long day of tailgating and rooting on the Patriots, there's nothing like having to do 8 miles on the elliptical. It wasn't a quick workout, but it was mileage in the bank.	8.2
Mon.	9/28/09	Had an appointment with a massage therapist. After working my legs for a few min she concluded that my leg issue is actually super-tight calves, not Achilles tendonitis. We've gone from Soleus to Achilles to calf. It's frustrating that professionals can't identify the body part that I point at when they ask, "where does it hurt?" In any case, she worked my calves so hard that they were sore all day. I stuck to the elliptical: 6 miles at 6:42 pace.	6.0
Tues.	9/29/09	Another hellish stair workout with Terry. Times were 2:58, 3:08, 3:08, 3:09, and 3:06 (15:29 total), an 8-sec improvement over last week. Terry averaged around 3:25 per set, a big improvement. We warmed down with 2 miles (16:12). Later we did drills at Harvard. 2.5 mile warm-up, then 8 sets of drills: high-knees (2 x 60yd, followed by 2 x 60yd strides), butt-kicks (2 x 60yd, followed by 2 x 60yd strides), hurdler strides (2 x 60yd, followed by 2 x 60yd strides), karaokes (2 x 60yd, followed by 2 x 60yd strides), lunges (30yd of lunges, followed by a 30-yd stride, followed by 30yd of lunges, followed by a 30yd stride), more high-knees (2 x 60yd, followed by 2 x 60yd strides), backward running (2 x 60yd, followed by 2 x 60yd strides), and frogs (full-squat leaps -- 30yd of lunges, followed by a 30yd stride, followed by 30yd of lunges, followed by a 30yd stride). After each drill we did 15 pushups. I remained strong throughout the workout, moving faster than last wk and leading most of the drills and strides. It felt good to open up the throttle again after a long hiatus from quicker workouts. More importantly, the calf/Achilles felt great.	10.5
Weds.	9/30/09	Another slow recovery run with Terry… (5.2 miles at 7:46 pace). I felt a *lot* better than I did last wk at this time. Considering I worked a bit harder this week, I'm very encouraged. My Achilles/Soleus/Calf has me most excited – I felt no pain in the leg today. This might be the first time since the beginning of training that I did anything fast and didn't feel it the next day. My massage therapist might be on to something…	5.2
Total		Averaged 6:58 per mile for the week	**47.0**

A number of cal-mag supplements are designed to buffer against acidosis: PowerStack, IntraXCell, and SportLegs are several that I found. According to RealAge.com, 400 milligrams (the RDA of magnesium) cannot be absorbed all at once. Apparently 200 milligrams is absorbed in about 6 hours, so they recommend taking 200 milligrams twice a day. If you take the full 400 milligrams, you can suffer digestion issues (because magnesium is the basis of laxatives, like Milk of Magnesia). Many competitive cyclists recommend varieties that contain vitamin D.

Based on the research, I started my experimentation with a simple test: I took a Tums every 30 minutes for two hours before a drill workout (Oct. 20th, 2009). The Tums were supposed to serve as lactate buffer; their basic ingredients are calcium and magnesium.

In my opinion, the experiment worked. We did two sets of 5 x 45-second drills, with each drill immediately followed by a 200-meter run, which was immediately followed by 15 pushups. (See the log entry for specific drills in each set.) During the drills and pushups, I kept pace with the group, but on the 200s I pushed the pace and led or co-led every one. I timed a couple of them. One was in 28 seconds and another was 31 seconds. I didn't time the rest, but I could feel that they were all in the same range.

Training Log Week 35				
Day	Date	Notes		Mileage
Thurs.	10/1/09	Low-mileage recovery day. 6 miles on the elliptical (6:24 pace). 15 min later, a yoga/Pilates class. My first in about a month but no worse than usual (no better, either!). Tomorrow, I'm going to try 10 miles on the road with Dino Dibiaso: another test for my leg...		6.0
Fri.	10/2/09	Dino and I did 10-miles around the Charles River at sub-7:00 pace. It reminded me of Coach Dave; he's a fan of the 70-min 10-miler. If I run like I did in high school, I will definitely contend for medals at Masters Nationals. Overall, I felt good. My legs were only a little worn from Tuesday's workout. Afterward, I took an Advil, iced my quads and drank an Endurox to speed my recovery. The real test will come when I wake up.		10.0
Sat.	10/3/09	Another painful session with my massage therapist. I swear she laid into my legs harder than last week. Later on, I did a brisk 6-miler (6:17 pace) on the elliptical. Like last week, my calves are sore from the massage, but hopefully I'll get the same results (i.e., a strong wk of work without straining anything).		6.0
Sun.	10/4/09	Did a long session on the elliptical while watching the Patriots game. Planned on doing 10 miles, but the game was exciting, so I ended up going 11 miles: 74 min (6:43 pace).		11.0
Mon.	10/5/09	Hit the roads for a pretty hard 6-miler. The course was an up-and-back past NU. I went out in 19:45 and came back in 18:57. Total time was 38:42 (6:27 pace).		6.0
Tues.	10/6/09	Terry was sick yesterday, so no stair workout. We did evening drills with the Black & Tan guys. Warmed up with a slow 4 miles. After, we hit MIT's football field for 8 sets of drills (high knees, butt kicks, jumping jacks, lunges, hurdler kicks, high knees again, twists -- jumping in place with your feet together but landing with your toes pointing left on one jump and right on the next jump -- and frogs). We started each set with a drill for 30 sec immediately followed by a 120m stride. After the strides we did 15 pushups to complete the set. Tough workout. Warmed down with a couple very easy miles.		7.0
Weds.	10/7/09	Did some light stretching at the gym. After 10 min, I hopped on the elliptical for the minimum 4-mile requirement. Finished comfortably in 27:28 (6:52 pace).		4.0
Total		Averaged 6:46 per mile for the week		50.0

I didn't *feel* like I was going all out at all, which is exactly what the buffer is supposed to do: delay the onset of acidosis. But this had a very unpleasant side effect. After the workout, my body broke down in exhaustion. I could barely muster a short warm down (less than a mile). I'm guessing that the buffer did its job during the workout, enabling me to run harder than I normally would. However, once the buffer was exhausted, my body felt exactly how one would expect to feel after an extra hard workout... like I had just run a very hard race.

Supplements are but part of the picture in the battle against acidosis. Diet also plays an important role in managing your pH balance. I found multiple sources itemizing which foods raise and lower your blood pH.[35]

As a reminder, hydrogen ions are a byproduct of lactic acid processing in the body. (Lactate is the other byproduct.) Lactate is a bodily fuel, but hydrogen ions acidify blood. If you start with less acidic (more alkaline) blood, it will take longer for you to hit the wall, because it will take longer for the hydrogen ions to acidify your blood.

I increased the amount of alkaline-forming foods in my diet, and I experienced accelerated athletic improvement. I also enjoyed better flexibility, recovery time, injury status, and overall health. One of the first dietary experiments I made in this regard? The addition of beet juice.

I believe that beet juice improved my workout performance by relaxing (and therefore opening up) the walls of my blood vessels. This enabled oxygen to more easily reach my muscles, improving workout times, fatigue recovery, and injury recovery. Supposedly, beet juice also decreases the production of lactic acid as well as the blood's need for oxygen. If true, these are two more reasons why beet juice improves performance. Similar to alkaline-forming foods/substances, beet juice seems to be capable of knocking seconds off an 800-meter time.

---

35 Sources: [Google: high-alkaline foods]

Day	Date	Notes	Mileage
Training Log Week 36			
Thurs.	10/8/09	Stairs today: I recorded 3:00, 3:02, 3:02, 2:59, and 2:59 (15:02 total) – a big 27-sec improvement versus last week. Terry also improved. I warmed down with 2 miles in 14:15. Hard to say why I had such a strong workout. Possibly more rest between sets (because time in the elevator can vary). Possibly last night's meal. Also, I'm likely getting stronger… Regardless of the reason, it was a great workout. In the evening, I did 2 miles on the elliptical (14:58) before hitting yoga/Pilates. Mercifully, the class started 15 min late.	7.0
Fri.	10/9/09	Ran Dino Dibiaso's 10-mile course and knocked 30 sec off the time (68:11; 6:49 pace). Definitely a tough run in the midst of a hard week. Took awhile to recover and my notorious calf doesn't feel right…	10.0
Sat.	10/10/09	Leg is definitely hurt, but only slightly. Today and tomorrow are elliptical days, so I'm sure it'll be ok. Today's session was 7.25 miles at 6:49 pace. It was effortless. The time passed quickly, thanks to NCAA football.	7.3
Sun.	10/11/09	Thankfully, the calf pain was gone this morning. Would have been nice to get it worked on yesterday, but I missed my regular massage therapy appointment. I deep-tissue massaged on my own before today's run. The NFL made it easy for me to put in a long session on the elliptical: 14 miles in 1:36:36 (6:54 per mile). Felt good start to finish. I'm getting the sense that my body could be making a breakthough.	14.0
Mon.	10/12/09	Easy 5-mile recovery run on the elliptical -- 34:57 (6:59 pace).	5.0
Tues.	10/13/09	Hard day of drills: 8 x 45-sec sets with quick 200m strides (untimed but around 30-35 seconds), then 15 pushups. The first seven sets were A-skips, high knees, butt kicks, twists, lunges, hurdler kicks, and jumping jacks. Eighth set was frogs (only 30 sec). I led every 200m, but Chris Simpson was right behind me. My calf felt a little strained, so I stayed off my toes and the strain didn't get too bad. I have a make-up date with my massage therapist tomorrow.	7.0
Weds.	10/14/09	Just a little 4-mile recovery run on the elliptical. I hammered the last mile at low 5-min pace though. Total time was 25:52 (6:28 per mile).	4.0
Total		Averaged 6:47 per mile for the week	**54.3**

Technical Tip – *I researched the use of painkillers as they relate to hard workouts or racing. Using painkillers is not a good idea before workouts or races. There is no evidence that painkillers decrease race-related pain. However, there is ample evidence that taking painkillers before workouts or races can have pretty significant negative effects, which include increased inflammation and increased time to recovery.[36] There is one potential exception: chronic cramps or stitches. In an Internet forum, Coach Tom Cotner advised a runner who suffered bad cramps to consume two Advil prior to longer races. (This advice was in conjunction with additional abdominal workouts and specific in-race breathing techniques to ward off the cramps as they came on.)*

Food Tip – *Caffeine activates fat reserves and encourages muscles to use that fat as fuel (instead of glycogen). This enables the body to conserve glycogen and therefore perform over a longer period of time before running out of energy. This can be helpful in getting through long Sunday runs or races exceeding 15 minutes in duration (probably the 5K and up for most runners). Glycogen is unlikely to be depleted during a short race.[37]*

Caffeine should only be used once in awhile (to avoid building a tolerance). It should be ingested an hour before performing to optimize its effect. More importantly, caffeine is a blood acidifier. As a result, in shorter races, where lactic acid has the greatest negative impact, caffeine may actually work with hydrogen ions to acidify the blood, causing an athlete to hit the wall sooner.

---

36 Source: www.tampabay.com; [Google: "tampa bay times" + "pain killers" + athletes]

37 It should be noted, I *did* find additional studies that indicated caffeine ingestion *could* improve performances at shorter races – but the researchers could not pinpoint the reasons why performances in those studies improved.

		Training Log Week 37	
Day	Date	Notes	Mileage
Thurs.	10/15/09	Turned up the mileage and pace: 8 miles on the elliptical in 50:55 (6:22 pace). Once again, I hit the last mile near 5:00. 30 min rest before yoga/Pilates, so I hit the hottub to loosen up and massage the calf. Feels like it'll be 100% tomorrow. Yoga is tough after a hard 8-miler.	8.0
Fri.	10/16/09	Was hoping to get outside for my Friday 10-miler, but it was cold and windy and my running partners cancelled. The calf is back to 100%, but all signs suggest I shouldn't push my luck, so I hit the elliptical. Pushed pretty hard… especially toward the end. Probably low 5-min pace for each of the last 2 miles. Definitely felt it.	10.0
Sat.	10/17/09	Another elliptical day. Planned to do an easy 4-6 miles, but I felt good, so I did 7 in 44:28 (6:21 pace, a little slower than yesterday's 10 miler).	7.0
Sun.	10/18/09	The New England Patriots kept me company for 14 miles on the elliptical. Workout was quite easy. Went through the first 8 miles in under 60 min and picked it up from there. Finished at 1:35:54 (6:51 per mile). Feel great. May have tweaked my calf by overworking it with The Stick. I'll see what the massage therapist thinks.	14.0
Mon.	10/19/09	Hit the elliptical for 6 miles in 40:14 (6:42 pace). Decent recovery run from yesterday and pre-cursor to tomorrow's drill workout at MIT.	6.0
Tues.	10/20/09	*Not* a fun day. Ran a great workout and didn't agitate my calf in the process, but I felt *awful* afterward. Experimented with cal-mag pills. We did two sets of five 45-sec drills, each immediately followed by a 200m run, immediately followed by 15 pushups. Set One consisted of 'A' Skips,[38] butt-kicks, lunges, jumping jacks, and high knees. Set Two consisted of 'B' Skips, twists, crunches, bunny hops (simply hopping in place), and a 30-sec set of frogs. During the drills and pushups, I kept pace with Chris Simpson, but on the 200s I pushed it and led or co-led each one. One was a 28 sec and another was 31 sec.	7.0
Weds.	10/21/09	Much-needed recovery day. Did an easy 5 miles on the elliptical in 37:36 (7:31 pace).	5.0
Total		Averaged 6:41 per mile for the week	57.0

I found a product made for pre-race consumption, aptly named PreRace. Each serving contains:

➤ 200 milligrams of caffeine – equal to two cups of coffee, which is half of the USOC's legal racing limit
➤ 3,000 milligrams of Taurine – a neuroinhibitory transmitter shown to reduce muscle damage (also found in Red Bull)
➤ 500 milligrams of Citrulline Malate – which supposedly stimulates nitric oxide and removes toxins, while reducing lactic acid and ammonia.

Rice University presented some research on caffeine use in endurance athletes:[39]

➤ Caffeine is more likely to assist in longer races and is unlikely to assist in sprints.
➤ Ideal dosing is under 1,000 milligrams (eight cups of coffee), due to rulebook restrictions on use (specifically IOC rules). Timing should be about three to four hours before the competition. Although blood levels of caffeine peak much sooner, the maximum caffeine effect on fat stores appears to occur several hours after peak blood levels.
➤ Consider decreasing or abstaining from caffeine for three to four days prior to competition. This allows for caffeine tolerance to decrease and helps ensure the maximum effect of the caffeine. Be careful though, because some people experience caffeine withdrawal.
➤ Make sure that you have used caffeine extensively under a variety of training conditions and are thoroughly familiar with how your body reacts to this drug.

---

38 The mechanical breakdown of the 'A' Skip is here: www.completespeedtraining.com/a-skip.html

39 www.rice.edu/~jenky/sports/caffeine.html

Training Log Week 38			
Day	**Date**	**Notes**	**Mileage**
Thurs.	10/22/09	Terry and I did stairs, as planned. Times were 3:08, 2:55, 2:54, 2:58, and 2:57 (14:52 total) – a 10-sec overall improvement with less effort. Walked 0.4 miles to Terry's office, then did a 3.6 mile warm down at 7:16 pace. Later, I did 3 miles elliptical (6:52 pace), stretched, did running curls, hit the hot tub, and headed to Ali's 1-hr yoga/Pilates class. Focused on arm strength, stretching, core, and abs. Perfect for what I need.	9.6
Fri.	10/23/09	Ran Dino's 10-miler again and knocked off another 10 sec per mile: 66:28 (6:39 per mile). Felt stronger than during the run 2 wks ago. Most importantly, the calf didn't act up (minor twinges as I picked up the pace during the final mile). My first mile was 6:30 and my last was 6:28. Feels like I might be reaching a new level of fitness. After the run, I drank an Endurox, iced, stretched, and took two Advil. After icing, I took a hot shower.	10.0
Sat.	10/24/09	Easy elliptical: 7 miles at 6:59 pace.	7.0
Sun.	10/25/09	The Patriots got me through another long elliptical session: 14 miles at 6:25 pace. The resistance level is adjustable, so I can simulate road resistance, but it doesn't simulate the pounding one's body takes during a long run, so it's easier to keep a quicker pace. Better to save the pounding for track workouts, which are more critical to my speed and development. Been dealing with side stitches a few times a week. To combat this, I've tried better breathing techniques. They have made a noticeable difference.	14.0
Mon.	10/26/09	Hit the roads for a 6-mile recovery run. Doubly wrong: first, until my injuries stay gone, the roads should be reserved for workouts; second, I have a hard time keeping slow on the roads. In any case, I did 15-20 min of stretching, slipped on my calf-sleeve, and ran. The first mile was 7:15. After that I picked it up: 6:30, 6:30, 6:15, 6:18, and 6:06 to finish in 38:54 (6:29 pace). Later I felt a small strain in my lower right leg, in the muscle just to the left of my Achilles tendon. This is a different spot than the injury that has dogged me for months.	6.0
Tues.	10/27/09	Stairs today because our track workout was moved to Thursday. Times = 2:59, 2:56, 2:54, 2:59, and 2:59 (14:47 total). This compares to Thursday's 14:52. A little quicker and more consistent. Later I attended yoga/Pilates class, then hit the elliptical. (I forgot how much harder an elliptical session is after class). Managed 7 miles in 49:57 (7:08 pace), starting above 8:00 pace and finishing at sub-6:00.	10.0
Weds.	10/28/09	Nice easy 4-mile recovery on the elliptical (27:57; 6:59 pace). This was my biggest wk of work since early August. More importantly, the work was higher quality, resulted in less injury, and I feel strong.	4.0
Total		Averaged 6:34 per mile for the week	**60.6**

Race Reports, Records, and Results

2009 Superhero 5K: I earned my first road race win *ever* at the Superhero 5K in Cambridge, Mass, on November 1st 2009! I wish I had more nice things to say about it. The concept was fun: Everyone had to wear a superhero costume. The competition and race management were terrible. The course wasn't even closed to traffic!

I was hoping to be pushed close to 5:00 pace, but there was no competition, so I hung behind the leader and kicked with about 800 meters to go. I finished in 18:02. The hardest thing about the race was dealing with my costume's cape, which I tripped over a couple times.

My winnings were as weak as the race management. After a $27 entry fee, I won an ugly medal and a $25 gift certificate. First prize was worth *less* than the entry fee! The 2009 race was the inaugural running, so hopefully subsequent years have been better. I noticed the winning times have improved, according to the race Web site.

Miscellaneous Research and Notes

During this stage of my training, I noticed my quadriceps getting sore again, so I implemented quad lifts and some biking. In the summer of 1989 I used to bike seven miles from Dorchester, Mass. to my part-time job in Braintree in the morning, then run home in the afternoon. The next day I'd run to work in the morning, then bike home that afternoon. Terry Pricher and I conjectured that this training worked because I would run twice on 12 hours rest and then not again for over 30 hours... lots of recovery time. I set a 10K PR that summer (31:08) and broke the Northeastern University 1,000-meter record that winter (2:24.5), so perhaps I was on to something.

Training Log Week 39

Day	Date	Notes	Mileage
Thurs.	10/29/09	Drills/track workout: two sets of 5 x 45-sec drills, each followed by a 300m run (instead of 200m like usual), immediately followed by 15 pushups. Set 1 consisted of 'A' Skips, butt-kicks, lunges, jumping jacks, and high knees. Set 2 consisted of 'B' Skips, twists, crunches, bunny hops, and a 30-sec set of frogs. I kept pace with Chris Simpson on the drills and pushups, but pushed the pace on the 300s, which ranged between 48 and 51 sec. Could have gone a little faster, but I found a good balance between working hard and not overdoing it. No sign of injury at all. Great day.	7.3
Fri.	10/30/09	Semi-recovery day: strong 10 miles in 1:04:30 (6:27 pace) on the elliptical instead of the roads. No sign of injury, but didn't want to risk it. May have turned the corner with the calf/Achilles!	10.0
Sat.	10/31/09	1-hr massage therapy then an easy 6.25 miles on the elliptical (43:10; 6:54 pace).	6.3
Sun.	11/1/09	My first road race win *ever*: the Superhero 5K in Cambridge, MA! Hoped for a fast pace, but no one pushed. Won in 18:02. Ran home (about 3 miles) and hopped on the elliptical for 8 miles so I wouldn't feel like the day was a waste. (More in the Race Reports section.)	18.3
Mon.	11/2/09	Did today's recovery session on a stationary bike: 15 miles in 45:23 (19.8 MPH), roughly equivalent to 6.5 miles at just under 7:00 pace.	6.5
Tues.	11/3/09	Drills/track workout: two sets of 5 x 60-sec drills (instead of 45 sec last week), each immediately followed by a 300m run, immediately followed by 15 pushups. Set 1 consisted of 'A' Skips, butt-kicks, lunges, jumping jacks, and high knees. Set 2 consisted of 'B' Skips, twists, crunches, bunny hops (simply hopping in place), and a 30-sec set of frogs. I was disappointed with my 300s, which ranged between 50 and 52 sec, until I realized we upped the drills by 15 sec each. Sunday's race and mileage didn't help either.	9.0
Weds.	11/4/09	Well-deserved day of rest. Did 4 miles on the elliptical at just under 7-min pace.	4.0
Total		Averaged 6:50 per mile for the week	**61.4**

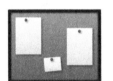

Bulletin Board Material – *I did some research on Tony Young and Jim Sorensen – world record holders at 1,500 meters or the mile in several Masters age categories. Young and Sorensen were the top dogs of over-40 middle distance running for quite a while.*

In Young, I found a similar story to mine. He actually ran slower than I did in high school (4:19 for the mile, versus my 4:17) and felt that he didn't do all he could to reach his potential when he was younger. According to interviews, that is what drove him as a Masters runner. Young put in pretty heavy mileage as a 40-year-old: 70-100 miles per week. I found that to be a bit intimidating (given that I averaged 55 miles per week) although to be fair, a lot of Young's extra mileage came from easy double-sessions.

With Sorensen, I was surprised to find that he only did 45-55 miles per week, usually erring toward the 45. This may be because he considered himself to be injury prone. Mileage aside, it was cool to see that his typical week looked a lot like mine:

- ➤ *Sunday:*   *11-14 miles, long run*
- ➤ *Monday:*   *4-6 miles, recovery pace*
- ➤ *Tuesday:*   *8-11 miles, harder workout*
- ➤ *Wednesday:*   *0-6 miles, recovery or day off*
- ➤ *Thursday:*   *5-9 miles, recovery or better*
- ➤ *Friday:*   *8-11 miles, harder workout*
- ➤ *Saturday:*   *4-8 miles, recovery*

The main difference is that I worked hard on Tuesday and Thursday instead of Tuesday and Friday. Sorensen also did core work once or twice a week (similar to my yoga/Pilates work). My regimen and mileage sat somewhere between that of Sorensen and Young, which I considered pretty good company.

Training Log Week 40

Day	Date	Notes	Mileage
Thurs.	11/5/09	Sticking with the stairs + track/drills weekly combo, Terry and I hit the flights. I logged 2:59, 2:58, 2:58, 2:55, and ended with a PR 2:51 (14:41 total), a small improvement over last week. I can't be plateauing, so the small improvement was probably due to my recently increased mileage. Was definitely tired during my afternoon session. After yoga I had very little left, so I did a short elliptical warm-down and called it a day.	5.4
Fri.	11/6/09	Recovery and rest day. Did 4 miles on the elliptical, alternating my speed every 0.1 miles (from 6:30-7:20 pace on the slow side, to 5:30-6:00 on the quicker side). The idea is to start incorporating more quickness into my training.	4.0
Sat.	11/7/09	Paced Terry through a 5K road race. Went through Mile 1 in 5:59 and Mile 2 in exactly 12:30 as planned. He ran a tough 3rd mile uphill in 6:25 and we finished in 19:29. Warm up and warm down added another 6.4 miles. Had just enough time to shower and change for massage therapy. My legs were tight from the run, and Dianne was intent on working it all out. Pain, pain, excruciating pain!	9.5
Sun.	11/8/09	After yesterday's road race and massage, I was concerned about today's 14-miler. I ate big in the morning to fuel up for the elliptical. Surprisingly, I felt strong from the get-go. Went through 10 miles in 63:32 and finished 14 miles in 1:25:59 – almost 4 min off my PR. Strong effort, but not exhausting. After a couple of flattish workouts this week, it's encouraging that yesterday and today came so easily.	14.0
Mon.	11/9/09	Rest and recovery day. Jogged to MIT's track (2.7 miles). To incorporate more speed into my daily routine, did 5 or 6 barefoot wind sprints (100yd) and some light jogging on the football field before heading home.	6.3
Tues.	11/10/09	Drills/track workout: two sets of five 60-sec drills, each immediately followed by a 300m run, followed by 15 pushups. Set One consisted of 'A' Skips, butt-kicks, lunges, jumping jacks, and high knees. Set Two consisted of 'B' Skips, twists, crunches, bunny hops, and a 30-sec set of frogs. My 300s are back to 48-52 sec.	8.2
Weds.	11/11/09	Simple 5.6-mile recovery session on the elliptical at 6:30 pace. Right on plan for weekly mileage. Previous two wks were over 60 miles each. "Smart training" requires easier days to follow hard days and easier wks to follow hard wks, so this was needed.	5.6
Total		Averaged 6:35 per mile for the week	**53.0**

Sorensen ran 48.6 seconds for 400-meters when he was 18 years old (a full second faster than I was at that age) and broke 4:00 in the mile. He also finished second at the 1996 Olympic Trials in the 1,500 meters – the race in which my Northeastern University teammate Erik Nedeau finished fourth. However, Sorensen's time didn't meet Olympic qualifying standards, so he didn't get to go. Apparently, that disappointment is what drove his Masters career.

Technical Tip – *Pre-race strides are critical. Moving at race pace is said to trigger bodily changes that you'll need during the race, including increasing your heart rate, breathing rate, blood flow to your working muscles, and oxygen consumption – and strides activate enzymes for aerobic energy production. If you do not warm up thoroughly, you put unnecessary strain on your cardiovascular system and produce more lactate.[40]*

Warm-downs are a little more controversial. An old Northeastern University teammate, Mark Cruz, sent me research that claims there's no clear evidence that warm-downs are necessary. Physiological evidence seems to show that warm-downs don't prevent muscle soreness or tightness, nor do they enable the cardiovascular system to ease back to normal in any beneficial manner versus the alternative (no warm-down at all). The researchers contest that blood continues to pump hard after a hard run, and the act of stopping greatly reduces the body's need for all that blood-pumping. Although this could produce effects akin to standing upside down – head rush, dizziness, or even unconsciousness – it doesn't justify a full traditional warm-down. Indications suggest that you can literally "walk it off."

Despite these findings, I continued to do warm-downs for the extra mileage and still recommend them – but if something prevents you from doing a traditional warm-down, you may not need to worry too much.

---

40 Source: RunningTimes.com [Google: "running times" + essential prerace preparation]

Chapter 6
You Must Learn

Weeks 41-50

I had an e-mail discussion with one of Coach Dave's guys, Ryan O'Connell, who began running for Springfield College in the fall of 2009. He seemed dissatisfied with his performances, and with good reason. At the time of our exchange, he hadn't hit a PR since arriving there. As someone who had started running only a couple of years prior, he should have been hitting PRs left and right, especially with the step up to college-level training. He may have been suffering from a weaker track program than he had in high school. He may also have been training inconsistently, as he adjusted to college life. I assumed the latter to be the case, so I offered this advice:

If you want to hit PRs, you have to train hard... and if you want to train hard, you have to train smart. Start by training constantly and consistently. The key to that is making everything an activity... and the key to that is figuring out what will help you enjoy it all (or at least not hate it).

My freshman year of college, I bought an old bike, a backpack, a cheap Walkman (the '80s version of the iPod), and some cheap rollerblades. The bike and rollerblades made it easy for me to travel everywhere on my own power. I used to bike or run from Boston to Braintree every day for work. That alone totaled close to 50 miles of running and 50 miles of biking every week. I'd also bike from Boston to Stoughton to visit friends and rollerblade wherever it made sense. This helped to improve my 10K PR by three minutes to 31:08.

The backpack had my books, changes of clothes, etc. The Walkman was my best friend. I would set my tape player to record the local hip hop radio show while I was in class, then I'd listen to the tapes on runs to discover new music. If I didn't like a song, I'd just fast-forward to the next one. I still do the same thing with my iPod Nano. Sometimes I discover a song I like so much, I just listen to it over and over and maybe even try to learn the words... and the next thing you know, eight miles have gone by. I love when that happens.

Nowadays, for my long workout on Sunday, I do up to 14 miles on an elliptical machine that has a TV, so I can watch football. I have multiple fantasy football teams, so I care about almost every game. Because of this, the first 10 miles usually fly by. The last four miles are tougher but not unbearable.

I also used to play a lot of football and basketball, but I was very careful not to do anything that would get me hurt. Nothing but fly-patterns, posts, and fast-breaks!

My point is, find a way to make it fun (or at least bearable) and then get out there every day. That's also why I have a training streak. If I take a day off, it's over. That keeps me motivated and keeps me from doing anything stupid (like diving for a pass in football and getting hurt – in fact, now I've taken a hiatus from all other sports to be safe). I'm hoping that my streak will be 900+ days before it ends. That will mean that I trained every day until the 2011 Masters Nationals.

FYI, I consider a day of "training" to be 30 straight minutes of non-stop aerobic activity (run, bike, treadmill, elliptical, Stairmaster, etc.) or four miles on the roads. I usually do the minimum once a week as a "day off." Let's face it, four miles at a pace that's a minute slower than my norm isn't really a workout.

By the way, you asked about Erik Nedeau and Brad Schlapak's PRs. You can see their college PRs here:

[Google: gonu.com + men's all time outdoor track performances]

p.s. Don't worry about not running early in high school. You're starting at a good time. A body can only handle so many years of hard running before it starts to break down. If you want, I'm sure you'll be hitting PRs for many, many years to come. Good luck!"

Here's another example of what a motivated athlete will do to maintain a training streak. Terry Pricher (one of my Boston training partners) needed surgery on his overworked hip. When he got the news, he had a training streak of 99 out of 100 days. The one missed day was because of the death of his wife's father. As it turned out, his streak did not end with the news that he needed surgery. Rather, he started working out for at least 30 minutes per day on a hand cycle. Yes, a hand cycle… but that's not where the story ended.

Terry's surgery was on a Thursday morning. To ensure his streak stayed alive, he decided to go to bed at 9 p.m. on the Wednesday before and wake up at midnight to do his Thursday workout on the hand cycle. He was advised not to drink fluid for a few hours before surgery – but by working out at midnight, he could rehydrate before going back to bed, without disobeying his pre-surgery protocol.

For this behavior, his wife called him crazy. I happen to agree, but I would add "ultimately dedicated" to the list of adjectives as well.

Training Log Week 41			
Day	**Date**	**Notes**	**Mileage**
Thurs.	11/12/09	Another fun-filled stairs session. Terry had to leave after our 4th set, but he established a PR. There was construction in my building and noxious fumes coming from the 28th floor. After our 1st set, our lungs were burning, but we pressed on. I logged 2:50 (PR), 2:52, 2:50, 2:53, and ended with 2:52 (14:17 total, 24-sec improvement from previous week). The final rest session was a little long.	4.0
Fri.	11/13/09	10-miler with Dino Dibiaso. We started at 6a (brutal) to accommodate his work/home schedule. I go to bed around 1a… so not fun. Luckily, we went 7:30-8:00 pace to run with Dino's 60-year-old friend. However, this guy was clearly capable of going faster. My time was 1:15:58 (7:36 pace), much slower than my usual pace, but I didn't feel any better at the end. It might explain why so many people believe in long slow distance.	10.0
Sat.	11/14/09	Started my day with the massage therapist, who was accidentally double-booked. As a result, I only got 35 min, but it was productive. Later I did a 7-mile recovery elliptical in 45 min (6:26 per mile).	7.0
Sun.	11/15/09	The New York Islanders were staying at the Boston Harbor Hotel, which houses my gym. Several of them showed up for a workout. Having them in the gym was fun and passed time, but physically I didn't think much of them. I looked in better shape than half of them. My elliptical was 1:26:30, 31 sec slower than last week.	14.0
Mon.	11/16/09	Rest and recovery day. Jogged to MIT's track for 5 barefoot wind sprints (100yd). The runs there and back (17:30 and 18:40) were 30 sec slower than last week. However, my wind sprints were much faster: 12 sec vs. 14 sec. My raw speed is coming back.	6.1
Tues.	11/17/09	Calf was a little sore, so I taped it up and went ahead with today's workout. The crew (including myself) is a little tired psychologically. After wks of 3-4 hard days per wk, our minds have hit the wall. The 40-degree weather didn't help. We decided to cut the drills to 30 sec and the intervals to about 250m, but to concentrate on proper form throughout. Our form had been deteriorating. I flew through the intervals for the first 6 sets. Unfortunately, about 200m into my 7th interval, I felt a tweak in my other calf. I immediately jogged to a halt and assessed. I decided that it was a new injury, but a slight one. Nonetheless, I shut it down for the night. My body finally adapted to 55+ mile wks, but my calves aren't ready for back-to-back days of sprinting… especially after a 14-mile elliptical session on Sunday and a 10-mile road run on Friday.	6.2
Weds.	11/18/09	Calf was still a little sore and my legs felt a little beat up. Time to take a step back and let the body recover. Did an easy 4 miles on the elliptical and an easier jog home.	4.2
Total		Averaged 6:39 per mile for the week	**51.5**

Training Log Week 42

Day	Date	Notes	Mileage
Thurs.	11/19/09	Terry and I canceled the stair workout in favor of recovery. For the next 2-3 wks I planned to stick with easy distance, mainly on the elliptical to recover from the 10 wks of hard work I just completed. It's time. I'm mentally tired, my calf is not 100%, and I move to Miami next wk to start winter training.	5.0
Fri.	11/20/09	Dino asked if I'd run an easy 10-miler at 7:15 - 7:30 pace, which didn't seem too threatening. *Wrong!* The run was easy, but it was too early for my calf and it ended up worse. Back to the elliptical.	9.6
Sat.	11/21/09	Did an easy 6 miles on the elliptical today (6:50 pace).	6.0
Sun.	11/22/09	Another 14-miler on the elliptical watching the NFL. My fantasy players and the Patriots played well, which made 14 miles easy! My time was 80 sec slower than last week, but still a respectable 1:27:50 (6:16 pace).	14.0
Mon.	11/23/09	Ripped 8 miles on the elliptical at 6:01 pace. I had no specific target going into the workout; thought I'd shoot for whatever pace felt right. After the first couple miles, I felt good, so I went with it. During this break from the roads/track, I've decided to play things by ear.	8.0
Tues.	11/24/09	Another strong 8 miles on the elliptical, finishing in 47:24 (5:55 pace). Jamie and I planned our winter move this week, so this may have been my last high quality workout until I get to Miami.	8.0
Weds.	11/25/09	Moved out of my condo, which made for a long workout but no cardio. Luckily, my cousins (where we're staying for a few days) have an elliptical machine. I did the minimum 4 miles.	4.0
Total		Averaged 6:36 per mile for the week	54.6

Training Log Week 43

Day	Date	Notes	Mileage
Thurs.	11/26/09	Thanksgiving!! I did an easy 4 miles on the elliptical before eating about 20lbs of turkey.	4.0
Fri.	11/27/09	Fueled with lots of Thanksgiving nutrition and rested, I set out to work hard. The result: my first sub-6:00 10-miler on the elliptical (59:30; 5:57 pace). I'm heading to Miami in peak condition. Later I talked to Coach Dave.	10.0
Sat.	11/28/09	Had my last massage therapy appointment before Miami. Afterward, I hit the elliptical for an easy 8-miler at 6:51 pace, much deserved after yesterday's tough workout.	8.0
Sun.	11/29/09	Today was my last day at my gym. Jamie and I went out with Jeff Baker, the Karnells, and a bunch of friends. We overdid it! I was completely hung over and only managed 4 miles elliptical. Thought I might get a second workout done later, but no...	4.0
Mon.	11/30/09	Hectic 39th birthday... We left Boston and headed for a hotel in Weehawken, NJ. Jeff Baker has some business there, so we decided that would make a good first stop. The hotel had a treadmill and bike, so I ran 7 miles at 7:00 pace and biked 2 miles at the same effort level. 365 days before I become a Master...	9.8
Tues.	12/1/09	Left NJ in the morning and stopped in Washington D.C. We stopped at the Holocaust Museum – a sobering experience that warrants description in something more than a training log. We drove on and settled into a Hampton Inn where I did 5 miles on an elliptical and 2 miles on a bike. This workout represented Day 300 of my training streak.	7.0
Weds.	12/2/09	Savannah, GA. The hotel had an elliptical, but it didn't work well, so I did 30 min on a stationary bike, then 25 min *very* easy jog on the treadmill at a 15-degree incline. I'm trying to minimize the pounding on my calf, so the incline allowed me to work hard without going fast or pounding. Logged the workout as 7.3 miles at 7:32 pace (which is probably conservative compared to the level of effort I put in).	7.3
Total		Averaged 6:50 per mile for the week	50.1

Injury Reports and Medical Findings

Massage and Flexibility: I knew I would need a massage therapist when I moved to Miami, and I chose Alex DaSilva, who works at the International Center for World-Class & Professional Athletes.[41] Alex works with several professional athletes, including players on the Tennessee Titans. (Each weekend, he flies to wherever they are playing). He's technically a flexibility therapist, but he incorporates muscle-releasing techniques, as well as aspects of Rolfing.

Rolfing massage therapy involves the aggressive realignment of muscles to where they belong. It also involves breaking down tissue. If that sounds painful, I've described it well. At one point, he was wrenching my lower legs, as if he was trying to "Indian Burn" the muscles under my shin. That was *the worst*. I could barely take it and my shins were still sore, several hours later. I asked Alex if pro football players grunt like I did during the experience. He said, "Of course not. They're NFL football players. If they make any sound at all, I know I got them good." After that, I did my best to not grunt or groan… to no avail. One more reason I never played in the NFL.

Most of the session involved motion-focused stretching. He'd move my legs into different positions, create some resistance, and have me activate certain leg muscles against his resistance. He would repeat that several times for the same for the same muscle group, but at five or six different angles (with each angle moving me into an increasingly stretched position). The latter angles were tough and painful to deal with, but I could tell that he was doing something good.

At the end of the first session, he advised me not to do a hard workout. After such an experience, a hard workout would put my weakened muscles at risk for injury. In other words, the session *was* a hard workout. When I got home, it was time to see how my body would handle an easy session on the elliptical. I was very pleasantly surprised. Right from the first step, I felt a lot faster and more powerful than in recent days. Nonetheless, I heeded Alex's warning and held back.

Alex thought he could eliminate my propensity for calf injuries by eliminating all the little things that contribute to them. I didn't doubt it. In Boston, my therapist did a great job of alleviating my problem. I wanted to see if Alex could make the difference between "alleviate" and "eliminate."

I also consulted with a chiropractor (Dr. William Moyal), who is known for working with Olympic-caliber athletes. I was sold on Alex, but I was skeptical of chiropractors in general. Dr. Moyal didn't do much to change my mind. However, he did enough to give him a chance. I told him that I'd need to see results in a few sessions or I'd be gone. He agreed.

After the first session, I felt rough. I was not a fan of all the cracking he did to my body – especially my neck. I had a headache that persisted through my workout later that day. Not a good sign. Dr. Moyal insisted that this was a normal first-time reaction and that things would get better. In our second session, he took some x-rays of my back. He saw two very explainable abnormalities:

➢ He said that my lower-back appeared to be in a seated position, even though I was standing at the time of the x-rays. (Explanation: I spend the majority of my day seated.)
➢ My right hip is very clearly higher than my left. (Explanation: when standing, I've always leaned on my right hip, positioning it higher than my left.)

Moyal believes that these imbalances were the ultimate cause of my calf troubles. It's possible that he's right. I didn't have calf problems in college, nor did I spend so much time in poor postural positions when I was younger. The toll one's career can take on the body…

---

41 www.miamiflex.com.

Moyal gave me some more adjustments in my second visit. He also scheduled an appointment for me to see his massage therapist. I paid a flat monthly fee to have him determine who I need to see and when. He was generous with his services.

My first appointment with a massage therapist in Miami was back at the International Center for World-Class & Professional Athletes. He was a Cuban guy and was a middle-distance runner when he was younger. He did a thorough examination of my legs and found several things that went along with what I was told by Dr. Moyal and Alex DaSilva. Basically, all of the muscles in my legs are too tight, including the ones in my shins. He found particular stiffness (and knots) along the outside of my upper calves. A lot of his work focused there. Needless to say, it was pretty painful although not as bad as what I experienced back in Boston or with Alex.

Afterward, he gave me a stretch to do for my calves/shins. It's basically a squat, with my feet/heels flat on the ground. Initially, this stretch will stretch the calves, but once the calves are loose, the same stretch will work on muscles in the shins.

Apparently, Alex and my massage therapist think alike. They both pinpointed my upper, outer calves as being a particular mess. The sessions were hard, but they alleviated decades of damage. However, after a few intense sessions, Alex determined I only needed to visit once every two-to-three weeks. Thank God. I don't know if I could have done that every week until Masters Nationals. In addition to the pain, there was a lot of resistance worked into the stretching routine, so I came out of there pretty tired each time.

The bottom line: My muscles remained tight, but my range of motion was noticeably better and less strained. (My research suggested I might be a naturally tight person, which isn't necessarily a bad thing.)

Training Log Week 44

Day	Date	Notes	Mileage
Thurs.	12/3/09	We left Savannah, GA and continued to Miami. Had dinner at my sister's place until around 10p. This gave us just enough time to get to South Beach by 11:15, so I could get my minimum workout completed before midnight. The run was pretty good. Once my lungs opened up, I picked up the pace and headed toward the more exciting areas of South Beach – Ocean Drive and Collins Avenue. (Adrenaline and excitement are potent performance enhancers.) I was a bit overzealous, and my recently injured calf flared up again. Afterward, I mapped the course, which Google measured to be 4.67 miles.[42] I was pretty surprised because that equates to a brisk 6:27 pace.	4.7
Fri.	12/4/09	My new building's gym has three TV-equipped LifeFitness elliptical machines. These are the exact models that I trained on in Boston, so at least one part of my training regimen wouldn't be changing. I acclimated myself to one of the machines with a long double. I started with 7.5 miles at 6:45 pace, then I took a 20-min rest before another 4 miles at 6:12 pace. The facility is better than the one I was using in Boston.	11.5
Sat.	12/5/09	Put in a hard 8 miles on the elliptical: 50:27 (6:18 pace). This gives me the flexibility to take it easier tomorrow because I'll be going to the Pats/Dolphins game. It has been harder to go as fast as I went in Boston. I don't know if it's my conditioning, the humid Miami weather, or slightly different equipment. It may be a combination, but my workouts have been noticeably sweatier, so it's probably the heavy, sticky air.	8.0
Sun.	12/6/09	A long day of eating, drinking, and sloppy Patriots football. We started tailgating at 11a, and we went to dinner after the game. By the time I got on the elliptical, I was over 160lbs. The gym closed at 11p, so I could only do 11.5 miles (versus my usual Sunday 14). I finished in 77:28 (6:44 pace) and weighed in at 157lbs, which is 8lbs more than usual. Between my slower times and extra body weight, I've got some work to do!	11.5
Mon.	12/7/09	The most important thing I did today was find a massage therapist. Afterward, I hit the elliptical for an uneventful 8 miles in 52:53 (6:37 pace). Tomorrow, I'll start evaluating Miami's local running clubs.	8.0
Tues.	12/8/09	Visited my new massage/flexibility therapist – Alex Da Silva. As expected, it was painful. In Boston, the sessions involved more *total* pain, but the worst pain from Alex was worse than the worst pain back home. He told me not to do a hard workout after. I completed a relaxed 5 miles on the elliptical in 32:54 (6:35 pace).	5.0
Weds.	12/9/09	Ripped 6.3 miles on the elliptical at 6:08 pace.	6.3
Total		Averaged 6:31 per mile for the week	55.0

---

42 You can see the course here: www.gmap-pedometer.com/?r=3353743

Dietary Research and Findings

Food Tip – *Bryan Huberty, a Miami training partner I met Week 49 (and still train with), extolled the virtues of bananas.* [43] *Incredibly, when we met, he was eating 30 bananas every day. That sounded like overkill, so I did some research. I found two articles that spell things out pretty clearly.* [44]

Potassium and salt (sodium) are very important minerals. Multiple sources recommend about 5,000 milligrams of potassium, daily. However, potassium should be balanced with salt to achieve maximum absorption. (2-3 milligrams of potassium for every 1 milligram of salt). Because bananas have 450 milligrams of potassium each, 30 per day are far too many, especially considering other common potassium sources in the typical diet, including the following:

- ➢ *1 cup of black beans = 800 milligrams*
- ➢ *1 cup of milk = 400 milligrams*
- ➢ *1/4 pound of ground beef = 275 milligrams*
- ➢ *1/4 pound of chicken = 260 milligrams*
- ➢ *1 orange = 250 milligrams*

Training Log Week 45			
Day	Date	Notes	Mileage
Thurs.	12/10/09	Calf still wasn't 100%, so I did 8 miles on the elliptical (6:20 pace). Thursday Night Football kept me entertained. Watched Pittsburgh (10-pt favorite), see their playoff hopes squashed by the lowly Browns.	8.0
Fri.	12/11/09	Massage therapist recommended that I stay off the road for a day or so, so I did 6 miles on the elliptical in 38:51 (6:29 pace).	6.0
Sat.	12/12/09	Still sore from yesterday's massage therapy session. Spent the day looking for rentals in Miami, so I didn't get to work out until late. Decided on an easy run to test the legs out. I ran up Washington St. to explore. South Beach is loaded with places to go... Could be a fun winter. The run went well. I took it easy and focused on staying loose. The course was 5.2 miles (36:27) After 2+ wks with my calf strain, it was nice to hit the roads and not feel hurt.	5.2
Sun.	12/13/09	My fantasy football teams were involved in playoff games, so my eyes were glued to the TV screen during my quickest Sunday 14-miler yet: 1:24:38 (6:03 pace). Elliptical times are not precisely comparable to road times – especially very short sessions, which undervalue your effort, and very long sessions, which overvalue your effort. However, this was my best long session on the elliptical to date. I may be back in business...	14.0
Mon.	12/14/09	Easy day (8 miles elliptical, 6:45 pace), but a tough day at the massage therapy office.	8.0
Tues.	12/15/09	After yesterday's session with Alex, my legs were sore. Wasn't sure I'd be able to hit the roads, but I spent the day trying to prep my legs for it. It's interval day with one of the running clubs. After a soak in the hot tub, I felt I could go. Easy warm-up: jogged 400m in 2:00, then picked it up through 1 mile (7:18), then 3:00 for 800m and some wind sprints... I was ready to roll. Workout was 5 x 500m, with 100m rest. I maintained 4:40 mile pace for all 5 reps; it was work, but comfortable. No injuries! 2.5-mile warm-down, and 2 miles at home.	9.1
Weds.	12/16/09	5 miles elliptical. Started at 8:00 pace and then dropped to sub-6:00for the remainder (31:22; 6:16 pace).	5.0
Total		Averaged 6:33 per mile for the week	55.3

43 Bryan Huberty lives in South Beach. He was a fairly serious soccer player, but he fell in love with running about two years ago. He has run sub-1:15 for the half-marathon and can challenge me on longer runs; hard to say who'd win in a 10K.

44 www.mcvitamins.com/vitamins/potassium.htm

Miscellaneous Research and Notes

Running Clubs: One aspect of training that I took for granted in Boston (and hoped to replace in Miami) was a club or team to run with. Finding a group to run with on a regular basis may be one of the most important elements you can build into your training cycle. The implicit commitment you make to a club greatly decreases the odds that you will skip a workout when you feel down, and having people to push you on days when you're meant to train hard greatly increases the odds that you will push yourself the way you should.

Based on some online research, I didn't expect much in Miami (especially compared with what I had in Boston). I also knew it would be hard to find any facility as good as MIT's outdoor complex or Harvard's indoor track.

After dropping in on a couple of clubs when they were scheduled to meet for intervals – and quickly realizing that in most cases the runners there would not be able to push me in any way – I settled on the Nike-sponsored Thursday night meet-up in South Beach.[45] About 25 people were there the first day I stopped by. They had male and female leaders, and the male leader had recently run 4:22 for the mile, so I felt he could make a good training partner. He also said that there were about 10 other good runners in the group, which sounded promising. When you're looking to join a group, it's best if you can find one with runners close to your ability. (However, I'd argue that even a group with no one at your level is better than no group at all.)

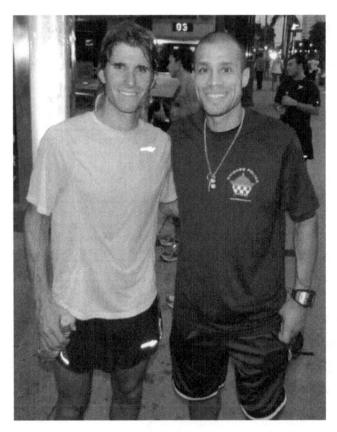

Indiana University's NCAA indoor one-mile champion Sean Jefferson (left) was one elite athlete who dropped by the Nike Run Club in Miami.

---

45 I found this group on www.meetup.com, which may be a good resource for people in other cities who are looking for a club to join.

Training Log Week 46

Day	Date	Notes	Mileage
Thurs.	12/17/09	Another painful session with Alex. Same as Monday, but with a few new stretches (some quad stuff) and w/out some other things. I met up with the Nike Running Club on Lincoln Road. Jogged over at 6:40 pace, stretched, and ran 5K with the lead group (6:30 pace). Calves were sore from Alex, but not hurt. Ran home slowly in a *downpour*! At home, I changed into dry clothes and did 4 miles on the elliptical at 6:28 pace. Not the best way to do 10.5 miles, but it'll do.	10.5
Fri.	12/18/09	Hit the roads again for 6.3 miles (41:10; 6:29 pace). Not bad, but for the way I felt, I should have been averaging 6:15. Could have been the humidity. Could also have been my lack of road work over the past several wks. Being healthy is more important, though.	6.4
Sat.	12/19/09	Same course as yesterday (38:37; 6:08 pace), and I had plenty left in the tank. It was cooler out and I was wearing flats instead of trainers. The extra 4.5 ounces per shoe makes a difference! Most importantly, no real pain. Some soreness between my right ankle and calf, but nothing major. I'll see what Alex and Dr. Moyal have to say about it. Tomorrow, I'll be on the elliptical, so I should be fine.	6.3
Sun.	12/20/09	Another good Sunday 14-miler on the elliptical: 1:25:13 (6:05 per mile), second only to last wk's session. However, I started last wk's training with 2 elliptical sessions and a road run, totaling 19.2 miles at 6:34 pace. This wk, I started with 3 road runs totaling 23.2 miles at 6:27 pace – so I've done more quality work.	14.0
Mon.	12/21/09	Went out for an easy 30-min run today. The course mapped out at 4.6 miles (6:39 pace).	4.6
Tues.	12/22/09	Ran 4 miles at 6:35 pace in the morning. My niece gave birth to a beautiful baby girl this afternoon. Both were in good health, so Jamie and I headed to Royal Palm Beach to meet my new great-niece, Avah Gomes. I was looking forward to hitting the track for intervals, but some things are more important than working out.	4.6
Weds.	12/23/09	Long day of work, visiting my niece, and taking my nephew out for his birthday. In the midst of it all, I was able to carve out 1 hr for myself for a long hard run: 9 miles in 56:23 (6:14 pace). I ran the second half of the run (which seemed slightly more uphill) in 6:03 pace. A great run. My hips and right lower-leg were sore afterward, but no worse than they've been. Need to make sure it stays that way, or preferably gets better. Was on the roads for 6 of 7 days for the first time since September. Average pace was 6:21, a PR.	9.1
Total		Averaged 6:21 per mile for the week	**54.8**

Training Log Week 47

Day	Date	Notes	Mileage
Thurs.	12/24/09	Ran for 33 min with Jamie rollerblading. Hard for her to keep a steady pace, but I enjoyed the company; went back out for 27 min solo later. Found techno remixes of some oldies (like "Major Tom" and "Everybody Wants Her"). Totaled 8.75 miles in 60 min (6:51 pace).	8.8
Fri.	12/25/09	Christmas = waking early and watching kids unwrap presents, then helping kids figure out how to use what they got. When the dust settled, I was tired. Ran 42:25, later mapped it out to be 6.65 miles (6:23 pace).	6.7
Sat.	12/26/09	Back in South Beach; back on my normal 6.3-mile loop. Started sluggish, but by Mile 1 I felt better and slowly accelerated throughout the run. By the end, I was easily sub-6:00pace and comfortable doing it. Finished in 40:26 (6:25 pace) to the sounds of 80s band, Ratt.	6.3
Sun.	12/27/09	Arduous 14-miler on the elliptical. Time was solid, but 3 min slower than my PR, set 2 wks ago. After 6 straight days on the road my body may be tired. Also possible that the time off the elliptical made me less proficient at it. Injury-wise, I feel great. Recently I've eaten a lot of pineapple (natural anti-inflammatory), spent time in the hot tub, and used an anti-inflammatory cream. Not sure why the leg feels better, but glad that it does. My only pain now is some soreness on the outside of my upper left calf. I think it's from Alex's rough grinding with the ultrasound wand. I'm fine with that.	14.0
Mon.	12/28/09	Ran to my massage with Alex (1.7 miles). It was a shorter, easier session but still pretty uncomfortable. Later, I did 6 moderate miles on the elliptical during Monday Night Football. Like yesterday, my time was slower than the effort implied, but my workout tomorrow will be a more relevant measure of my fitness.	7.7
Tues.	12/29/09	Worked out at an asphalt track on Alton and 11th. I jogged over and did long warm-up. The workout was 6 x 600m with 200m rest in between. I ran the first in 1:48 (4:48 mile pace) and the rest in 1:44-1:46 (4:40 pace). Basically I ran my 600s at the same pace as my 500s 2 wks ago. This was only my 2nd workout since Nov 17th. It was an improvement from 2 wks ago and that's good enough for now. The calves held up great, but my right leg took a little step back. We'll see how it feels tomorrow.	8.5
Weds.	12/30/09	Easy 4.3-mile, 31-min jog today (7:13 pace). I could feel a little pain in the leg at times during the day, not on the roads at all. It's clearly a "going fast" injury.	4.3
Total		Averaged 6:32 per mile for the week	**56.2**

Training Log Week 48

Day	Date	Notes	Mileage
Thurs.	12/31/09	Hectic day at work (last trading day of the year) and looking for better digs. Managed an easy 50-min jog before heading out for NYE festivities; 7 miles (7:09 pace). I finished 2009 with 330 straight days of training.	7.0
Fri.	1/1/10	Went out for a leisurely 10.2 mile run in 73:20 (7:11 per mile). I may have a pinched nerve or muscle in my lower back on the left side. Hopefully it takes care of itself.	10.2
Sat.	1/2/10	Been thinking of modifying my training regimen to be more like Johnny Gray's (i.e., less LSD and a lot more speed work). Today, I did a little of both. Started with 5.5 miles at 6:30-6:40 pace. At the track on Alton, I ran 8 x 100m on the field. I went easy on the first few sets, but picked it up from there. Everything felt fine. I ran back to my condo at a quick clip and called it a day.	6.5
Sun.	1/3/10	My pinched nerve hurt all day. I felt it when seated but really feel it when I tried to move. I did the minimum (30 min; 6:54 pace). Felt ok on the roads; not great. I don't think I worsened it by running, but I'll have to see the trainer first thing in the morning. I want to be good to go for Tuesday's intervals.	4.4
Mon.	1/4/10	Back pain has moved to my hip. I limped to the chiropractor's. Despite my skepticism, Dr. Moyal made adjustments that gave me 50% relief in about 5 min. I was impressed, but I wonder if he played a part in the injury. I was pretty fast my whole life with uneven hips. Now, I'm just injured. Next I had a stretching session with Alex. That loosened me up a little more, which enabled me through 4.4 miles in 32:27 (7:28 per mile). I'm not optimistic about tomorrow's interval workout.	4.4
Tues.	1/5/10	Hip still sore. I was limited to a minimal workout (4.4 miles in 30:00). My pace was quicker (6:49), but that is small consolation for missing intervals. Not happy.	4.4
Weds.	1/6/10	Hip *still* sore, but improving. Managed a rigorous 5.1-mile elliptical (30:00; 5:54 pace). Definitely moving fast, but the new LifeFitness elliptical may be easier at the same resistance (Level 13). Oh well.	5.1
Total		Averaged 6:51 per mile for the week	41.9

Training Log Week 49

Day	Date	Notes	Mileage
Thurs.	1/7/10	Had an appointment with a physical therapist named Bruce Wilk,[46] who specializes in runners. He does *not* believe that I'm seriously injured; more likely I jammed the hip during my 8 x 100m workout. He took me through a battery of exercises, which did a great job of loosening it up. After the appointment, I was able to run with the Nike Running Club. Total was roughly 5.3 miles in 35:30 (6:42 pace). Hopefully, I'm back on track.	5.3
Fri.	1/8/10	Hip still sore, but improving (about 85% now). I met up with a new training partner, Bryan Huberty. We did 11.4 miles in 1:28:24 (7:45 pace) up and down the boardwalk, with a stretch of packed-sand running on the beach. Hit the gym for military presses, pull-ups, and pull-downs, final set to exhaustion. I overdid it today.	11.4
Sat.	1/9/10	Hit the elliptical for a hard 30-min session to get some leg turnover back. 5 miles (just under 6:00 pace).	5.0
Sun.	1/10/10	The Patriots made my long elliptical session even longer as they got bounced out of the playoffs. I worked hard and completed 14.7 miles in 1:24:00 (an obviously exaggerated 5:43 pace). I may have to boost the resistance to Level 14 to get a more accurate workout.	14.7
Mon.	1/11/10	Met Bryan for an easy 5.1 miles (7:16 pace). Later I met Matt Kiss, another guy from my running group, in the gym. We worked biceps, triceps, and abs and did some runner curls to simulate the home stretch of a race.	5.1
Tues.	1/12/10	Work-wise, this is my busiest time of year, but I pulled out all the stops for intervals: extra sleep, pasta for lunch, cal-mag and finally some sugar-free coffee-bean chocolate about 20 min before the start. Basically, my current pre-race routine. Warmed up with stretching, followed by 400m in 2:00. Did a couple more quick stretches, followed by a 400m (6:40 pace), then 800m (5:50 pace), followed by a 6:30 mile. Workout was 6 x 400m with 200m rest. I focused on form and breathing and stayed off my toes to protect my calves. First 4 sets were 64, 65, 65, and 65 sec. I was more tired after each rep but didn't overdo it. My body wasn't breaking down, so I got up on my toes for the last 2 sets and finished each in 62 sec. After, I did 3 miles easy with Matt.	7.3
Weds.	1/13/10	No ill effects from intervals. Matt and I hit the gym at 10a. Then I hit the elliptical at 8p. 6.5 easy miles (42:37, 6:33 pace). Learned Chris Simpson ran a 4:30 mile. That ranks him #1 among U.S. Masters this year.	6.5
Total		Averaged 6:38 per mile for the week	55.3

Training Log Week 50			
Day	Date	Notes	Mileage
Thurs.	1/14/10	Restarted the stair routine and dragged Matt and Bryan along. After a warm-up, we did 5 sets. A full set here is only 16 flights, compared with 32 in Boston. We adjusted by running a faster pace. I averaged under 60 sec per 16-flight set (versus 3:00 per set in Boston). Times were 58, 57, 61, 62, and 56 sec (total 4:54). 2-mile warm-down. The sets were shorter, but I felt just as fatigued. Later I joined Robb Falaguerra and his girlfriend Amy for a slow 5 miles. Robb is a friend from Chicago who also winters in Miami.	10.0
Fri.	1/15/10	Hit the weight room in the a.m. in the evening, I led a drill workout. We started with a 5-lap warm-up, then did 8 x 30-sec drills (high-knees, butt-kicks, A-skips, lunges, bunny hops, frogs, jumping jacks, and crunches then 15 pushups and 50m strides). Got the legs turning over, and the pushups added up. 30 min later, I went out for a brisk 4-mile warm-down, starting at 7:00 pace and dropping under 6:30 in the middle.	6.5
Sat.	1/16/10	Led a drill encore at 11a. We started with 2 miles and did 6 sets of drills. After, I ran a 5-mile warm-down with Bryan. Later I ran an easy 4.7 miles with Robb and Amy. I ran the final 0.7 miles alone at close to 6:00 pace. This wk has been an interesting experiment. The aerobic mileage has been very slow, but I've done a decent workout each day. My legs are sore and a little tired, but I feel 100% healthy. I don't know if adopting the Johnny Gray routine is advancing my cause, but Tuesday's track workout may provide some insight.	12.7
Sun.	1/17/10	In Miami people run distance runs slower than I'm used to. It may not be a bad thing because I probably run distance runs too fast for my own good. I've been doing more speed-type workouts but running my distance at a slower pace. I feel a little more sore (from the speed), but I'm quicker and I'm not injured. This strategy may work. I jogged 8 miles with Matt at 8:00 pace. Later, I did 4.7 miles (elliptical) at 6:25 pace.	12.7
Mon.	1/18/10	Rest day 5-miler before 45 min of weights. Bryan uses a GPS watch to track time and mileage, but I question it. 8:26 pace is *very* slow and I'm sure we were going faster.	5.0
Tues.	1/19/10	Interval day. Basically same warm up as last week: 400m (2:00), stretch, 400m (1:30), stretch, 800m (3:00), stretch. Workout was simple, but effective: 2 x 1 mile with 5:00 rest. Mandatory negative half-mile splits and the second mile had to be faster than the first. For Mile 1, I passed 800m in 2:29 and came back in 2:27 (4:56 total). For Mile 2, I went out in 2:29 and came back in 2:26 (4:55 total). 2-mile warm-down. These were my first two sub-5:00 miles since 1996.	7.0
Weds.	1/20/10	5 miles with Bryan (7:05 pace), then I met Matt at the gym for a 40-min workout. My average mile pace this wk was over 1 min slower than usual. However, I did more quality speed work. Most importantly, I feel pretty healthy.	5.0
Total		Averaged 7:42 per mile for the week	58.8

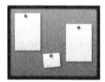

Bulletin Board Material – *I finished 2009 with 330 straight days of training, averaging 7.7 miles in 53:55 (7:01 pace). I totaled 10 miles or more 53 times, and 14 miles or more a dozen times. My most common workout was eight miles – 80 times, close to 25 percent of my workouts. My fastest eight-miler was 49:20 (6:10 pace) on the roads and 46:46 on the elliptical (5:51 pace). For the year, my total was 2,545.8 miles in 12 days, 8 hours, 32 minutes, and 16 seconds.*

Chapter 7
Brass Monkey (That Funky Monkey)

Weeks 51-60

Consider this social science experiment:

➢ Take one or more group(s) of highly trained athletes
➢ Add generous portions of fearlessness
➢ Add moderate portions of eccentricity and disregard (sometimes bordering on disdain) for established social norms
➢ Add numerous established or contrived-on-the-fly competitive challenges
➢ Add alcohol

What is the likely result? In a word, nudity. In two words, public nudity.

I would not be so bold as to suggest that 1990s New England track nerds invented streaking. According to Wikipedia, the first recorded U.S. incident occurred in 1804 at Washington & Lee University (by George William Crump, who later became a Congressman).[47] However, I *would* be so bold as to suggest that few eras or geographies produced as many variants of the event performed by as much athletic talent. Mr. Crump was no four-minute miler.

And although the on-track rivalries could be vicious, the common interest in throwing a good old-fashion drunkfest off the track brought together athletes from Northeastern University, Boston College, Boston University, Brandeis, even Harvard. Occasionally the kids from Providence College would make the trek up I-95 for a change of scenery and a few socials… But in off-campus apartments packed to the gills with type-A alpha dogs, the "socials" were just warm-up laps before the trash talking started and the challenges were put forth – challenges that involved drinking fast and running faster, almost always sans clothing. Not surprisingly, each school seemed to have its own variant on the same activities.

At Northeastern we played Anchor Man (a relay performed with two four-man teams and two pitchers of beer and a simple premise: each relay member drank as much as he could as quickly as he could and passed the pitcher down the line until it reached the Anchor Man – who would be responsible for completing it.) The runners at BC seemed to enjoy a more "civilized" game called Century Club, in which you'd drink but one ounce of beer – but you would do so every minute for 100 minutes in a row. Not surprisingly, the rules to these games shifted occasionally based on how many beers the competitors had consumed at the time. The less inventive, or less team-oriented drinking games like keg stands and quarters were also typical pastimes – but they all led to the night's eventual finale, the naked run.

Locale often determined the type of naked run, for pure logistical reasons. Out in the seclusion of Western Mass, colleges were known to organize full-blown naked one-mile runs around the college tracks – complete with water stops stocked with beer. At Boston University, one enterprising undergrad figured how to trip the lock at the field house to set the stage for naked games indoor-track style. In the late 1980s/early 1990s, the University at Albany allegedly held naked road races – albeit short ones. The most notorious naked run of them all might have been the Nude Relays at University of Florida, which – following one running of the prestigious Florida Relays – received local and national press coverage.[48]

Because the only track near Northeastern's campus was a cinder-based public track in the Fens – with year-round lighting and frequent police presence – most of our naked races were away-games… most frequently up the road at Boston College.

One event I still remember was a Northeastern versus Boston College naked 4 x 400-meter relay. The object was simple; our four best quarter-milers would face theirs, abiding by only two rules: 1) competitors were allowed to wear nothing but shoes, and 2) each contestant had to drink three pints of beer before the start of the race.

Because of Rule #2, an ancillary game was born: The Drinking Relay. The Drinking Relay started with six contestants from each school standing on opposing sides of a long table. Two pints of beer were placed in front of each contestant. At the starter's command, the first member of each team would race to complete one pint. When the cup was finished, the next team member would start. The sixth member of each team would finish both of their pints back-to-back before "passing the baton" back up the line, eventually back to the leadoff man. The first team to finish all 12 pints was of course the winner. From the pool of six players, each team captain would select four members to complete one more pint to fulfill their three-beer quota for the naked 4 x 400.

To say that school pride ran as deeply on tap as it did on the track would be an understatement. When it came to drinking games, there was no easy escape. You couldn't false start your way out of competing, nor could you fake an injury. You might feign sickness, but even that didn't always get you excused – and if anyone thought you were faking, you would be booed and ridiculed. I wasn't the best drinker on the team, but I could drink just fast enough and run more than fast enough to be a fixture on Northeastern's naked relay squad.

One night during cross country season, the Northeastern team hopped the 'T' to Chestnut Hill. Brian "Murph" Murphy[49] was hosting a post-meet party at his off-campus apartment. When the party got started, it didn't take long for the BC and NU runners to start jawing. Once the beers were lined up, we selected a presumably impartial starter/judge. In this case, we agreed on an attractive young lady we'll call "Zoe" – mostly because I forgot her real name. Zoe happened to be the daughter of a BC dean. In hindsight this inherently made her biased, but she was attractive and the BC guys argued that as the daughter of a dean, she would be more impartial than any other bystander. After a few beers, this logic made sense. Did I mention she was attractive?

Zoe said go and the debauchery began.

I led off The Drinking Relay for NU. With a couple of gulps I downed my first pint and slammed the empty cup, upside down, to the table. In a single motion, my teammate Dennis Shine lifted his cup, swallowed the entire pint in one gulp, and returned his cup to its original position. Our third man finished his pint before BC's second man. The rout was on. The frenzied BC crowd urged for a home-team comeback, but it wasn't to be. I had barely finished a preparatory burp when I saw Shine reach for his second pint on the way back up the line.

We were way ahead, but that didn't disrupt our precision – we were trained competitors, after all. Shine's hand dropped and mine went up. As I finished my beer, I peeked across the table. BC still had three beers to go. I saw an opportunity for humiliation. I still had to drink one more beer to qualify for the naked 4 x 400, and that seemed like as good a time as any. I reached across the table, grabbed one of their remaining beers, and tossed it down before they could finish their penultimate pint.

---

48 Source = [Google: "Sports Illustrated" + Nude Relays]

49 As of this writing Brian Murphy still holds Boston College's outdoor 3,000-meters record (8:08.6) and once ran a 2:23.3 1,000-meters – one second faster than my best.

With a collective home-team moan, the drinking relay ended... and the trash-talking began anew. BC couldn't wait to avenge their loss. Murph ordered an underclassman to refill their cups, while everyone dropped down to their boxers and tightened their shoelaces.

A quick qualifying pint later, several dozen of BC and NU's finest role models scurried out to BC's track (sadly now removed as part of renovations to the football stadium). Everyone was fired up, but the air was crisp. After three cold pints, the 40-degree breeze had a sobering effect. The sooner we got things done, the sooner we could get back to Murph's warm apartment (and more cold beer).

The contestants dropped trou as Zoe, our starter, positioned herself just beyond the starting line. You could always tell a lot about a guy from the ceremonial pants dropping. Some were proud. Some were sheepish, and some were all business. Some were just eager to show the ladies their stuff. Whether or not they had good reason to was irrelevant.

Zoe's rushed "ready, set, go" command caught some folks off guard and left something to be desired... but did I mention she was attractive? Either way, the race was on.

In the pitch dark, we could barely make out the shadowy forms as they negotiated the first turn. By the time they reached the back straightaway, we couldn't tell who was in the lead. That didn't stop the rabid home supporters from bellowing encouragement. Soon, the figures came back into view. NU held a slight lead into the hand-off zone.

At this point, I was already feeling pretty cold. I could see my breath. I could see everyone else's too. The collective respiration cast a fog. I did a quick stride and kept moving in place to stay warm. The shaking forced a belch, which I actually appreciated. Across the track, we could see BC's third runner double over in full stride. Most of the spectators didn't know what was going on, but anyone who had ever sprinted 400 meters on 48 ounces of beer did. He threw up a fair amount of beer but never broke stride. A true competitor. Nonetheless, his momentum was disrupted and NU's lead increased. Shine, our third man, wasn't the fastest 400-meter runner, but he had competitive spirit to spare. He held the lead, rounded the final turn at a good clip and executed a clean baton exchange. I took off like a shot.

I had to. Murph was BC's anchor leg. Not only could he handle his beer, he had run a 3:45 1,500-meters the prior spring. I had a good head start, but I was naked and carrying three pints of beer in my belly. Luckily, everything stayed where it belonged. Rounding the final turn, I could see two small beams of lights up ahead. "Where did they find flashlights?" I thought, going into my final kick. A few more steps and I had my answer. They weren't our flashlights. They belonged to the two BC police officers lured to the track by the cheering mob.

I continued sprinting through the finish line and kept going. There's no doubt the officers saw me, but they had plenty of fish to fry. After I was safely out of view, I doubled back along the darkness of the stadium stands and quietly grabbed my clothes. Just within earshot I could see one of the runners, still naked, explaining himself to the police. One of the cops lowered his flashlight to waist-level and said, "I wouldn't be doing this if I were you."

I had to bite my bottom lip to keep from laughing. One last insult to cap BC's night. I tiptoed off the track and rendezvoused with everyone who had escaped. Murph was among us, still naked. He had sensed the danger and aborted his leg of the relay. As we headed back to Murph's place, all I could think about was whether someone got my split time. More twisted than that? Someone actually did: 53 seconds – a new naked relay record. The record didn't last long though. A year later, Erik Nedeau ran 49 seconds. It was bad enough that he had broken my Northeastern University 1,000-meter run record... but my naked relay record too?

Back at Murph's apartment, we thought it best to gather our things and head to a local bar. A few of the BC folks were still missing, including Zoe, which proved unfortunate for Murph. Being a dean's daughter, I guess she was compelled to rat him out. As punishment, he had to write a 5,000 word essay entitled, "Why It's Not a Good Idea to Get Drunk and Race Naked." I never did get to read that essay. I wonder if Murph kept it...

In Hindsight – A*t no point will I attempt to discourage the college readers of this book from drinking alcohol – that would be as effective as advising fish to stop swimming. However, physiological research has illuminated multiple specific ways in which alcohol impedes athletic performance. Women's Health posted a very succinct article bullet-pointing these effects.*[50]

The most interesting aspects of alcohol consumption and its corollary effect on training, at least to me, were the effects on recovery time and sleep quality. Few athletes, especially college athletes, recognize that most muscle development happens not during training sessions but during sleep – so catching forty winks after a race or hard workout is very important. Disrupting this sleep cycle with a booze session can be very deleterious.

Training Log Week 51			
Day	Date	Notes	Mileage
Thurs.	1/21/10	Stairs at noon: 2-mile warm-up, 5 sets, 2-mile warm-down. Matt Kiss was consistent. Bryan Huberty and I died at the end. I logged 55, 56, 58, 1:02, 1:20 (5:11 total). A combination of factors contributed to my breakdown. Later we joined the Nike Running Club for a brisk 3.5 miles. I ran to the meet-up then completed the 3.5-mile course in 21:41 (6:12 pace). Bryan was right with me until the final 400m.	10.7
Fri.	1/22/10	Easy day. Slow 50-min run with Robb Falaguerra at 5:30p. After that, I led a drill workout (see Jan. 15), but with frogs instead of squats, so this was a little easier.	6.8
Sat.	1/23/10	Drill workout in the morning. Basically the same workout as yesterday (total 6 miles). I was hoping to do more in the afternoon, but the day didn't play into my hands.	6.0
Sun.	1/24/10	Easy 7 miles (60 min) with Matt in the morning. That served as a warm-up for my third drill workout in as many days. I'm definitely feeling stronger during drills. My sprints are faster and my pushups are easier. New shoes felt pretty good. Later I loaded up my iPod with hard, fast songs and hit the roads for a stiff 4-miler (23:52; 5:58 pace).	12.0
Mon.	1/25/10	Recovery day. Roughly 6 miles at 8-min pace with Bryan.	6.1
Tues.	1/26/10	Great interval session with Track Club Miami.[51] Standard easy 400m/400m/800m/1-mile warm-up with stretching and strides. Workout was a downward ladder: 1,000m (2:54), 800m (2:18), 600m (1:38), 400m (63 sec), 400m (63 sec), with 200m rest after each. I jogged an easy 1,200m then my quads cramped up. After that, I walked for 10 min, shaking the cramps out and stretching. Doing slower distance runs has prevented injuries but hasn't hurt my overall development.	5.6
Weds.	1/27/10	Recovery day: 6.5 miles (7:11 pace) with Bryan. Felt rough.	6.5
Total		Averaged 7:34 per mile for the week	**53.7**

Injury Reports and Medical Findings

Colon Cleansing: I did some research on colon-cleansing products. These products claim that excess waste builds up in the colon and can add up to several pounds of unnecessary weight – depending on age and diet. I'd have been happy – well not happy, but motivated – to use one of those products to rid myself of a few extra pounds, but unfortunately (or maybe *fortunately*), my research indicated these products to be more marketing BS than anything else. A variety of articles aggregated on the Web site everydayhealth.com – including one by Dr. Ed Zimney – indicate no benefit to colon cleansing at all.

---

50 Source = www.womenshealth.com; [Google: "women's health" + alcohol and exercise]

51 Track Club Miami (www.trackclubmiami.com) was founded by former MIT runner Dave Afshartous PhD. He captained the MIT cross country team and was All-New England in the 10,000 meters.

Training Log Week 52			
Day	Date	Notes	Mileage
Thurs.	1/28/10	This morning I taught Matt my typical interval warm-up routine. After that, we did some 100m strides. Later, I ran 3 miles at 6:20 pace, then I joined the Nike running group for a 5K run (6:00 pace) and jogged home.	10.4
Fri.	1/29/10	Miami Tropical 5K is tomorrow. I have no idea what to expect, so I'm just gonna do my best. In preparation, I got extra rest today and only did 4 miles (elliptical), my first time on it in over two wks. I haven't been injury-free that long since last April, so I'm feeling great about my new regimen.	4.1
Sat.	1/30/10	Today I was the *overall* winner in the 2010 Miami Tropical 5K – my 3rd 5K victory during my Masters training. (See Race Reports.) My time was 16:51 – fastest since college, but still pretty slow.	7.1
Sun.	1/31/10	Today was Marathon Sunday in Miami. My job was to wake up at 6:30a, show up at Mile 18 by 8a, and help Bryan Huberty through the final 8.2 miles. When I got home, I was pretty amped, so I grabbed Matt and did an easy sprint/stride workout to shake out yesterday's race residue: 5 x 75m with 125m rest, walk 1 lap, then 5 x 75m. We then did two sets of 3 x 50m. After that, we jogged home.	14.0
Mon.	2/1/10	An "off" day. Morning weight work with Matt. Later it was raining, so I did an easy elliptical session (5 miles in 37:17; 7:27 pace), followed by calf stretches. I also worked on a drill where I do squats with an object placed between my knees. The object keeps my legs from collapsing inward, which has been a significant contributor to my pesky calf-strain issue.	5.0
Tues.	2/2/10	As usual, Tuesday is interval day; 7 miles total.	7.0
Weds.	2/3/10	Recovery day. Planned on 5-6 miles at 7:00-7:30 pace with Bryan, but we felt good early, so we went faster. After 3 or 4 miles, yesterday's intervals caught up to me. Next, we took a wrong turn and ended up running 6.75 miles (45:28;6:45 pace), a little fast for an off day, but no big deal. Also today is Jamie's birthday!	6.8
Total		Averaged 7:07 per mile for the week	54.3

Dietary Research and Findings

Nitric Oxide (NO): NO is a vasodilator: it opens blood vessels by relaxing the muscle cells within the vessel walls. This results in more blood traveling to your muscles at a faster rate, presumably improving athletic performance. Many body builders take L-arginine supplements to stimulate NO production. (L-arginine is an amino acid, which breaks down in the body, releasing NO into the system.) Based on my research, stimulating NO production appears to be a *very* good thing to do.

However, studies greatly favor natural NO production over supplements. Apparently, there is little evidence that supplements produce any beneficial impact on NO production. Meanwhile one side effect of L-arginine supplementation pertaining to growth hormone production may be negative. In *active* subjects (i.e., athletes), one study showed that working out increased growth hormone production by 300-500 percent. L-arginine supplementation seemed to *decrease* that number to 200 percent. In *non-active* subjects, L-arginine use resulted in a 100-percent increase in growth hormone production, so the supplements are probably best left to the inactive.

All that being said, an increase in fruit and vegetable consumption was found to increase natural NO production. Fruits and vegetables are high in *nitrates*, which easily convert to *nitrites*, which convert to NO. (Confused yet? It's a little hard to keep straight...) The result is lower oxygen demand at an equal workload. In other words, increased nitrate/nitrite consumption will increase your maximum performance.[52] Unlike L-arginine, *nitrite* supplements appear to be as effective as natural sources.

Taking this research a step further, beet juice has been found to be an excellent source of nitrate/nitrite, displaying incredible results in a University of Exeter (UK) study.[53] To make a long story short, 500 milliliters per day of beet juice increased stamina (how long the subjects could perform) by 16 percent. This was calculated to translate into a 2 percent improvement in the amount of time required to perform an athletic task.

---

52 Source: [Google: pponline.co.uk + nitric oxide + truth]

53 Sources: [Google: pponline.co.uk + dietary nitrate; Google: webmd + truth about beet root juice]

For 800 meters, this would cut a 2:00 time down to 1:57.6!

Beets, celery, turnip greens, radishes, seaweed, and spinach are among the richest sources of nitrates. My diet was woefully low in all of the above, so I had a lot to gain. Beet juice seems to be the nitrate champ, delivering 140-160 milligrams per 100 milliliters... but it is hard to do much more than sip it, because the taste is pretty strong.

Aside from taste, a potential downside is that high-nitrate foods are sometimes suspected to cause headaches. I started ramping up my nitrate/nitrite intake and had a headache the following day. In addition, high-nitrite diets are linked to a high incidence of gastric cancer. However, high-nitrite diets are also usually high in salt and fried foods, while lacking in nutrition. All three of those attributes have been closely linked to gastric cancer, so high-nitrite foods may not be the source – or at least not the sole source – of increased cancer risk.

<u>Vitamin D</u>: I explored the benefits of Vitamin D. An excellent article from the *New York Times* summed up its attributes.[54] If you read the article, take notice of two key points:

First, in one study, a group of four Russian sprinters were doused with artificial, ultraviolet light. A control group wasn't. Both trained identically for the 100-meter dash. The control group lowered their sprint times by 1.7 percent. The radiated runners, in comparison, improved by an impressive 7.4 percent.

Second, one online comment on the article came from a 51-year-old runner who was taking ibuprofen every night to deal with muscular pain. He started taking "2,000 mg of vitamin D and 1.5 capsules of wild salmon oil from Costco" and has subsequently felt that he has "knocked 10 years off" his running and hasn't taken ibuprofen since.

First off, a 7.4-percent time improvement for the sprinters (or anyone) is *sick!* For the 100-meter dash, that's pretty close to a full second for most people. If that improvement carried through to 800-meters, we'd be talking about knocking nine seconds off of a 2:00 half-mile time... down to 1:51. Insane! At the risk of taking the 51-year old commenter's proclamation too literally, if you look at the Masters All-American records, you'll find that the average differential between the 40-year-olds' standards and the 50-year-olds' standards is... you guessed it: 7 percent.

I was doubtful that the results presented would occur across a broad sample of runners, but an improvement of even 1 percent would knock more than a full second off of my 800-meter time. That potential was too high to ignore. However, proper vitamin D absorption by the body is among the trickiest things I have seen. Despite its presence in everything from multi-vitamins to milk to sunlight, vitamin D deficiencies are common, even among people who take D supplements and spend a lot of time in the sun.

---

54 Source: [Google: new york times + vitamin d + performance]

Training Log Week 53

Day	Date	Notes	Mileage
Thurs.	2/4/10	Morning track work with Bryan Huberty. Brief warm up, then a 35-35 workout: as many 200m repeats as possible at 35 sec each, with 35 sec rest. We finished most of the 200s in 32 sec and took 38 sec rest. (I liked that better!) That night, I joined the Nike group for our usual run. We started slowly because people wanted to hear about Bryan Sharkey's 2:39 4th-place finish in the Miami Marathon.[55] I picked up the pace after 3-4 min; final time was 19:37 (3.2 miles; 6:08 pace). Today was my 365th straight day of training!	10.5
Fri.	2/5/10	One year ago, I laced up a pair of Nike cross-trainers and ran a "hard" 3.5 miles in 27:00 (7:43 pace). Today, I laced up a new pair of Brooks trainers and led a drill workout. It was pretty easy. Go figure.	4.5
Sat.	2/6/10	Started the day with an easy drill workout. Later I completed a hard 6.4 miles in 39:13 (6:07 pace). Between this and my recent workouts, I feel I'm taking another step forward in my conditioning. I'll get to test it in a couple of wks in a 1-mile track race.	9.9
Sun.	2/7/10	Bryan Huberty won a 5K this morning in 16:59. He won a cool crystal plaque and a $100 gift certificate to a running store. I've won two races and come away with less than I paid to enter! At noon I met him for a 10-miler. Finished with 10.5 miles in 72 min (6:55 pace).	12.5
Mon.	2/8/10	Easy day. Bryan and I ran about 5.5 miles at 7-min pace in the morning. At 2p, I had a tough session with my flexibility trainer. The hard work of the past few days left me pretty stiff, so his routine was painful and exhausting. I felt great afterward, though.	4.8
Tues.	2/9/10	Interval session: Standard warm-up; 400m (1:45), 400m (1:15), 800m (2:45), 1 mile (5:23), easy 400m with strides; all with stretching in between. Workout was 2K with 5-min rest, followed by 2 x 400m with 200m rest. For the 2K, I planned on 75 sec per lap. I went out a little quick (68-sec 400m), then settled in (4:51 through 1 mile) and gutted a 78-sec last lap for a total 2K of 6:09. I wasn't excited to run the remaining 400m segments. In the first, I heard footsteps behind me and pushed to a 62-sec finish. That pumped me up, and I ran 61.5 sec for the final 400m. I felt a twinge in the center of my calf, so I limited the warm-down, but after icing it at home I could tell it would be fine.	7.7
Weds.	2/10/10	Rest day; 30-min elliptical (5 miles).	5.0
Total		Averaged 6:36 per mile for the week	**52.4**

Training Log Week 54

Day	Date	Notes	Mileage
Thurs.	2/11/10	Skipped morning speed work due to the calf. Did 6 miles (elliptical), gradually increasing the pace. In the evening, I joined the Nike crew for a 4-miler. We took the pace out moderately (2 miles in ~14 min). Bryan Huberty and another runner picked up the pace. Bryan Sharkey and I rested our injuries, but with about 1,200m left, we gave chase and passed them. Sharkey finished 2 sec ahead of me. He thinks we closed with a sub-5:00 mile. Total time was 24 min, so it's possible. Hard finish to a solid run. Calf held up fine.	11.9
Fri.	2/12/10	Despite the fast finish, yesterday felt easy, so I did an extra 2 miles today. I planned a jog around Miami Beach, but at Mile 2 it poured rain. I stretched and did some exercises under an awning until I could dash home at 6:00 pace. I hit the gym for a quick 3-mile elliptical.	7.0
Sat.	2/13/10	Morning drill workout (minus pushups). Matt showed up and I helped him with intervals. I assigned him 2 x 1,600m, 1 x 800m, and 2 x 400m. I paced him through in 6:15, 6:00, 2:54, 84, and 84 sec. We did a 160m sprint to make an even 5K. Matt was excited by the results. We hit the gym for 20 min elliptical, ab work, and foam rollers on the legs (painful, but good for the calf). Looking forward to Valentine's dinner at Palme D'Or.	9.5
Sun.	2/14/10	Calf needed rest, so I logged 12.5 miles (7:12 pace) on the elliptical. Needed TV, iPod and a comic book to entertain me for the 90 min.	12.5
Mon.	2/15/10	Rest day before intervals tomorrow. 36 min (elliptical) at 7:35 pace. Choked down some beet juice. Tough to drink, but I've noticed a real difference in endurance and recovery. Hoping it will get my calf close to 100%.	4.8
Tues.	2/16/10	Evening intervals. Standard warm-up: 400m (93 sec), 400m (89 sec), 800m (2:38), 1 mile (5:41) – stretching and jogging in between. Workout = 6 x 400m with 200m rest. I wanted 65 sec across the board and logged 65, 66, 65, 63, 62, and 60 sec . (The 66 sec rep pissed me off, so I picked it up.) I was never going all out. I warmed down at home, after icing the calf, so I could use the elliptical. I added weights, including runners' curls.	7.7
Weds.	2/17/10	Jogged to a morning session with the flexibility trainer. He worked on my calves, and they didn't feel too bad. Golfed nine holes and picked up Rick Miller at the airport.	5.0
Total		Averaged 6:57 per mile for the week	**58.3**

---

55 Bryan Sharkey was a standout in high school and ran 8:59 in the steeplechase for Princeton University.

Some tips/hints for maximizing your vitamin D absorption are as follows:

➢ Vitamin D is fat-soluble, *not* water soluble. This means that you should eat some sort of fat (olive oil or nuts would be a healthy choice) with your dose of vitamin D in order to ensure absorption into your system. Vitamins A, E, and K are also fat-soluble. FYI, all of these get stored in the liver and are therefore not essential to take daily (assuming your liver is pre-loaded).

➢ You can get vitamin D from sunlight, but this is more complex than it sounds. Specifically, vitamin D can be synthesized via direct exposure to the proper wavelength of ultraviolet light. We're talking about the summer sun in southern Florida, not the winter sun in Boston. The latter is near useless. The closer to the equator and the closer to summer, the better.

Ultraviolet D requires somewhat oily skin to be properly absorbed. Dry skin can be an impediment. Also, vitamin D from ultraviolet light takes a while to absorb, so showering can wash it away, especially if you use soap. In other words, what a pain the ass... It's much more practical to get vitamin D from food sources.

➢ There are multiple types of vitamin D. D3 is more effective in most ways than D2. The former is more naturally-occurring and is almost never the type found in supplements. Your best bets are cod liver oil, egg yolks, and sunlight.

➢ In addition to fat, optimal absorption requires magnesium and calcium. In the absence of available calcium, the vitamin D will simply strip it away from your bones and teeth... so make sure you're ingesting some calcium with your vitamin D!

My conclusions: Considering how hard it is to absorb vitamin D, I believe doing it right can differentiate you from most competitors. I focused on eating eggs and taking cod liver oil pills (with some nuts and calcium/magnesium supplements), thus improving absorption rate by timing my vitamin D intake to correspond with my intake of fats.

Food Tip – *Although fat-soluble vitamins get stored in the liver for extended periods of time, water-soluble vitamins are not stored in the body and must therefore be replaced daily. One strategy is to take a mega vitamin at different times of the day (e.g., one in the morning, to enable absorption of the water-soluble vitamins – mainly, B and C – and then one at night with a fatty meal or fish-oil supplement to ensure absorption of fat-soluble vitamins A, D, E, and K).*

Race Reports, Records, and Results

2010 Miami Tropical 5K: On January 30th, I outran 2,000 competitors in the 2010 Miami Tropical 5K Road Race – my third 5K victory in as many attempts (two on the roads and one on the track).

My time was 16:51, faster than I had run since college, but still pretty slow by good runners' standards. All I did was hang and kick, so I could have gone faster, but not by very much. Wind was the primary cause of the slow time. The course was unidirectional (one way, point-to-point), and a stiff headwind greeted us every step of the way. Times were slow across the board. Elva Dryer[56] (a two-time Olympian) won the female division but ran only 18:09, a full minute slower than the time she sought. That indicates a stiff wind!

All things considered, I was happy with the time and ecstatic about the result. The pace was hard from the start, driven by five or six guys who took it out too fast. All but one dropped way back before the halfway point. Just after the two-mile mark, three of us congregated and it became a one-mile war of wills. At one point, the other two guys

---

56 Elva Dryer competed in the Sidney Olympics in 2000 at 5,000 meters and in the Athens Olympics in 2004 at 10,000 meters. Her bests are 15:03 for 5K and 31:21 for 10K.

Side Track: The Kenyans, Nitrates, and Beet Juice

My research into nitrites caused me to investigate what Kenyan runners eat. I figured I could do a lot worse than mimic their diet. I found the results to be kind of funny. As it turns out, my diet – especially once I focused on nitrate/nitrite consumption – was getting very close to that of the Kenyans.

The typical Kenyan diet is roughly 80 percent carbs, 10 percent protein, and 10 percent fats. Their primary source of carbs comes from "ugali," which appears to be the national staple in Kenya. Ugali is essentially cornmeal porridge (white corn flour and water). My sense is that ugali can be substituted with any number of other healthy carbs. Most Kenyans' protein and fat comes from whole milk, which they use liberally in the relatively large quantities of tea they consume, and modest amounts of roasted meat (usually beef). Kenyans also eat a healthy amount of greens (e.g., collard greens), which clearly provide them with an ample source of nitrates.

Speaking of nitrates, I became convinced that beet juice works minor wonders. After one of my many calf injuries, I tried drinking beet juice, and one day later my calf felt 100-percent better. For good measure, I drank some more beet juice the next day at lunch. To dilute the strong flavor, I tried mixing it with V-8 Juice, but that only prolonged the agony. I tried heating the mixture to make it like tomato soup and added rice – still no good. Next, I added frozen mixed vegetables and it was *still* tough to swallow. I ultimately arrived at one-ounce shots so the suffering was over quickly. I eventually figured out that beet juice is easier to drink when you use a chaser. I would do a four-ounce shot of beet juice and chase it with five ounces of cranberry juice. About 90 percent of the taste and aftertaste was eliminated. To further boost my nitrates, I also introduced some celery and parsley to my morning protein smoothie. I expected it to be gross, but it was actually pretty good.

I did some additional research and discovered that only drinking a few ounces of beet juice at a time was probably a good thing. Beet juice is so potent that only small servings are recommended. I also learned you should not drink beet juice at the same time that you plan to consume anything high in calcium (like milk or broccoli). Beet juice is high in oxalic acid, which combines with calcium to create an indigestible compound.[57] The Web site Juicingbook.com warns that oxalic acid should be avoided by people who suffer from or are at risk for kidney stones, gout, rheumatoid arthritis, osteoporosis and those whose stomach is easily irritated.

I cannot stress the benefits of this dietary change strongly enough. I realized immediate performance and recovery improvements once I upped my nitrate consumption.

(Jeff Zickers, a 36-year-old Georgia Tech grad, and David Ramirez, a 17-year-old high school standout) exchanged elbows and words. I sat back and let them beat each other up while they blocked much of the wind.

The final hill was the bridge into South Beach. Zickers faded near the top, leaving me and "the kid" to battle it out. I hung on his shoulder until the bottom of the bridge before testing him with a surge. He didn't respond, so I was off to the races. I was definitely tired and still had 800 meters to go, so I didn't know if he would come back on me or not. Luckily, he did not, and I cruised the last 200 meters without a fight.

The Miami Herald interviewed me for a few minutes after the race but still managed to spell my name wrong and fabricated a few quotes for good measure. Oh, well... After posing for some pictures and doing a video interview, I hung out with Matt Kiss and Zickers until the awards ceremony. Matt had turned into a personal project for me; he needed more speed work and better race preparation, but he clearly had potential. I was amused by my award for winning: No cash. No gift certificate; just a big medal.

---

57 Source: www.juicingbook.com/vegetables/beet

2010 Founders Mile at Tropical Park: On February 21st I woke up before my alarm sounded, but I still got six hours of sleep. I believe getting *extra* rest is important two days before a race, but I find *less* sleep the night before is okay – even preferable.

My co-author Rick Miller, who had been visiting Jamie and I and enjoying the Miami nightlife for the previous three nights, summoned the strength to emerge from our guest room and accompany me to the race. I benevolently made a stop at McDonald's so he could grab some breakfast. When he got back to the car, he told me that some of the runners were in there eating, and we joked that that might actually give me a chance to win. It was tongue-in-cheek though. A 4:21 miler would still be able to run 4:25, even weighed down by a McDonald's breakfast. I didn't think it was reasonable that I could run a 4:24 mile yet, so the joke quickly ended.

We got to the track at 9 a.m., 90 minutes before the mile was scheduled to go off. That gave me 30 minutes to check in, settle in, and get the lay of the land. It was already 72 degrees with about 75 percent humidity. At 9:30 I started my work-in-progress warm-up routine (described initially in Week 51), and by the time I was done it was 10:10 and only 20 minutes until race time.

As I headed toward the stands, where Miller was watching the meet, I was surprised to see Dave Afshartous, who ran one of Miami's running clubs. He offered to provide 200-meter splits on the far side of the track, which I thought might be critical. At the stands, I found another surprise – Kevin Carberry[58] and his family. Apparently Miller and Afshartous weren't the only third parties curious to see what an aging athlete could turn for an all-out mile.

With 20 minutes to go, I went into my final routine. It was time to strap on the spikes and play my battle hymn, "Neue Regel" by Queensrÿche. (Don't judge. Everybody has a song that gets the adrenaline rushing, and that had been mine since college.)

I moved onto the track and tested the spikes with a quick stride. The shoes were a little loose, but with a quick re-tie everything felt great. It had been 14 years since my last one-mile race, but based on my training I felt I might bust out something decent – maybe even 4:30. There was just one problem… I jogged over to the race clerk, only to find that the meet was behind schedule because of an awards presentation. "No problem," I thought. "A couple extra strides will keep me loose, and I'll listen to 'Neue Regel' one more time."

The awards presentation lasted 30 minutes! Then the officials had trouble rustling up the 400-meter contestants for the heats that would precede the mile. When it was all said and done, 45 minutes had passed. I was cooling down and getting tired of "Neue Regel." I knew the other runners faced the same dilemma, but I wanted to run a good time more than compete for place. I did my best to remain warmed-up and hyped-up.

Disorganized as the meet was, there were no lane assignments. At the line, someone was already in Lane 1, so I parked myself Lane 2. The announcer rattled off our names and even said something about me training for the 2011 Masters' National Championships. The last thing I remember hearing was, "Let's see if he can give these youngsters a run for their money." I thought that was funny.

When the gun went off, the kid in Lane 1 went out quickly. The wind was blowing hard, so I was happy to let him have the lead. I felt very comfortable through 200 meters, but I heard Dave Afshartous shout, "30, 31, 32."

That was a quick opening for our talent level. Simultaneously, everyone reacted. Like synchronized swimmers, the entire field immediately turned it down a notch. We went through the next 200 meters in 36 seconds, giving us a 68 for the first quarter. Three more of those would give me a 4:32 – not what I wanted.

During the second lap, I thought the pace was picking up again, but the third 200-meter split was another 36 seconds, taking us through 600 meters in 1:43. I figured the leader thought he could win a tactical race, but I wanted

---

58 Kevin Carberry was a pole vaulter on Northeastern University's track team. He and his wife have been close friends of the NU track guys for many years.

Training Log Week 55

Day	Date	Notes	Mileage
Thurs.	2/18/10	Stairs with Bryan Huberty: 6 x 16 flights (59, 60, 61, 61, 62, and 61 sec; 6:05 total) with about 2 min rest. Much better than the last stair workout where we tanked the final flight. In the evening, Rick Miller and I ran 4.5 miles with the Nike group. I picked it up each mile to finish in 29:38 (last mile about 6:00).	12.0
Fri.	2/19/10	Wanted some morning track work because tomorrow is a rest day. A half-mile into my warm-up, the shin started to hurt, so I backed right off. After some stretching, I was able to do 5 strides. I decided to warm down (1 mile) and try again later. Midday I hit the track and warmed up with an easy mile. I ran strides on the grass instead of full-out 200s on the oval: 5 x 50m, 6 x 75m, and 1 x 100m. The shin was ok, but not great, so I jogged a half-mile to the gym to hit the elliptical for 30 min with a number of short pick-ups.	7.7
Sat.	2/20/10	Did an easy pre-race drill workout: six sets of standard drills, no pushups. 50 min total work, then a very easy 30-min elliptical. Indonesian food for dinner with friends. A little beef and lamb, but mostly rice and vegetables. I also had 2 glasses of wine. Popped 2 Cal-Mag tablets aimed for 6-7 hrs sleep.	4.0
Sun.	2/21/10	Race day: I won the Founder's Mile at Tropical Park and broke 4:30! (See Race Reports section.) Standard warm-up, w/out the 1-mile leg. The race started tactically, and I had to run negative splits – 2:18 + 2:10 – to finish in 4:28. Meanwhile, Bryan Huberty, won the Fort Lauderdale Marathon in 2:44, a 12-min PR!	13.0
Mon.	2/22/10	Sore, but I hit the gym for a light 30-min workout (bench, runners' curls, chin ups, and light calf lifts). I also hit the legs with the foam roller. Weighed in at 148lbs. Met Bryan for a victory jog: 8.6 miles at 7:44 pace.	8.6
Tues.	2/23/10	Bryan Sharkey attended intervals. He can kick my ass, but I welcomed being pushed by a stronger runner. Bryan Huberty came as well. The workout was 3 x 1,000m with 200m rest. After my standard warm-up, we decided we'd do the first interval at 5:00 pace and work from there. Sharkey led us through the first one in 3:05 (4:57 pace). It felt too easy, but I didn't know if the 200m recovery would be enough. I led the second rep in 3:00 (4:49 pace) – still easy. We did the third interval in 2:57 (4:45 pace), then added a fourth: 2:50 for Sharkey; 2:52 for me (4:37 pace). Easy 1.5-mile warm-down.	6.8
Weds.	2/24/10	Recovery day: 4.1 miles in 27:06 (6:37 pace). It was pouring, but the pace was easy.	4.1
Total		Averaged 7:02 per mile for the week	**56.2**

Training Log Week 56

Day	Date	Notes	Mileage
Thurs.	2/25/10	Noon stair workout with Bryan Huberty. Again we did 6 x 16 flights with an easy 2-mile warm-up and warm-down. We went 59, 61, 61, 59, 59, and 59 sec (total 5:58), which bettered last wk by 7 sec. I was wiped out though. Bryan, being a marathoner, was fine. That night, I met the Nike group for our Thursday jaunt: 4 miles at low 6-min pace. I jogged home and worked every inch of my legs with the foam roller.	11.2
Fri.	2/26/10	Easy day: 6 miles on the elliptical in 44:00 (7:20 pace).	6.0
Sat.	2/27/10	Morning drill workout; *not* easy, because Jamie and I were out until 4a. Michael[59] wanted to do more sets when the beginners finished. We settled on 3 x 50m karaokes, a set of bunny hops, and 2 x 100m strides. It woke me up but didn't stop me from going back to bed afterward! Later, I did 8 hard miles on the elliptical (51:00; 6:22 pace), runners' curls, and 20 min on a foam roller.	11.0
Sun.	2/28/10	With the U.S. Hockey Team in the Olympic gold-medal match, I hit the elliptical for my long day. Logged 12.5 miles, and although the U.S. lost, it was a valiant game. Iced down and drank a protein drink.	12.5
Mon.	3/1/10	Easy day: 4 miles at 8:00 pace with Matt, then a couple of strides after the run. I registered to run the 800m at the University of Miami's Hurricane Invitational. It'll be my first 800m in more than 13 years. Despite that, I don't feel the same buildup over this race. I expect to run between 1:57 and 1:59, assuming I run well.	4.0
Tues.	3/2/10	Started the day tired and still sore from Sunday's elliptical. I lucked out because our interval workout was 8 x 200m with 200m rest. My natural speed handles the 200s with ease while my endurance makes a 200m rest nearly a full recovery. Bryan Sharkey and I targeted 31-32 sec for the first set because the workout demanded the last 4 reps be 3 sec faster than the first. In a stiff wind, we started with a 30, 31, 29, and 29 sec. The second set, with the wind at our backs, we did 27 and 27, then I opened up a 26.5 and 25.9 on the field (including Sharkey). We shared some track war stories over a 3.5-mile warm-down.	7.5
Weds.	3/3/10	Went for 4 easy miles in the morning with Matt. After, we did a few strides and 30 min of weights, stretching, drills, and the foam roller.	4.2
Total		Averaged 7:11 per mile for the week	**56.4**

---

59 Michael Strout is originally from Maine. He's 47 years old and I was shocked to hear he runs with very little consistency. I have a feeling he is dripping with natural talent and has no idea.

a fast time. On the home stretch, approaching the 800-meter mark, I got up on the leader's shoulder. The wind was blowing down the straightaway, but I had to make a move. I was hoping he'd respond, but he didn't. He left me with no choice, and I took the lead with just over 800 meters to go. Our half-mile split was 2:18.

I figured I was probably going to end up running something like 4:34… but I wasn't going to go down without a fight. The next 200-meter split was just under 34 seconds, giving me a 2:52 for 1,000 meters. I focused on staying relaxed. If I could pick it up just a little more and get to the 1,200-meter mark without feeling fatigued, I'd still have a shot at 4:30. I cranked out a 33-second segment into the headwind and crossed the 1,200-meter mark in 3:25.

With the wind at my back on the backstretch, I opened up the throttle and a solid lead on the pack. A few seconds later, Dave Afshartous fed me my final split: 3:57 flat. I had thrown in a sub-32-second 200-meter split, and now I had about 33 seconds to break 4:30. For the first time in the race, I liked my chances. I leaned forward and prepared for 32 seconds of pain.

I urged myself down the final straightaway. My prior surge and the headwind conspired to slow my pace. I could feel myself slowing ever so slightly. I could hear the crowd getting louder. Someone was making a run at me. I had 50 meters to go, and I had one last surge left in the tank. I used it and crossed the line victorious. My young nemesis crossed a second later.

I immediately dropped to all fours on the infield. I didn't hear my time so I turned to Miller in the stands and held two fingers up with a puzzled look on my face. He knew what I what was asking. He nodded his head in the affirmative. Then he flashed eight fingers… 4:28! It took an eight-second negative split (2:18 + 2:10), but I broke 4:30 in a one-miler more than a decade after running anything even close to that.

I pumped my fist and started to shuffle across the track, but my body rejected my command to move. It expressed its displeasure by feeding me a generous helping of pain. I dropped back to my knees and tried to ward away the agony, but at that moment my brain finished processing what had just transpired… I was crying like a baby.

I could understand if this were the Masters' Nationals, but this was a low-level meet against mostly high school kids. I guess I had underestimated how much effort and emotion I had put into getting to that point. Luckily, it was a hot day and the sweat pouring down my face disguised my embarrassing tears. Once the official results were posted, Miller, the Carberry's, and I headed back to South Beach for a victory lunch: burgers, sweet potato fries, and a chocolate shake. That was something to cry over.

2010 Hurricane Invitational: March 20th, 2010 was another big day for my Masters comeback: my first 800-meter race since 1996.

According to plan, I woke up after seven hours of sleep. I was a bit tired, but that's par for the course when I wake up on race days. What was worrisome was that I still felt some fatigue from the previous week of work. My confidence was a little low, but I talked myself into a more optimistic mood. I set a modest goal for myself – 2:00 – and felt I could pull that off regardless of residual fatigue.

When I got to the track, I discovered that the 800-meter run would be run in three heats. I was ranked eighth (last) in the second heat. I was okay with that. With the top guys running the first heat, there would be no temptation to go out too fast. The second heat would probably be fast enough for me, but not over my head. My concern was getting out at the right pace from Lane 8.

I went through my typical warm-up routine and listened to some Queensrÿche. After that it was show time. I tried to stay relaxed as I watched my competition. One taller white kid with a head full of dirty-blond dreadlocks looked intimidating. I stopped thinking about him and focused the job I had to do: Go out in 28-point for the first 200 meters, go through 400 meters in 58 seconds, then come back as hard as possible.

Training Log Week 57

Day	Date	Notes	Mileage
Thurs.	3/4/10	Still feeling Tuesday's 200s, but Bryan Huberty and I did stairs (6 x 16 floors) as usual: 62, 62, 60, 60, and 56 sec (6:00 total). Roughly same as last week, but I felt better today. 2-mile warm-up and 4-mile warm-down. I skipped the p.m. Nike run to watch the Heat/Lakers game and went out for 4.75 miles and 10 x 75m strides.	12.8
Fri.	3/5/10	Fridays are "off" days, but without an up-tempo Nike run last night, I felt good. Ran 7 miles with Bryan Huberty at noon (7:00 pace), then 4 miles with Matt at 8:00 pace and a few strides later in the afternoon.	11.0
Sat.	3/6/10	Led a morning drill workout; we moved up to 100m strides instead of 50m. It made a difference. Later Mike Dennehy and Robb Falaguerra asked me to teach them drills, so I did 6 more sets but with 50m strides. I then helped Matt through the second half of a 1-mile interval and then a full 1 mile after his rest (6:00 pace)	6.8
Sun.	3/7/10	Went for a 12-mile jog around Miami and South Beach. Matt came along for the first 8 miles (8:00 pace). He's getting more serious and wants to make the FIU cross country and track teams next year. I picked up the pace for the final 4 miles (sub-7-min pace).	12.0
Mon.	3/8/10	Bryan, Matt, and I went for a leisurely 5-mile jog. After yesterday, it took a couple miles to loosen up (even after 10 min stretching). By the end, I felt loose and rested.	5.0
Tues.	3/9/10	Intervals: Standard warm-up, then 6 x 400m with 100m rest. Given the short rest, I wasn't sure what pace to run. The first 400m was 68 sec. It felt easy, so I ran 66 sec for the next 2. At that point, the workout was half over and I knew what to expect, so I ended with 65, 64, and 63 secs.	6.8
Weds.	3/10/10	Easy day: Matt and I ran 4 miles (7:30 pace). After, we did a few strides and hit the gym for runners' curls and foam roller work. Generally speaking, I have a growing feeling that I'm not working hard enough, but as long as I keep improving and not getting hurt I'll take that as a good thing. I feel fast and healthy!	4.1
Total		Averaged 7:27 per mile for the week	**58.4**

Training Log Week 58

Day	Date	Notes	Mileage
Thurs.	3/11/10	Bryan, Michael, Matt and I started the day on the asphalt-paved Flamingo Track. We did different workouts, all involving 200m intervals. I tried to see how many times in a row I could run a 28-sec 200m in a 60-sec cycle. I completed 3 reps in 28, 27, and 27 sec. I rested for 90 sec, then ran three more in 28 sec. My next was 31 sec, so I shut the workout down. The idea was to run at faster than race pace, so race pace will feel more comfortable. That evening, still a little tired, I jogged to the Nike run. As usual, we started at 7-min pace and accelerated. I dropped the group at the 3-mile mark, running the final 3/4 mile alone. Finished with 22:05 (5:53 per mile).	10.0
Fri.	3/12/10	Easy day: 4.5 miles on the elliptical at 6:44 pace.	4.5
Sat.	3/13/10	Started the day at 7a and walked Matt through the process of preparing for and running a 5K race. After a warm-up, I played pacesetter. Matt ran a gutsy race into a headwind, and I'm sure he'll PR next time out. We warmed down then hit the track for a drill workout: 8 x 30-sec drills, with 100m strides then 15 pushups.	8.0
Sun.	3/14/10	Last "long" run (8 miles) before Saturday's 800m race. Matt and I ran up the Venetian Causeway and back over the McArthur Causeway. We coasted through it (7:40 pace) and Matt even tacked a little on at the end. For me, it was business as usual. The right knee got a little sore, but no big deal.	8.0
Mon.	3/15/10	Hit the gym to loosen up on the foam roller before the run. After that, I went for an easy 4-miler, but I struggled a bit. Toward the end, I figured out why. I was running 6:10 pace. My perception of "fast" is changing for the better. After the run, I did 4 short, quick strides, then had a recovery drink, and iced up.	4.2
Tues.	3/16/10	Sticking with a plan I culled from Sebastian Coe and Peter Snell, I prepared with my pre-race warm-up, then hit the track for 4-6 x 300m with plenty of rest (2 min). This was straight from Coe's '84 Olympic training log. He did his at race pace, so I targeted 44 sec for mine (1:57 pace). I was right on pace, finishing my reps in 44, 43, 43, and 44 sec, but after four reps I was beat. There are a few possible reasons: the 43s may have been a bit quick for me; the asphalt track is awful, and my "easy" Monday jog was more like a 4-mile tempo run. Excuses aside, I completed 4 strong reps, which was within the bounds of what I set out to do. The rest of the wk will be easy. My legs feel a little fatigued. They probably need to catch up on recovery.	4.0
Weds.	3/17/10	Bryan joined me for an easy 4-miler in 29:24 (7:21 pace) – much smarter than the 6:00 pace I ran two days ago – followed by some strides.	4.2
Total		Averaged 6:47 per mile for the week	**42.9**

Training Log Week 59			
Day	Date	Notes	Mileage
Thurs.	3/18/10	Last workout before Saturday's race. Sticking with the Coe/Snell plan, I did a typical pre-workout warm-up, followed by 6 x 150m at race pace with 2 min rest. I ran 21, 20, 22, 21, 21, and 22 sec, which equates to between 1:49 and 2:00 pace for 800m. Not easy, but not too hard either. My running form is different during faster reps than slower ones. During the faster reps, my head is down and my body leans further forward. I'll be sure to remember that Saturday. Did a light warm-down to end the day.	4.0
Fri.	3/19/10	*Very* easy day: slow 30-min elliptical and some stretching on the foam roller. My legs still feel tired from this week's work. I'm struggling to maintain my confidence. However, I know that the Alton track is slow, and I know I'll be well-rested for tomorrow.	4.0
Sat.	3/20/10	My first 800m race since 1996! Same pre-race routine as last month: an easy 400m, followed by a 400m, 600m, and 800m, all at 5:20 pace. Stretching between each interval to loosen up and catch my breath. 25 min before race time, I ran 4 short, quick strides. When the gun went off, things went almost perfectly. (See Race Report section.) I stayed in the pack until the second lap, then pulled away and ran fairly even splits to win in 1:57.5 – the fastest time for an American my age this year.	4.5
Sun.	3/21/10	More sore this morning than after last month's race. Must be the higher intensity of the 800m distance. Yesterday's race ended my "winter" season, so I took it easy today: 4 miles at 6:42 pace (most closer to 7:00 pace). My body deserves a few days of recovery!	4.0
Mon.	3/22/10	Still tired and sore. At 2p I visited Alex, who confirmed that I was a mess. Even had some fluid in my left calf. He worked on the trouble spots, and I felt a lot better afterward, but far from 100%. About 30 min later, I went for an easy 4-miler with Dennis Shine. Afterward I iced everything from the knee down.	4.5
Tues.	3/23/10	Slept late, hoping to induce a recovery. When I awoke, I still wasn't quite right. Intervals were out of the question. Recovery is Job 1. I failed in that regard. No post-race ice, no bananas, and lots of alcohol. *Dumb!* At least this was the end of a training cycle. I hit the gym for 4.5 miles on the elliptical. I felt better, so I did some core work and runners' curls then worked the foam roller from head to toe. Around 6:15p, I jogged to the Alton Street track and did a couple miles with Frank Green. I felt good, so I assisted the group by serving as a pacer. We did 3 x 1 mile with 400m rest. I paced Dan Krawiec, who ran 6:00, 5:35, and 5:50. That felt pretty good too, so I joined Matt for a 2-mile warm-down. A mile into it, I felt some pain in my calf, so I stopped. Home, I went through my complete recovery routine and the calf felt fine.	13.0
Weds.	3/24/10	After yesterday's mileage, today started rough. Matt and I jogged our normal 4-mile loop at a sluggish 8:15 pace. Afterward, he torched me in a couple of strides. Too risky to push it on an "off" day. Later, I hit the elliptical and felt much better: 4.25 miles in 26:00 (6:07 pace). After the elliptical, I did a bunch of dumbbell twists for my core, and a bunch of runners' curls. I hit the foam roller, iced, and called it a day.	8.3
Total		Averaged 6:50 per mile for the week	42.3

I noticed a fairly stiff wind cutting diagonally across the track. My Lane 8 assignment would limit the amount of wind I'd have to take in the first turn. It would also be directly at my back when the time came to cut into Lane 1. If I played my cards right, my competitors would take on most of the headwind until the home straightaway.

When the gun went off, things went according to plan. My pace felt right, and the headwind felt minimal. When the time came to cut to Lane 1, we had a tailwind. I settled into fourth place.

At the 200-meter mark I listened for a split time. I thought I heard "28." It felt like about 28: quick, but not *too* quick. I was very comfortable. As we hit the front straightaway, I started getting antsy. The pace was starting to feel a little slow, but we still had 500 meters to go. I didn't want to take the headwind if I could avoid it. I hung on the third-place runner's shoulder and stayed patient. It wasn't easy.

As we approached the 400-meter mark, I looked up at the clock that loomed above the track on the facility's scoreboard: 56… 57… 58. My second 200 meters was just under 30 seconds, getting me through the halfway point in just over 58 seconds. Perfect. I felt great. In fact, I thought I might come back faster than I went out.

Halfway around the turn, I stepped on the accelerator and made a bid for the lead. If anyone contested the move, I don't remember it. I stayed relaxed and maintained the faster pace. I hit 600 meters in 1:28 flat, so my third 200-meter split was just under 30 seconds. I picked it up a little bit more. I didn't feel anyone on my shoulder, but I

Training Log Week 60

Day	Date	Notes	Mileage
Thurs.	3/25/10	As I started a new training cycle, I wanted to increase my weight lifting and distance running. Started the day with easy/moderate weight work, followed by a fairly easy 30-min elliptical. Later I ran with the Nike group. It's almost exactly 1 mile to the meet-up and I got there effortlessly in 5:40. Must be almost recovered from last week's race. The actual run was a different story. It was hot and humid, and I was dying. I felt a side stitch early, but I got it under control. Everyone else was hurting too -- I was alone before the halfway point. I completed the 3.7-mile run in 21:25 (5:47 pace). No wonder it felt hard! I walked home with Jamie, who also came out to run. She had a rough time but finished the entire course. We both iced up, and I did some drills and called it a day.	9.0
Fri.	3/26/10	Scheduled easy day after yesterday's hard work: 4.3-mile elliptical (30:00; 7:04 pace).	4.3
Sat.	3/27/10	Well-rested, I hit the track for Saturday drills. Six others showed up. We did 8 sets of 30-sec drills with 100m strides and 15 pushups. One guy (Lee Cotton) beat me on the final 100m stride. It hurt my pride a little, but I was proud to see these workouts have helped him build his speed. Later, I did a moderate 5.3-mile elliptical.	8.3
Sun.	3/28/10	Ran 8 miles with Matt over the causeways. No sun, no traffic jam, and lots of wind. Not fun. I continued for another 4.3 miles, which was tough. Soaked in a cold Epson salt bath then iced. Not my idea of a great Sunday, but while I was running, the Masters were battling at the USATF Indoor Nationals. Hoping Chris Simpson tore it up in the 800m.	12.3
Mon.	3/29/10	Chris Simpson ran 1:58.2 to take the silver medal in the Masters 800m. A guy named Nick Berra won it all in 1:56.26 – 1.24 sec faster than my time last week. Getting the news about Berra fired me up. Instead of an easy Monday, I did a moderate 7-mile elliptical session. Afterward, I did some core work, weights, and foam roller.	7.0
Tues.	3/30/10	As is the norm on Tuesdays, I hit the track. I'm in base building mode now, but this was my last chance to see my Miami training mates before Jamie and I leave for our next big adventure. The workout was two "miracle miles" – jog the turns and run hard on the straightaways. Each straightaway is faster than the last until you complete 1 mile. Your time should be about 5K pace (pretty good considering you run the turns slowly). I ran 5:23 and 5:09, which was fairly easy. Afterward, I paced Karl Ross in a 400m in 63 sec. After saying good-byes to the crew, I did a 3.5-mile warm-down at sub-7:00 pace.	8.9
Weds.	3/31/10	Hit the elliptical for a low-impact 7.4 miles in 55 min (7:26 pace). In the evening, I did my newly-established routine of core, curls, lunges, squats, and foam rolling. The thought of Berra's 1:56 800m is still on my mind. How can I get stronger without risking injury? The new routine seems like a nice fit. Only the squats and lunges could cause injury – and even those are low-risk because I don't do them too hard.	8.7
Total		Averaged 6:57 per mile for the week	58.3

assumed they were there. Halfway through the turn, I thrust my shoulders forward, exaggerating my stride slightly. I was reaching for my last bit of anaerobic power, hoping it would whip me into the final straightaway with enough momentum to get home without rigging up.

It was a decent surge. I hit the straightaway and went into survival mode. I put my head down and leaned forward, conjuring gravity to push me toward my destination. I expected someone to challenge my lead. No one came. My race was against the clock. With about 20 meters still to run, I looked up.

1:55 – What a beautiful sight! A 1:58 or quicker was all but assured.

1:56 – Assured indeed. I lurched toward the line with all I had left. With a step to go, it was safe to take a final peek.

1:57 – The six turned to seven a split-second before my chest crossed the finish line. With nobody ahead or beside me, my arms launched skyward in exaltation… Then gravity took its pound of flesh. As is usually the case, my full effort left me completely taxed. I stumbled toward the fence at the edge of the track. During the next 10 or 15 minutes, I struggled to regain my composure with a modicum of success and grace.

A little awhile later, I got my official time: 1:57.5. This was the fastest time by an American my age or older since Jim Sorensen (former World Record holder) ran a 1:55.78 the previous June.

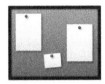 **Bulletin Board Material** – *While trolling around the Internet researching times and records, I found some more competition. The first adversary was a guy named Nick Berra. Berra is from Philadelphia and ran a 4:24.7 mile in January of 2010 to overtake my Boston friend, Chris Simpson, as American's number-one Master that year. He supposedly hadn't worn spikes in the 18 years before his Masters comeback. Just before New Years Eve, Berra and three other Americans joined forces and broke the Masters 4 x 800-meter relay world record.[60]*

That got me fired up, because I knew Chris Simpson and I could find two more good runners and crush that record. I was also fired up because Berra's 4:24 mile was better than my recent attempt. I would have to take things up a notch if I wanted to be the top American Master at the middle distances.

I also stumbled across results from the February 6th 2010 Reebok Indoor Challenge in Boston, which added more fuel to my fire. Chris Simpson ran the mile and was beaten by two familiar names from my college days: Chris Teague, a former standout at Providence College, and Ray Pugsley a former top guy at Dartmouth. Their Masters Mile results were as follows:

➢ *1. Chris Teague - HFC Striders 4:29.05*
➢ *2. Ray Pugsley - Potomic River Running 4:29.43*
➢ *3. Chris Simpson - Eliot Track Club 4:30.56*

Lastly, my research yielded one more important competitor. His name was Charlie Kern and he was not exactly new to the Masters racing scene. Kern was the American and World Masters 1,500-meter champion in 2009. He coached track near Chicago, and at one point he was an assistant coach under the legendary Joe Newton.[61]

Clearly there was no shortage of talent among the old guys; I had my work cut out for me.

Miscellaneous Research and Notes

Matt Kiss: On the last day of March, I got an excited text message from Matt saying that he had a tryout with the St. Thomas University cross country team. The tryout was a 12 x 300-meters workout. Matt told me that he lagged a few seconds behind the leaders during the first six reps... but after that, he "turned on the jets" and led each of the final reps by a few seconds.

At the end of the workout, the coaches and team got together and decided that they would offer him a spot on their squad. Not only that, but they also offered him a $15,000 scholarship! They were impressed with his ability, considering that he had only been training seriously for a few weeks. Between his work ethic, initial talent level, and grades, they felt he would make a great addition to the team.

I was greatly excited for him. A month prior, he was running three-to-four days per week, totaling 20-25 miles. I put him on a plan that involved training seven days per week (including one very easy day) and totaling 40 miles, including two or three workouts. After just a few weeks on that program, he was granted a big payday. It felt pretty good to have contributed to such a great accomplishment!

Training Cycles: Between hard workouts and races, putting yourself through two or three grueling days per week definitely takes a psychological toll. I found my threshold to be about two months. After researching this, I learned that most elite runners establish specific training cycles leading up to a key race or racing season – not unlike what Johnny Gray did with his base training cycle and speed cycle going into race season.

---

60 Race recap at: www.letsrun.com/2009/masters1231.php

61 Joe Newton won 26 Illinois state titles, four National Cross Country Coach of the Year awards, and was an assistant manager for the 1988 Olympic marathon team. He's also the subject of an acclaimed documentary, called *The Long Green Line*.

Based on a great deal of reading, I'd say there are actually four cycles:

➢ The base training cycle
➢ The interval training cycle
➢ The race-season cycle
➢ The post-season cycle (a.k.a. time off).

This made sense, physically and psychologically. Physically, a change in routines allows the runner to strengthen different aspects of his or her game while allowing taxed parts of the body to recover from the previous cycle. Psychologically, the benefits were clear to me. After two months on an interval routine, my mind started to go. On Mondays, I was dreading the Tuesday torture. On Tuesday, I was enduring the Tuesday torture. On Wednesday, I was recovering from Tuesday and already dreading the Thursday torture, etc.

Chapter 8
Check Yo Self (Before You Wreck Yo Self)

Weeks 61-71

At the one-year mark of my training, with the 2011 U.S.A. Track and Field Masters Championships still more than a year away, it seemed like a good time to reflect and reexamine my training philosophy. I probably learned more about training in that year than I learned in all my years of high school and collegiate running.

Older and on my own, I leaned heavily on outside counsel: my old coaches, ex-teammates, and other runners I befriended over the years. I conducted countless hours of research, with the corresponding experimentation on the track or in the gym, and discovered new techniques that accelerated my progress.

At the high level, my training philosophy boils down to three simple rules:

1.   Don't get hurt!
2.   Find ways to keep it fun.
3.   Train as hard as possible, without breaking rules #1 and #2.

Rule #1: Don't get hurt!

Disregard the obvious pain factor for a minute and consider the further downsides to injury: First, injuries keep you from training. Time away from training is time you're not applying toward your goal (and time your competitors may be applying toward theirs). Second, injuries can crush your motivation. Remember my story from Chapter 1 about my adventures with the steeplechase in college? Once I got hurt, I never regained the momentum I had from my early successes. My reaction reflected my immaturity. The remainder of my collegiate career was a waste.

My bid for a Masters championship was a shot at a small measure of redemption and some payback for the people I let down all those years ago. Because of this, I was maniacal about avoiding the straw that broke this camel's back in 1991. That is why "Don't get hurt!" is Rule #1.

So, what are the best ways to avoid injury? Here are some tips:

Stay loose. Before a run, I got loose through static stretching (e.g., toe touches) and dynamic stretching (e.g., walking; light jogging/bouncing around). Often I would take a hot shower before working out. Experts often debate which methods are best, or even effective. After a lot of research, I decided to hedge my bets and do a little bit of everything.

During a run, staying loose means keeping every inch of your body as relaxed as possible. If you pay extra attention during a run, you'll notice excessive tension in many parts of your body. Some people hold their arms too high and tight. Others tense their calves just prior to foot-strike. I happen to fall into the latter category, a habit which has surely contributed to the lower-leg ailments I dealt with through much of my early training. Running loose/relaxed requires good form, practice, and lots of mental concentration. Watch top marathoners, like Robert Cheruyiot to get the right idea. Taking a class in ChiRunning is another good idea.[62] I had a natural tendency to tense up when I ran.

---

62 You can gather general information about ChiRunning at www.chirunning.com. If you live in the Miami area, you can work with one of my training partners, Bryan Huberty, who is a certified ChiRunning instructor: www.runwithbryan.com.

Running tight increased my risk of injury *and* it hurt my times. I got a *lot* better at practicing good form and staying loose.

Even between runs, staying loose is important. Tense muscles injure more easily. During the day, if you focus on keeping your entire body as relaxed as possible, it will carry over into your running. Again, it requires a great deal of self-awareness and concentration. I spend most of my days typing on a computer and making high-pressure financial decisions. This type of work life is a perfect recipe for muscle tension. I often catch myself hunching over, furrowing my brow, and committing many other tell-tale signs of tension. The key is catching myself and quickly returning to a position of good posture and relaxation. Sitting correctly and taking a few deep breaths can go a long way. Standing up for an occasional stretch can also make a big difference when it's time to hit the track.

In addition to focusing on staying loose, massage makes a difference. Many top athletes get multiple massages per week – although for folks without access to collegiate or professional-level resources, that is probably not realistic. But if you can schedule massage once per week or once every couple of weeks, I'd recommend doing so. I'm also a big fan of finding a good physical therapist. My savior was Alex DaSilva in Miami. Alex virtually eliminated my calf and Achilles issues, and whenever issues arose, he quickly put them in check.

While staying loose and employing massage when I could may have been the biggest factors that kept me mostly injury free, I also paid heed to rotating my running shoes regularly, icing muscles and joints at the first sign of soreness, and wearing protective sleeves and braces on any trouble spots to alleviate pain and prevent any overcompensation in my stride.

Rule #2: Find ways to keep it fun.

Unless you *love* the physical sensation of running (or are clinically addicted to endorphins), training at an elite level will wear on your mind. Sunday runs seem to last forever. Track workouts are self-inflicted torture... literally. The same goes for Fartleks, tempo runs, stair workouts, repeat hills, drills, weight training, etc.

Because of this, it's important to find ways to package the same old routines in fun new wrappers. For me, keeping it fun was all about making the time pass quickly. On cross-training machines, I had an arsenal of pastimes: my laptop, cell phone, comic books, movies, televised sports, etc.

On the roads, most people like to have a variety of courses to run. I preferred to run the same *few* courses over and over. It made it easy to compare times and track my progress or detect trouble. Because of that, my iPod was critical. My library consists of 8,000 songs, and I seek out new music all the time. My running routes didn't vary much, but I never suffered from musical monotony.

I did a lot of visualization, a mental training technique used by most Olympic and professional athletes. Techniques vary from athlete to athlete, depending on the specific goal; I used visualization to inject positive thought into my training regimen. Virtually any positive or happy thoughts would do. My favorite was simulated winning. During runs (especially hard solitary runs), a decent chunk of my mileage would be spent pretending that I was in the middle of a race, always leading, always with a crowd involved, and I was always feeding off of that crowd's energy. I can't prove that it impacted my racing ability, but I'll say two things: My training runs passed by faster, and I seldom succumbed to the pressure of leading a race.

During interval workouts, fun was a lot more elusive. For me, training partners were an absolute must. Unless the workout consisted of short distances (like repeat 200 meters), I had a hard time getting the most out of a workout. I kept things fun in intervals by hooting and hollering to keep my adrenaline level high, similar to how a football team revs up before a game. Running is very primal, so primal behaviors made sense to me

Rule #3: Train as hard as possible, without breaking rules #1 and #2.

This is a more complex rule than it appears at face value. Training as hard as possible does *not* mean doing as many hard workouts as intensely as possible, just below the injury threshold. Rather, it means training hard enough that you're maximizing your workload but *also* maximizing your recovery. Recovery may be one of the biggest differences between collegiate training and Masters training, but most athletes of any age don't understand two key facts:

1. Working out *breaks you down.*
2. *Recovery* is what makes you stronger.

When you finish a tough workout, you are nowhere near your physical peak. In fact, you are in worse condition than when you started. You are broken down. As you recover, your body rebuilds itself stronger than before. (This is known as supercompensation.)[63] The goal of a hard workout is to trigger this rebuilding process. Thus, it stands to reason that the next hard workout shouldn't take place until your body has not only recovered, but is also stronger than it was before the previous workout.

It's not the hardest working athlete who improves the most – it's the one who supercompensates the best.

The trick is to optimally balance recovery with training (because too much time off is lost workout time). Your recovery days should include heavy doses of easy aerobic work. I do a lot *more* work on these days, but at a much lower intensity level. This allows my body to recover *while* increasing my aerobic base.

The optimal recovery time for supercompensation varies from person to person, and the average is unknown. For me, and I suspect for most Masters, 24 hours is simply not enough, but 72 hours might be more than enough – depending on the intensity of the previous hard workout.

The chart on the following page shows a rudimentary visual of how supercompensation takes place.

Rule #4: A bonus rule?

As I've said, there are only three rules… However, one additional rule I placed on myself was: Train *every* day.

Millions of people disagree with this rule – and for many reasons they may be right – but this is something that worked for *me*. By training every day, I built a streak. I took great pride in that. It represented overcoming many days of bad weather, illness, injury, and better things to do. Through it all, I knew that a day off would take the streak all the way back to zero. Long training streaks I achieved earlier in my career were always accompanied by great improvements and success on the track.

As a result, I defended my streak vigorously, and the bigger it got, the more I defended it… and the more I defended it, the smarter I trained. For example, I started training earlier in the day to avert unforeseen events. I did a better job preventing injuries (see Rule #1). I also eliminated any chance that I would take a day off out of sheer laziness.

In my opinion, there are only two arguments against training every day:

1. Everyone needs rest. I agree with this argument; however, I did this by taking easy days. My self-imposed measure of a "training day" was a minimum of four miles running or 30 minutes of some sort of cardio. At my level of fitness, if all I did was the minimum, it was basically equivalent to a day of rest. This was especially true if I did the four miles or 30 minutes at a very slow pace.

---

63 Source: [Google: wikipedia + supercompensation]

2. The psychological impact of a streak is detrimental. A runner can burn out mentally, or conversely, the streak can become more important than the desired result of the training (i.e., race performance), leading to poor training decisions. This is a valid argument and my main reason why "Train *every* day" is not one of the core rules. It's an approach that should be considered on a case-by-case basis. For me, it worked great. It kept me motivated and focused on living to run another day. I couldn't be happier with the results, but that doesn't mean that training every day is the right move for everyone.

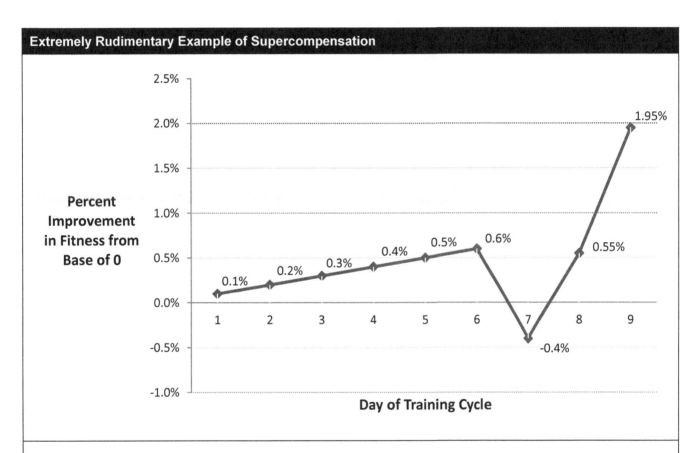

The above table shows the fitness level of "Average Joe" – a guy who has never run a step in his life and decides to embark on a workout program. His base fitness level is 0. He has done some reading, so he knows to start very slowly. His first six days he runs a couple of miles per day and runs well below his lactic threshold. He improves his fitness level by 0.1% each day.* On Day 7 he decides to try an interval workout. He runs all-out and breaks his body down to the point where his fitness level is actually below where he started. On Day 8 and Day 9, he rests – and as he does so his fitness level improves. Were he to try and run hard (or even moderately) on Day 8 or Day 9, not only would he struggle, he would actually be breaking his body down further and decreasing his fitness level.

* Note: These are *not* real percentages. We did not research the actual percentage improvement from day to day because it would be very hard to measure without a large-scale longitudinal study – and it would likely vary from person to person. Also, in the real world the percentage improvement is not linear. The fitter you become, the harder it is to achieve each additional percentage of improvement.

Training Log Week 61

Day	Date	Notes	Mileage
Thurs.	4/1/10	Easy 8 miles today; first 5 miles with Matt Kiss (7:21 pace) then picked it up for the last 3 miles. Total time was 55:10 (6:54 pace). I read an article on Nick Berra, the reigning U.S. and World Masters 800m champion. I learned he trains on a HydroWorx underwater treadmill, so he can work with extra resistance without added injury risk. I suspect that this gives him the leg strength needed for the 800m. I need to counter this tactic.	8.0
Fri.	4/2/10	Moderate 6 miles on the elliptical. Feeling fresh and recovering better.	6.0
Sat.	4/3/10	Final drill workout in Miami for the year. Lee Cotton beats me again on the final set, but he wasn't near me for most of the workout. Hard 100m runs!	9.3
Sun.	4/4/10	Final Sunday 12-miler with Matt and Michael. Matt went 9 miles; Michael and I continued on, but Michael's knee flared up at 10 miles, severely slowing our pace. I felt a lot better this wk and didn't take a cold Epson salt bath afterward (though I did my regular icing).	12.0
Mon.	4/5/10	8-mile elliptical on a machine at Disney World. 53 min (6:37 pace), 7 sec faster per mile than last Monday's elliptical. Still feeling fresher/recovering better. Did foam roller and dumbbell drills.	8.0
Tues.	4/6/10	Squeaked in the daily requirement with 5.25 miles at 11p in Lake City, FL	5.3
Weds.	4/7/10	8 miles at 7a on the elliptical at the Fairfield Inn in Lake City, FL	8.0
Total		Averaged 6:58 per mile for the week	**56.6**

Training Log Week 62

Day	Date	Notes	Mileage
Thurs.	4/8/10	45-min elliptical session in Chattanooga, TN. Spoke to Coach Dave on the phone for most of the run.	6.8
Fri.	4/9/10	*Not* a good day: Before leaving Chattanooga, I squeezed in 7 miles on the elliptical (47:15; 6:45 pace). Good thing I did. Jamie got word that her dad suffered a heart attack. I drove all day and night to try and reach Boston before Jack's surgery. I won't admit to breaking any laws, but we covered 1,300 miles in 17 hours. It wasn't enough, and we could only hope Jack made it through OK. I crashed at my cousins while Jamie went straight to the hospital.	7.0
Sat.	4/10/10	We were allowed to see Jack at the hospital. I can't say he looked good, which was no surprise. The doctor said the operation was successful but there were still some near-term risks. I did a 10-mile elliptical at my cousins' (7:00 pace). Tomorrow is usually long-run day, but it's unclear what will happen with Jack, so I wanted to get some extra mileage while I had the chance.	10.0
Sun.	4/11/10	Jack made it through the night, and his progress continued apace. He looked and sounded a lot better, and we learned he would be moved out of ICU. Running a strong pace over a good distance always feels good, but Jack's progress was the true definition of a *great* day. I did a 10-mile elliptical (7:00 pace) instead of going long because I did extra yesterday. I tried reading a comic book while on the elliptical, and the time flew. Some comic books are very well-written now. I'll try that again!	10.0
Mon.	4/12/10	Jack took another leap forward. His voice (and wit) is coming back. It's time to start planning his rehab and return to "normal" life. I planned to run with Rick Miller, who is in Boston for several months on business. However, Miller has been battling a foot injury, and when I got to his place, he just couldn't go. As if things weren't bad enough, my GPS battery went dead a few min into the run. Luckily, I had just checked my watch, so I used my iPod Nano to keep time and simply did a 25-min out-and-back near Miller's apartment in Newton. I knew I could check the distance later, using G-Maps Pedometer. The course was very hilly, which didn't help my knees any, but the cool dry air made for easy running. I later confirmed the distance was 8.1 miles. My time was 49:35 (6:07 pace). If correct, that beat my old 8-mile PR by 3 sec per mile.	8.1
Tues.	4/13/10	Sore from yesterday. Consecutive days on the elliptical followed by a hard tempo run will do that. Jamie and I visited Jack, and I'm officially astounded by modern medicine. Jack went from heart attack to triple bypass to walking around in 4 days. That beats any athletic achievement in my book. Later I visited my aunt and uncle. They live 5.25 miles from my cousin's house – a perfect distance for a run, a visit, and a run back. I got there in 36:15 (6:54 pace). After about 45 min, I headed back. I pushed the last mile, but still ran a little slower than the first run (36:37 - 6:58 pace). The run back was more uphill, giving me some solace. Of course, solace shouldn't be needed on a recovery day. When I got back, I worked with 8lb dumbbells and foam roller. I weighed in at 147lbs – 3lbs below my norm.	10.5
Weds.	4/14/10	Typical elliptical: 7 miles in 48:00 (6:51 pace). A comic book (*Preacher* by Garth Ennis) kept my mind busy.	7.0
Total		Averaged 6:47 per mile for the week	**59.4**

Injury Reports and Medical Findings

Joint and Tendon Health: By Week 64 of my training, it had been seven weeks since my quick 800-meter run at the Hurricane Invitational. Since that time, I adopted a training-cycle approach and went into base-building mode to get ready for the spring/summer season. I was averaging 58 miles per week and didn't get hurt. However, my right foot and knee became a minor annoyance. I suspected that the foot issue was an overuse injury, related to the elliptical machine. I adjusted my form a little to lessen the strain.

As for the knee, between pounding the asphalt track in Miami and pounding the pavement when I returned to Boston, I had been doing a lot of hard running on hard surfaces. I did some research to see if any foods or supplements might help with the recovery. By chance, I may have found the answer the book, *Eat Smart, Play Hard*, by *Runner's World* Nutrition Editor Liz Applegate:

> *Glucosamine is an amino acid sugar that acts as the structural component of tendons, ligaments, and cartilage. Chondroitin is a component of cartilage. According to the manufacturers' claims, when taken together, these two supplements protect joints and tendons and relieve osteoarthritis pain... According to several studies, about 1,500 milligrams each of supplemental glucosamine and chondroitin daily helps soothe pain, possibly by stimulating cartilage growth. Animal studies also suggest that supplemental glucosamine may speed the repair of injured joints.*

> *Glucosamine also helps produce substances in ligaments, tendons, and joint fluids called glycoproteins, so it may speed healing in those areas as well. Research has yet to test that theory, however.*

My personal experience with glucosamine was only moderately successful. I noticed some decrease in discomfort, but not enough to call it a Godsend. The panacea came after I began training with New Balance Boston. After several weeks under the tutelage of Coach Kevin Curtin, my condition actually worsened to the point where it was visible in my stride.

Coach Curtin took notice and asked me what was wrong. After explaining the situation, he asked how my glutes were. I found the question odd, but answered, "tight." He told me that tightness in one area of the body can impact areas that aren't even near the afflicted muscles. Sure enough, after three days of hot tubs and aggressive stretching, my knee pain miraculously disappeared!

My next workout was great and the knee problems never returned.

Dietary Research and Findings

More on pH, and Lactic Acid: Back in Chapter 5, I introduced the idea that manipulating your pH levels might produce a beneficial effect on race performance. In addition to my personal experiments, I had another willing guinea pig to test this theory. In his first year at college, Ryan O'Connell's times had been very inconsistent. He mentioned that he often felt strong through the first three-fourths of a race, only to "hit the wall" hard. I thought that might be indicative of acidosis.

He ran a leg on Springfield College's 4 x 800 relay team at the 2009 Division III New England Track & Field Championships at Tufts University. In an outing prior to this important race, he took Cal-Mag pills to raise his pre-race pH. It worked like a charm, yielding a PR in the 1,500 meters (4:05). O'Connell tried it again at Tufts and the result was another PR: 1:57 for his 800-meter leg. My race results and those posted by O'Connell – although anecdotal – implied that higher pH could lead to less lactic acid buildup. Given the potential of this finding, I wanted to learn more about blood pH and why it can give you an edge in race situations.

Day	Date	Notes	Mileage
Training Log Week 63			
Thurs.	4/15/10	Today Coyle & Cassidy High School (Coach Dave's team) raced Abington, which is coached by my high school teammate, Brian Lanner. Brian was a sub-50-sec 400m runner in high school, and I wanted to pick his brain. I needed more raw speed to improve my 800m time. The meet took place 4 miles from my cousin's house, so I packed a backpack with some gear and ran there. I reached Abington High School in 27:19 (6:50 pace). I watched a few events and helped out with a few others, then I changed back into my gear, strapped on the pack, and ran home. My pace was a little slower coming back (7:04).	8.2
Fri.	4/16/10	Gave my body a break from impact and hit the elliptical for 8 miles (54:00, 6:45 pace). It was a hard session, but not physically. Friends and family members had come to my cousin's for a get-together. Sometimes dedication means missing 1 hr of fun. Fortunately, when that hr is over, there is still much fun to be had. That is a metaphor for my Master's comeback in the context of life.	8.0
Sat.	4/17/10	Jack was moved to a rehab facility in Braintree, just 5 miles from my cousin's house. I killed two birds with one stone by running to the facility. I tacked on extra distance to reach 8 miles, which I completed in 52:36 (6:34 pace). Jack continues to recover at an astounding rate.	8.0
Sun.	4/18/10	Sunday is 'funday,' a.k.a. 12-mile-elliptical day. I brought a movie, a running magazine, a comic book, my iPod Nano, and my cell phone. At the end of 90 min, I felt great. Built my base and my injuries were non-existent. Keeping my mind occupied is half the battle on long days. Today, it was an easy one to win.	12.0
Mon.	4/19/10	Today was Patriots' Day, a.k.a. Marathon Day in the city of Boston. Rick Miller's temporary apartment is about 800m from the course, near Mile 18. Around 11:30a we headed out to catch some of the race and cheer on Bryan Huberty, who flew in from Miami to run. After a couple of high fives, Bryan continued on his way while Miller and I raced back to his place to watch the finish. Later, we ran 4 miles, which gave Miller and his bad foot about 6 miles for the day. I ran 3 more miles at a solid pace, giving me 9 miles total.	9.0
Tues.	4/20/10	I planned an elliptical session. However, a sunny, 60-degree day in Boston in April is too much to turn down. I put on my knee sleeves and hit the roads. I ran 5 miles to visit Jack and 5 miles back about 1 hr later. I took it easy on the way to the rehab center (6:53 pace) and pushed harder on the way back (6:31 pace). The total was 10.5 miles at 6:43 pace. Ample icing afterward!	10.5
Weds.	4/21/10	After a hard wk of work, I felt I had earned a rest. I only needed 4.2 miles to hit 60 for the week, so I hit the elliptical for 30 min. I was on track for my biggest month of mileage since last April. Of course, that preceded the calf injury that doomed me to months of elliptical work, so I needed to keep that in mind.	4.5
Total		Averaged 6:52 per mile for the week	**60.3**

For starters, the "p" stands for potential, and the "H" stands for Hydrogen. pH represents a substance's *potential* to attract Hydrogen ions by virtue of how many Hydrogen ions already exist in the substance. The fewer ions in the substance, the greater potential the substance has to attract more. The numbers that represent pH are on a logarithmic scale. This means that a substance with a pH of 7 has 10 times *fewer* Hydrogen ions as something with a pH of 6 – and therefore has 10 times the potential to attract Hydrogen ions. (That's a somewhat simplistic definition, but it's good enough for this discussion.)

Based on this, if your natural blood pH was one point higher than everyone else's, you could produce significantly more lactic acid before hitting "the wall." Imagine running at your best 300-meter pace for an entire mile! Under that scenario, an average college runner could break the world record by a comfortable margin.

The problem with the above example is not so much the accuracy as it is the feasibility. The average pH of human blood is between 7.35 and 7.45. Anything over 7.7 can kill you in a few hours. Anything over 8.0 can kill you almost immediately. So you can't break the mile world record by messing with your blood pH... Sorry if I got your hopes up. However, you don't need to raise your blood pH by a full point to knock a couple seconds from your 800-meter or mile time.

As noted in Chapter 5, you can optimize your blood pH with proper sodium bicarbonate loading before your race. Your body also produces sodium bicarbonate in your stomach as part of the digestive process. In fact, your body will produce extra sodium bicarbonate if you consume acidic substances.

Training Log Week 64

Day	Date	Notes	Mileage
Thurs.	4/22/10	55-min elliptical while finishing up the movie *A River Runs Through It*. It was a long, somewhat-boring movie, but it got me through a few elliptical sessions…	8.2
Fri.	4/23/10	I figured out how to affix my laptop to the elliptical machine – a game changer! 50 min passed like 15 min. I completed 7.3 miles (6:54 pace). Later, watching the NFL draft, I did drills with 8lbs dumbbells: runners' curls, upper-body twists, and lunges. I celebrated with Thai food and Bertucci's pizza.	7.3
Sat.	4/24/10	Very sore (but not hurt) from yesterday. Love it! The lunges should lead to increased leg strength, key to improving my sprinting ability. I'll definitely do that workout again. Started today with a 1-hr, 8.5-mile elliptical (7:04 pace). After, I did some light dumbbell drills and worked on the foam roller. Later, I was still sore, but felt strong, so I ran the 5 miles home from Jack's rehab center (32:28; 6:29 pace).	13.5
Sun.	4/25/10	Still tight and sore from Friday. I loosened up a little after stretching, but not totally. Yesterday's double-session went well, so I decided to do it again. I hit the elliptical for 61 min – easier than yesterday – completing 8.5 miles at 7:11 pace. A few hours later, I hit the road for 5.1 miles. I blasted through the last 3 miles at sub-6:00 pace (total = 31:38; 6:11 pace). After, I iced, stretched, and took a hot shower. Rather than gaining my usual 5lbs this weekend, I *lost* a pound – but it felt like a well-balanced weekend. The fewer road miles kept my aches and pains in check, but I did plenty of cardio.	13.6
Mon.	4/26/10	A much-needed rest day: 4.25 miles in 30:00 (7:04 pace)	4.3
Tues.	4/27/10	Long elliptical: 9 miles (65 min; 7:13 pace). I felt like I needed some time away from road pounding.	9.0
Weds.	4/28/10	64th consecutive wk without missing a day of training! This was my 6th biggest wk in terms of total training time – 6 hrs 24 min. The elliptical gets most of the credit, saving me the punishment of the roads.	9.0
Total		Averaged 6:55 per mile for the week	**64.8**

Taken a step further, eating a lot of fruits every day may train your body to become better at producing sodium bicarbonate. If so, that could come in handy on race day, when you're not likely to be eating an orange – but your body might be producing extra sodium bicarbonate simply because it's accustomed to doing so. I've not found any studies that confirm this theory specifically, but nutritionists maintain that eating certain fruits (specifically lemons, pears, and apples) does contribute to a higher blood pH, which is good for general health, as well as performance.[64] One more thing: Stress stimulates a biological reaction that lowers the pH of your blood. So, in addition to eating more fruit, you should do your best to control your stress levels. This is true on a daily basis, as well as on race day.

Lactic acid isn't the only substance that produces Hydrogen ions during strenuous exercise. Carbon dioxide (CO_2) is another. As you exercise, your lungs work harder, inhaling oxygen and exhaling CO_2. Of course, there comes a point where the lungs just can't breathe any harder. The body starts to produce lactic acid as an alternative means of fueling the engine. Lactic acid breaks down into two things. One is lactate, which is a fuel your body uses to continue performing at a high level. The other is Hydrogen. The takeaways are two-fold:

1. When racing or doing intervals, feeling a shortness of breath is very common. CO_2 builds up fast, and it doesn't take long before your lungs can't work fast enough or hard enough to keep up. This can be painful and mentally debilitating. However, you most likely are not in any medical danger. Lactate production increases to pick up the energy slack while heightened blood pH helps to keep you safe from the Hydrogen ion production. For the sake of performance, athletes train to ignore the discomfort.

2. Some clever thinkers may posit that hyperventilating before a race could clear out any lingering CO_2 in advance. However, I have seen no evidence this works. This might be due to the fact the CO_2 and H_2O combine in the body to form H_2CO_3, which then breaks down into HCO_3-, which is carbonic bicarbonate (a lactic acid buffer) and H+ (a Hydrogen ion). Therefore, expelling excess CO_2 from your system may also prevent the formation of the carbonic bicarbonate. So basically, you lose as much as you gain. In addition, decreased CO_2 can cause your blood vessels to constrict, which is the exact opposite of what you want before a race!

---

64 Source: [Google: prevention.com + "Kimberly Snyder" + alkaline foods]

Training Log Week 65

Day	Date	Notes	Mileage
Thurs.	4/29/10	In this base-building phase, I'm doing more of my cardio on the elliptical instead of roads. I got the idea from Nick Berra, who trains on an underwater treadmill. His treadmill is a *much* cooler machine than what I have, but a machine nonetheless. Nothing simulates running like running, but nothing injures like running, either.	8.6
Fri.	4/30/10	Back on the roads today. Wasn't long before I realized my new apartment is at one of the lowest points in Braintree! Every direction I ran was uphill. Reminded me of the cliché uphill-to-school-both-ways story. If you start and finish at the same point, every uphill gets a downhill, but I wasn't doing that. I was running to visit Jack. According to my GPS watch, I ran 8 miles in 54:45 (6:51 pace). Not bad for all uphill.	8.0
Sat.	5/1/10	I decided to have a rematch against yesterday's course. It was hotter out today, but I was mentally prepared for the uphill trek. I felt worse than yesterday, but I was running faster too. I shaved off the last half mile, finishing 7.5 miles in 49:36 (6:37 pace). I was exhausted and dehydrated after but felt good about the work.	7.5
Sun.	5/2/10	After two tough days in a row, I hit the elliptical for 90 min of Sunday fun. My laptop kept me distracted and entertained enough to help the time pass quickly.	12.5
Mon.	5/3/10	Today was Jack's birthday *and* his last day at the rehab clinic! Jamie and I spent the day getting him home and setting up his place. He's under strict order not to overexert himself, so every daily task needs to be optimized to take least amount of total effort. Put in 9 miles elliptical at 7:07 pace.	9.0
Tues.	5/4/10	Started with a jog around the apartment complex that Jamie and I have settled into for the summer and fall. A full loop was nearly a mile. After that, I headed to Pond Meadow Park, which has a number of wooded trails. Once I got into it, I got the feeling I'd be awhile before finding my way out. So much for keeping the distance short today! The GPS watch kept score: 7.2 miles in 48:32 (6:44 pace). I was tired and hungry afterward.	7.2
Weds.	5/5/10	Finally took it a little *easier* today. I headed back to the park to map out some distances for future runs. I started out at 7:00 pace and determined (via GPS watch) it's about 0.75 miles to the park. Once at the park, I picked up the pace. According to my watch, it was a 1.75-mile loop around. I did another loop and headed back, logging 5.1 miles at 6:29 pace. Easier than most days, but the last 4.1 miles was at 6:21 pace, so not exactly a day off.	5.1
Total		Averaged 6:55 per mile for the week	**57.9**

Training Log Week 66

Day	Date	Notes	Mileage
Thurs.	5/6/10	After a couple days on the roads, I gave my body a break by hitting the elliptical for 1 hr (8.5 miles; 7:04 pace).	8.5
Fri.	5/7/10	Started my transition away from base building. Ran a mostly uphill 3-mile warm-up to Braintree High School's track and added a few laps for an even 4 miles (26:20; 6:35 pace). Next, I loosened up and noticed that the football field's shaggy, soft bed of grass looked perfect for 100m strides, so I did 8 x 100m in 2:00. Not a bad way to reacclimatize myself to race pace. Next, I did 4 x 50m lunges and headed home in 20:25 (6:24 pace).	7.2
Sat.	5/8/10	Needed an easy day after yesterday's workout, and the weather was bad; perfect for 1 hr on the elliptical with my laptop and Pandora Internet radio. (8.5 miles in the books.)	8.5
Sun.	5/9/10	Sunday fun day: 90 min of cardio work. Session #1 took me back to Pond Meadow Park for 1 hr and a supposed 8.4 miles. I could have run the path that circumnavigates the pond, but the trails are more fun. I just bounce from trail to trail and let the miles rack up. The only problem is, I'm not sure my GPS watch is accurate there. At times, deep in the woods, the watch will report my pace is much too slow; at other points it says I'm running sub-5:00 pace. (I wish!) Back at my place, I logged 30 min on the elliptical. That added 4.1 miles of cardio, giving me 12.5 miles for the day.	12.5
Mon.	5/10/10	After a hard weekend of work, today was an off day: 5 miles on the elliptical (35:00; 7:00 pace). I also worked on the foam roller to get a core workout and to loosen up my muscles which are *still* sore from Friday.	5.0
Tues.	5/11/10	I planned on speed work in Boston with the Brandeis crew, but the team needs one more wk to rest, heal, and get mentally prepared. Interval/drill workouts start next wk. It may be for the best. I felt pain directly under the arch in both feet, which could be a strain of the plantar fascia. I will be *very* careful with this. When my calf hurt, I could still use the elliptical. This injury seems provoked *by* the elliptical (perhaps because I've been using a relatively high incline). My options will be limited if this turns into a full-fledged injury. Plantar fasciitis takes forever to heal. I hit a stationary bike for a low-impact 35-min spin (equivalent of 5 miles) to take it easy.	5.0
Weds.	5/12/10	Tried the elliptical but opted for mostly a bike session – a long bike session.	13.0
Total		Averaged 7:04 per mile for the week	**59.7**

Training Log Week 67			
Day	Date	Notes	Mileage
Thurs.	5/13/10	Feet still hurting; bike/elliptical combo.	13.0
Fri.	5/14/10	One foot feeling better, but can't risk anything. Bike/elliptical combo.	8.0
Sat.	5/15/10	Started the day with the foam roller and dumbbell drills. I delayed my workout until the afternoon for additional rest. The body's recuperative powers increase up to 50% between 24 and 36 hrs after a workout. So, by waiting until the afternoon, I gave myself 30 hrs of rest. The foot is *slowly* getting better, but still not 100%, so I hit the stationary bike again (1 hr; 8-mile equivalent).	8.0
Sun.	5/16/10	Hit the elliptical. The plan was to work as much as possible without inflaming my foot. I was ok for about 1 hr, then I decided that discretion was the better part of valor and called it a day at 9.4 miles (68:00; 7:14 pace). Later I did dumbbell drills, including deep lunges. The foot continues to get better. In other news, Ryan O'Connell notched his 4th straight PR, (4:03 for 1,500m).	9.4
Mon.	5/17/10	Morning stationary bike (35 min, 4.7-mile running equivalent). In the afternoon, I tested the foot with 3.7 miles on the roads. I started slow but couldn't resist dropping the hammer and finished in 22:52 (6:11 pace).	8.5
Tues.	5/18/10	Standard 35 min on the stationary bike in the morning. Standard 35 min on the elliptical in the afternoon. Total work: 9.9-mile equivalent at 7:04 pace. The foot is getting better but still hurts. May have to back off on the mileage if it doesn't get to 100% soon. It doesn't seem to react well to any kind of cardio work (roads, bike, elliptical, etc).	9.9
Weds.	5/19/10	Easy day. Standard 35 min on the stationary bike in the morning. That makes 8 wks of base-building. It's past time to build speed, but the foot may not be ready.	4.9
Total		Averaged 7:14 per mile for the week	**61.7**

L-Carnitine: I visited the local GNC to inquire about a supplement I researched called L-carnitine, which stimulates production of carnitine in the body. I had stumbled on a Web site that claimed that carnitine helps your body use fat as fuel, giving you a greater aerobic capacity. It also said that carnitine inhibits the production of lactic acid. That sounded like a great one-two punch. Unfortunately, my research uncovered a handful of studies in which carnitine was found to do very little or nothing at all. From what I gathered, your body almost certainly produces enough carnitine on its own. Therefore, supplementing your natural production is likely a waste of time and money.[65]

By chance, one of the workers at the GNC I visited was a student at Northeastern University. He had run track for BC High, one of the better high schools in Massachusetts, and took it upon himself to research and add some supplements to his training diet. We traded notes and both thought there was a very low probability that L-carnitine was of any value. He said that some old-school gym rats swear by it, but that most people he had spoken with reported no effect.

Food Tip: *What can a skinny middle distance runner learn from MMA behemoth Brock Lesnar (a UFC World Heavyweight Champion)?[66] Lesnar completely changed his diet after a run-in with a bacterial infection that ate a hole in his colon. He believes his old, beef-heavy, Midwestern diet may have contributed to his downfall. He said, "For years, I know I ate a whole cow in one year, easy."*

That's a lot of beef! The punch line to Lesnar's story – at least for me – was when he said, "But now I'm eating a lot of fish, a lot of chicken, some pork, and mixing in red meat here and there. And then on top of that, a lot of fruits, a lot of vegetables — just a well-balanced diet." He continued, "I got rid of pretty much all processed sugar. I'm eating just natural sugars from fruit and whatever… I cut out my dairy a little bit. I've really cleaned it up."

These are very similar to the changes I made to my diet, which helped me shed 40-something pounds and regain a facet of athletic prominence. Lesnar also spoke of another seldom-thought-of dietary strategy: grouping foods together to ease the digestive system's job and get the most nutrients out of each and every meal. I started doing a little of this, mostly in the morning, when I ate almost nothing but fruits, plus some whey protein powder.

---

65 Source: [Google: "Dr Bill" + Carnitine review]

66 Source: [Google: "brock lesnar" + diet + "muscle and body"]

Mark Gomes Supplementation Stack, Year One

By the end of one year of research and training, I felt my supplementation strategy was complete. I was taking the following supplements daily:

➢ Two GNC Mega Men Sport multi-vitamins (one morning; one evening)
➢ Two recovery drinks – Whey protein shake, with banana, strawberries, and blueberries, and/or one Endurox workout drink (for decreased muscular breakdown and increased protein synthesis)
➢ 3,000mg of HMB for better endurance, decreased protein breakdown and increased protein synthesis
➢ 3,200mg of Beta Alanine, plus a few ounces of beet juice, for vasodilation
➢ 2,550mg of L-Citrulline Malate for vasodilation and ammonia cleansing (decreases muscle fatigue)
➢ 1,500mg of Glucosamine and 1200mg of Chondroitin for stronger/healthier tendons, cartilages, and ligaments (these were unproven, but anecdotal testimonials appeared favorable.)
➢ Three cod liver oil pills for omega-3 fatty acids and vitamin D-3.
➢ 5,000mg of branched-chain amino acids (BCAAs) for decreased muscular breakdown and increased protein synthesis

The May 2010 issue of *Muscle & Body* magazine had an article about which supplements should and shouldn't be used together. Nothing in the article suggested I was taking any combination that is redundant, mutually neutralizing, or potentially dangerous.

Miscellaneous Research and Notes

Nixon Kiprotich: I stumbled upon 800-meter great Nixon Kiprotich's old workout regimen.[67] Kiprotich's 800-meter PR was 1:43.3, and in 1993 he was rated the top 800-meter runner in the world by *Track & Field News*. Interestingly, his training regimen was similar to Johnny Gray's (i.e., a *lot* of interval training).

Kiprotich started his training cycle by building a base for two months. On weekdays, he did nine miles in the morning and five miles in the evening, all around 6:25 pace. During this phase he took the weekends off, so his weekly total was 70 miles. Impressive for five days of work… especially for an 800-meter runner. He credited this phase of training with his ability to run great times at several meets in a single season.

Looking at his training pace, 6:25 pace must have felt pretty easy for someone of his caliber. If you add 10 percent to his 800-meter PR, the equivalent time is 1:53. So, all else being equal, if someone did everything exactly as he did, but 10 percent slower, that person should be able to run something close to 1:53. I incorporated that logic into some of my training – 10 percent slower than 6:25 pace is 7:00 pace.

After Kiprotich's base building phase was done, he would incorporate two hill workouts per week. One would replace his Monday distance training and one would replace his Saturday day off. The hills were generally 200 meters in length. He would do 20 hard sets in each workout. This routine would continue for two months. (Sounds like fun!) This would build his strength to power through 800 meters like a 400-meter runner.

After the hill-training phase, Kiprotich would cut way back on mileage and get interval happy for two months. His warm-up was similar to mine. It took 30 minutes and featured a mix of jogging and stretching. The big difference was that his warm-up included more 100-meter strides than mine. (I adjusted mine accordingly, especially on race days.) The table on page 112 shows what his workout schedule looked like during interval season. I've added the equivalent times for a runner training to run 1:53 in a separate column.

---

67 Source: [Google: kiprotich + pponline]

Training Log Week 68

Day	Date	Notes	Mileage
Thurs.	5/20/10	My cousin Danny is 35 and plays in a local baseball league. He bats well, but he thinks he needs more speed, so he joined me for a drill workout. My foot still bothers me, but I can't tell if it's hurt or just sore. Drills weren't the smartest litmus test, but I proceeded with caution. We did a standard drill workout: 8 x 30-sec sets with 50m sprints (no pushups). Danny handled 6 sets well. After a few tweaks to his form, he was running much faster. I jogged 3+ miles home, then hit the elliptical for 5 more miles. The foot didn't feel any worse than it previously did.	10.3
Fri.	5/21/10	Really sore after yesterday's drills. The foot was ok – not bad, but definitely not good. Time to take it easy for a few days… I did an easy 4.5 miles on the elliptical, taking extra care to step lightly on my bad wheel.	4.5
Sat.	5/22/10	Hit the roads/trails for 4 moderate miles. I realized later that my knee felt better than it has in months. Perhaps the glucosamine is kicking in? Most people I know that have taken glucosamine have had positive results after 3 wks. It's been about 1.5 wks for me. We'll see how I feel on my next run. My foot remains my gating factor. I'm in great shape and can't wait to do speed workouts, but I have to let the foot heal. Can't risk a full-blown case of Plantar Fasciitis.	4.0
Sun.	5/23/10	42 injury-friendly min on the stationary bike (5.6-mile equivalent).	5.6
Mon.	5/24/10	Started with 30 min on the stationary bike (4-mile equivalent), then my cousin asked me to take him through a drill workout. My Rule #1 is to stay healthy, but rules #2 & #3 (have fun & work hard) are hard to ignore sometimes. We hit the Braintree football field for 6 sets of drills (with pushups). After, I did 8 x 100m in 2:00. On the track this is easy, but on an overgrown football field it's a little tougher. I got my body going fast while minimizing risk on a soft surface.	5.6
Tues.	5/25/10	35 injury-friendly min on the stationary bike (4.8-mile equivalent). Foot feels ok considering yesterday's work. I'm icing and stretching it more. I am pent-up, but at least the rest of my body is getting a chance to heal. That's what I tell myself when I look at my training log and see that I'll end the wk with about 40 miles…	4.8
Weds.	5/26/10	34 min on the stationary bike (4.75-mile equivalent). I worked the foam roller, which I should probably do every day, but because I'm hurt I'm sort of taking a semi-vacation.	4.8
Total		Averaged 7:10 per mile for the week	**39.6**

Training Log Week 69

Day	Date	Notes	Mileage
Thurs.	5/27/10	Steering clear of the bad foot, I did 30 min on the stationary bike (4.2-mile equivalent). I also added some dumbbell drills. The foot is noticeably better. I want it back to 100%, because I never want to deal with this again! Some research showed I'm not the only one who has gotten hurt by overusing an elliptical machine.[68]	4.2
Fri.	5/28/10	32 min on the stationary bike (4.5-mile equivalent).	4.5
Sat.	5/29/10	30 min on the stationary bike (4.2-mile equivalent). This injury has sapped much of my enthusiasm. I know my attitude will turn around when the foot is 100%.	4.2
Sun.	5/30/10	30 min on the stationary bike (4.2-mile equivalent). I also did extensive dumbbell drills.	4.2
Mon.	5/31/10	30 min on the stationary bike (4.2-mile equivalent) plus extensive dumbbell drills. The pool in my complex opens this weekend, which may offer a reprieve from boring bike training.	4.2
Tues.	6/1/10	My condo complex started renting bicycles. I decided to see how the foot would respond to a real bike instead of stationary. I worked a hilly 10-mile loop, finishing in 34:23 (17.5 mph). The foot felt pretty good. My friend Dr. Jeff Baker, one of the nation's top sports podiatrists, believes I have a mild case of Plantar Fasciitis and recommended ice, stretching, and *no* flat shoes or bare feet. Walking barefooted feels good, but Plantar Fasciitis requires arch support, so I'll abide by the doctor's word.	5.2
Weds.	6/2/10	Hit the stationary in the morning for 30 min. In the evening, I felt the need to do real work, so I biked to the high school for a 6-set drill workout. The ride there was an uphill 5K, which I pushed pretty hard. At the track, I did some stretching and a couple of laps. Afterward, I biked back at a breakneck 20 mph to cap the workout – pretty fast considering I was riding a fat-wheeled mountain bike. I hit the gym for some dumbbell drills and foam roller work. The foot felt ok throughout. Strong day (8.3-mile equivalent).	8.3
Total		Averaged 7:01 per mile for the week	**34.6**

---

68 Source = [Google: peertrainer + numbness + balls of feet]

Kiprotich's two-month interval cycle would take him to the beginning of race season. During race season, he would ease back to two interval workouts per week. The first workout was typically 6 x 200 meters at 25-26 seconds. The second workout was usually 5 x 400 meters at 51-52 seconds or 5 x 600 meters at 78-80 seconds. On his off days, he would "jog for 30-40 minutes on a grassy surface" and run a few 300-meter repeats at race pace. After racing season, Kiprotich would take one or two months completely off... then start the whole thing over again.

Weight training was absent from Kiprotich's regimen. Kenyans believe that hill training is all the weight work they need... Hard to argue with a system that produces several of the world's the top 800-meter runners every year.

One thing to note if you're a younger runner: In a Peak Performance Online article, where Kiprotich provided much of this great info, he said the following:

The high school and college kids should be patient and wait for their time to come. If they try to train the way I do now, they will definitely get injured. When high school runners come to me and ask what to do, I tell them 'Just do two difficult workouts per week. Do not attempt to train hard every day...' Young 800-metre runners should avoid the temptation to try to progress too fast.

Nixon Kiprotich's Interval Workout Schedule (With Conversions for 1:53-Level 800-Meter Runners)

	Workout	Kiprotich	1:53 Runner	Notes
Monday	5 x 1,000m w/2 min rest (2 sets; 10 min btw sets)	2:45-2:55 per rep (66-70 sec per 400m)	3:00-3:15 per rep (72-77 sec per 400m)	Training to run fast when tired; the last 200m of each rep is at race pace
Tuesday	8 x 200m w/5-10 min rest	25-27 sec per rep	27.5-30 sec per rep	"Speed endurance" training
Wednesday	4 x 600m w/2 min rest; 5 x 300m w/2 min rest	83-86 sec per 600m; 40-41 sec per 300m	91-94 sec per 600m; 44-45 sec per 300m	Training for a finishing kick; the 300m should be run at increasing pace
Thursday	4 x 400m w/2 min rest	49-50 sec	54-55 sec	Pure speed
Friday	4 x 500m w/2 min rest	66-68 sec	73-75 sec	"Speed endurance" training
Saturday	Easy 40-min jog	40 min	40 min	Recovery
Sunday	Rest			Recovery

Training Log Week 70

Day	Date	Notes	Mileage
Thurs.	6/3/10	Back to my injury-friendly routine of 30-min on the stationary bike. Yawn.	4.2
Fri.	6/4/10	Spoke with Dr. Baker. He made it clear that I should not be doing *any* running for the next wk to let the foot heal... 30 min on the stationary bike.	4.2
Sat.	6/5/10	30 min on the stationary bike.	4.2
Sun.	6/6/10	As usual, 30 min on the stationary bike. Also did weight work (dumbbell drills, squats, lunges, leg extensions, bench press, pull downs, etc) and foam roller work.	4.2
Mon.	6/7/10	30 min on the stationary bike, then dumbbell drills, lunges and weight work (upper and lower body).	4.2
Tues.	6/8/10	32 min on the stationary bike. I was sore and slow from yesterday's weight workout, which makes me think I'm progressing despite my injury. My foot continues to improve. It's an odd injury. Two wks ago, I thought it was 90% normal. It has steadily improved since then, but still seems about 95%.	4.2
Weds.	6/9/10	32 min on the stationary bike. Afterward, I did my normal routine of dumbbell drills and foam roller work. I also did some lunges and core exercises.	4.2
Total		Averaged 7:11 per mile for the week	29.8

Training Log Week 71

Day	Date	Notes	Mileage
Thurs.	6/10/10	Tempo ride on the mountain bike. Before the ride, I taped up my bad foot. After prodding it with my thumbs, I pinpointed the problem area and the motion that causes pain. The tape-job was designed to minimize the straining motion. The ride was hilly and tough. I did 10 miles at 18.5 mph and was pretty winded afterward. It felt good to let loose. More importantly, the foot felt ok.	4.2
Fri.	6/11/10	Stationary bike (30 min). Afterward, I did dumbbell drills, lunges and weight work (upper and lower body). I taped the foot again, which seemed to help. It felt better than expected.	4.2
Sat.	6/12/10	30 min on the stationary bike. The foot felt a lot better, so hopefully this is the beginning of the end of this stationary bike nonsense.	4.2
Sun.	6/13/10	The foot felt great again, but just in case, I did 30 min on the stationary bike.	4.2
Mon.	6/14/10	30 min on the stationary bike. I also coached my cousin and girlfriend through a drill workout, during which I did foot-friendly exercises (stretching, pushups, dumbbell drills, and easy lunges). The foot is better than it was last wk but not as good as the past couple of days. I didn't tape it yesterday or today, so maybe that's the missing link. I'll get back to taping it tomorrow.	4.2
Tues.	6/15/10	A little sore from yesterday. That dull pain is my only solace these days. Despite my frustration, I still feel the biking, lifting, and drills will pay dividends when I get back to a normal training regimen. Today was recovery. I taped the foot and took the mountain bike out for a couple of easy rides: the first one was 30 min at 16.7 mph; the second was 5 miles at 17.8 mph. The foot acted up but is still improving.	6.6
Weds.	6/16/10	30 min on the stationary bike. Ready or not, I race tomorrow: the Bay State Games Trials. The steeplechase isn't hotly contested in the trials, so I may be able to coast. I can race hard if need be. The Bay State Games Finals may be my last steeplechase before the 2011 Nationals. My time will determine if I race it for a national title next year.	4.2
Total		Averaged 7:12 per mile for the week	**31.8**

Chapter 9
Once You Step in the Arena

Weeks 72-80

One key factor that separates the elite runner from the hobbyist is a laser-like focus – especially during a workout. In a workout, the elite runner is monitoring myriad data presented by his body in absolute real time and making immediate decisions based on this data. Success or failure and terrible pain versus slightly less terrible pain are determinant on his decisions. But the body's clues can be subtle, and the data can change based on the slightest adjustments to pace, form, terrain, and other factors. Consequently, this ability to focus – often called "the zone" – day in and day out, is often the differentiator between good runners and great runners.

Because the elite runner doesn't just practice his sport, he lives it (sacrificing all manner of creature comforts and societal pleasantries during the course of normal life), the workout rises in importance to a level that's nearly spiritual. The track is his temple, his Mecca, his sanctuary. And because the elite runner is more often than not a physical badass who is usually ill-tempered due to the aforementioned sacrifices, woe be the person or thing that disrupts the sanctity of the workout.

At Northeastern University, an institution located almost solely in an urban area, day-to-day workouts took place on the busy Boston streets, and more often than not a seven-mile recovery day would turn into a tempo run when a member of the pack was aggrieved by an errant motorist, pedestrian, homeless person, or any number of other quasi-innocent types of bystanders sharing the streets and sidewalks.

(I recall one such recovery day where a few of my mates and I were chased the wrong way down a one-way street by a black Mercedes that had nearly hit us when it failed to stop for a stop sign. The fact that two of us stepped on the hood and trunk while one guy pulled off the hood ornament as we jumped over or slid past the vehicle surely played a role in the ensuing chase.)

One of Coach Lech's most challenging jobs was finding places and means to conduct our hard workouts where the typical city distractions did not exist. One such place was Larz Anderson Park in nearby Brookline. Larz Anderson had a perfect grassy loop for cross country-style interval workouts. The park was serene, somewhat secluded, and offered little likelihood of interference. It was a gem Lech hoped to utilize many times, and he probably invested a noteworthy amount of time scouting it and measuring the loop for accuracy.

One afternoon he presented us with the directions to get to Larz and sent us out. It was during Northeastern's fall break, and the crew was small – maybe five guys or so. We jogged the four miles to the park, where Lech was waiting in the parking lot next to the school van.

"Eight times the loop, with a jogging rest," he said, tapping on his ever-present clipboard. "Let's get started."

He explained the landmarks and distances of the loop in most basic detail, making sure we understood, then away we went. About three-fourths the way into the first rep – maybe 600 meters or so – a small mop-haired dog decided to join us for the ride, yipping and nipping at my teammate Matt's heels as we ran. Matt did his best to keep his focus while shooing the dog away as gently as he could with his fast-moving feet. We reached the top of the hill on the far side of the loop, turned for home, and spied the dog's owners: a middle-aged couple – a diminutive woman and a very large man.

"Keep tabs on your dog before I punt it," Matt growled at them as we cruised along the perimeter of the park.

In reply, the large man bellowed, "Hey, you touch my f-ing dog, I'll wring your f-ing neck!"

Back by the parking lot, we shuffled through our rest period and started into the next rep. Halfway through the loop, the dog was back and made a beeline for Matt's ankles. This time he kicked it away with more force – not enough to hurt the dog but enough to show it he meant business. The dog yelped and recoiled.

We reached the top of the hill on the far side of the loop and started home again. Sprinting across the grass toward us was the man, arms out-stretched and aimed straight at Matt as he approached. We stopped in our tracks, and in less than a second it was over. Matt hit him square in the face with three quick jabs and down he went – and off *we* went, straight across the center of Larz Anderson Park at full clip.

"You all are gonna burn in hell!" the man's wife screamed at us as her husband rolled around on the ground.

We headed straight for the parking lot and the Northeastern University van.

"Hey!" Lech demanded, knuckles whitening around the edges of his clipboard. "What the hell do you think you're doing?"

"Coach, we gotta go," someone urged.

Lech glared at us for a second.

"Coach, Matt just knocked a guy out," someone else offered.

This was something Lech didn't have to contemplate for more than a second. He knew what he was dealing with. All at once, he shook his head in resignation, muttered something incomprehensible about a good location wasted, looked as his clipboard and its incomplete workout notes, and grabbed the van keys from his pocket.

The sanctity of the workout was broken. Day over. Lech never brought us back to Larz Anderson for the remainder of my collegiate career – which meant more trips to Summit Hill (a steeper, nastier fate, from a pure workout perspective).

Training Log Week 72

Day	Date	Notes	Mileage
Thurs.	6/17/10	The Bay State Games Trials were held today. The 5,000m doubled as the steeplechase qualifier and was pretty predictable. Nobody gave it much effort, except for Ryan O'Connell who treated it like a workout. He ran about 16:30 and lapped everyone in the field except for me. I treated the race like a brisk jog, clocking 18:30 (6:00 per mile).	4.0
Fri.	6/18/10	Ran some laps in the swimming pool, then did 35 min on the stationary bike; added miscellaneous weights (legs and lats). Foot felt better than usual.	4.9
Sat.	6/19/10	This was Training Day #500. It should have been a celebrated milestone, but it's hard to be fired up about doing 30 min on the stationary bike again. At least, the foot felt good.	4.2
Sun.	6/20/10	The weather and Father's Day conspired to keep me off the roads. We visited Jamie's dad, who looked great, then hit my uncle's for his traditional Father's Day Lobster-Fest: The picnic table buckled under the nachos, pizza, yogurt-covered pretzels, beer, wine, cake… and of course, lobsters. After this feast, I'd be lucky to stand, much less run. When we got home, I hopped on the scale to survey the damage: 160lbs. I hadn't been 160lbs in well over a year. Shamed, I shuffled to the gym for 30 min on the stationary bike. Later I did some light weight work. Will need to work to make 150lbs by Friday.	4.2
Mon.	6/21/10	Received my pair of Recovery Socks. (See Injury Reports section.) I expected to flash back to the 1986 Celtics, but they looked pretty good, all things considered. After 60 min I felt a slight tingle in my feet, like a thin layer of menthol had been applied. Can't say for sure if the socks worked, but they didn't hurt. I made my return to the roads (85 degrees and humid). I ran to the track (where I joined Jamie and Julie in drills) then continued 10 min more to make an even 30:00. Weighed in at 150lbs, all water weight loss.	5.0
Tues.	6/22/10	Nice and sore after yesterday's return to action. A little pain in the foot, but not bad. Regardless, I took it easy: stationary bike for 30 min.	4.2
Weds.	6/23/10	Foot felt ok, so I tried another drill workout. Everything was identical to Monday's workout.	5.0
Total		Averaged 6:48 per mile for the week	31.5

Training Log Week 73

Day	Date	Notes	Mileage
Thurs.	6/24/10	Wearing my Recovery Socks close to 24 hrs per day. Take them off to work out and shower. The foot feels very good, so I assume the socks are legit. Today was a recovery day, so I was back on the stationary bike for a 30 min.	4.2
Fri.	6/25/10	Jamie, Julie, and I planned a noontime drill workout. I got sidetracked by work and had to drive to the track. I cranked out a sub-6:00 mile to warm up and got into the drills. Julie has been developing shin splints, so we focused on lower-impact drills. This didn't make them any easier because I made each set encompass a full trip up and down the football field. Later, I hopped on the stationary bike for 30 min.	6.0
Sat.	6/26/10	30 min on the stationary bike.	4.2
Sun.	6/27/10	Approximately 4-mile run (6:30 pace).	4.2
Mon.	6/28/10	Did 30 min on the stationary bike and a ton of upper- and lower-body weight work. Also I paid a visit to a podiatrist. (See Injury Reports section.)	4.2
Tues.	6/29/10	Started easing back into things with 4 miles (7:00 pace), then I did a very easy barefoot mile around the football field, followed by 5 barefoot 50m strides. After, I stretched for 10 min, laced up the shoes, and did 2 miles closer to 6:00 pace. (A cheap path to 7 miles, but a step in the right direction.)	7.2
Weds.	6/30/10	Recovery day. My hamstrings were sore from yesterday's return to full training. The foot felt fine though. I ran 4 miles in 26:23 (6:36 pace), followed by 6 sets of light drills/stride. Afterward I iced myself up and down.	4.3
Total		Averaged 6:53 per mile for the week	34.2

Injury Reports and Medical Findings

Foot Structure: At the 2010 Bay State Games Trials (see Race Results section), the trainer[69] checked out my foot and identified it as non-acute plantar fasciitis. She proffered that the condition was probably spurred by my right Achilles being out of alignment, caused by the presence of scar tissue where the top of my foot meets my ankle. The scar tissue – built up over many years of ankle turns from my high school and college days – is on the right side, which forces my ankle to the left, thus accentuating my pronated gait. As a result, certain areas of my lower leg undergo more stress than the rest -- most notably, the upper right side of my calf and my plantar fascia.

The trainer gave me the name of a local podiatrist and recommended that I purchase a Recovery Sock from recoverysock.com. The Recovery Sock is a compression sock designed to increase blood flow to the area, which aids in healing. It's also designed to help keep one's foot well-aligned. It appears that I'm destined to look like Chris Solinsky[70] on the track from here on out.

I sought the counsel of a podiatrist in Boston, named Dr. Dan Riley – a great guy who understands running. He was a 4:40 miler in high school, and I could tell that he still took fitness at least somewhat seriously because his physique and face belied his 60 years of age. I could also tell he knew his stuff. He x-rayed my lame hoof before inspecting both feet, up and down. Afterward, he talked me through every nuance and oddity he found. He explained how each facet played a part in injury. A lot of the terminology went over my head, but I understood enough. Based on what I experienced in training, I could tell that he was spot on.

Dr. Riley believed that my issue was a strain – not a big deal. Because of this, he gave me the green light to get back to a full training regimen. However, he said that I needed special shoe inserts from a running store... and possibly orthotics if I wanted something custom tailored for my feet.

He pulled out his prescription pad and jotted down two things in capital letters: GENU VARUM and FOREFOOT VARUS HYPERPRONATOR.

Genu varum simply means "bow-legged." Varus is the "condition in which the metatarsals have an inversion misalignment; the first two metatarsals are in a more dorsiflexed position than the third to fifth metatarsals. Needless to say, that did little to enlighten me... Eventually, I figured out the layman's translation is: "Your foot is twisted in an abnormal alignment... You need orthotics."

The term hyperpronator rang a bell. When I had my gait analysis done in Florida, the video showed that with each stride, my leg collapsed inward – violently. Hyperpronation is usually caused by a congenital defect. In my case, it was more pronounced in my right (injured) foot, likely because of the scar tissue on the top, right side.

Shoe inserts helped to correct the condition by raising my arch. Stuck between one barrier (the scar tissue) and another (my raised arch), my foot had little choose but to move forward, instead of collapsing to either side.

Dr. Riley's diagnosis and recommendations gave me a renewed excitement. The foot had been a hindrance for two months.

---

69 The race trainer was Debby White-Lyons, one of the trainers for Northeastern University's track team when I ran there. She has many, many years of experience with top-class runners.

70 Chris Solinsky became the first American to break 27:00 for 10,000 meters and did so wearing compression socks – spurring an immediate interest in the product. [Google: Solinsky + socks + photo]

Training Log Week 74

Day	Date	Notes	Mileage
Thurs.	7/1/10	Ryan O'Connell and John Mantia came to train for the day. We did a 4-mile warm-up and 6 x 100m drills in the morning, followed by weights and the foam roller closer to noon. That evening we did a 3-mile warm-up and steeple drills at MIT. Stopped at Marathon Sports to buy new trainers and insoles for my feet. Tried to stress to the young guys (especially Mantia) to "just do what Coach tells you." He responds like I would at his age.	8.8
Fri.	7/2/10	Set out for a super slow 5-miler. It started out that way (8:00 pace), but it felt different – comfortable; not cumbersome. I kept going all the way to my aunt and grandmother's house, an undulating 5 miles, at 7:30 pace. No one was home, so I trekked back in the same manner: an 8:00 first mile and 7:29 total pace. Afterward, the scale displayed an integer below 150. The weekend is mine... I'll watch Joey Chestnut provide a demo in consumption at Nathan's 4th of July Hot Dog Eating Contest.	10.0
Sat.	7/3/10	After yesterday, it was time for some rest. I hit Pond Meadow Park for a hot 4-miler at just under 7:00 pace.	4.0
Sun.	7/4/10	Happy Independence Day! Jamie and I headed to my Uncle Louie's beach house on Cape Cod. Between the sun tanning and the BBQ, I snuck out for 7 miles at 6:50 pace.	7.0
Mon.	7/5/10	Leveraging the injury-prevention benefits of cross-training, I took the mountain bike out for 8.9 miles at a pedestrian 15 mph. Total time was 35:45, which I logged as the equivalent of running 4.5 miles at 7:57 pace.	4.5
Tues.	7/6/10	Went to check out the New Balance Boston Running Club and meet coach Kevin Curtin. Most NBB runners take much of the summer off, which is problematic for my goal to peaking in late July next year. I had hoped to do a track workout, but due to my schedule, I had to settle for 30 min on the elliptical.	10.0
Weds.	7/7/10	Drove into Boston for a lunch run with Terry. We ran 35 min, and I added another 10 min alone. Later, I did 10 min of drills (high knees, butt-kicks, etc) in the swimming pool.	8.8
Total		Averaged 7:13 per mile for the week	**45.7**

Training Log Week 75

Day	Date	Notes	Mileage
Thurs.	7/8/10	1.5-mile warm-up. Drills (6 x 100m). 2.1-mile warm-down.	4.3
Fri.	7/9/10	Tomorrow is the steeplechase at the Bay State Games Finals. For pre-race day, I did the bare minimum: 30 min or 4 miles, whichever came first. Surprisingly the 4 miles came first, albeit by a mere 6 sec. It appears 7:30 pace is the slowest I can comfortably run.	4.0
Sat.	7/10/10	Ran the steeplechase at the Bay State Games Finals (race report below) The weather was awful, and I finished second to Ryan O'Connell by 1 sec (10:35 to 10:34). I ran 1 sec faster last year, but no one ran fast all day.	4.8
Sun.	7/10/10	Woke up sore from the race but felt good overall. I ran to Braintree High, with Jamie following on a bike. Did some light stair work, then we had to scramble. Jeff Baker came to town for the 311 concert, and halfway home from the track, he picked up Jamie while I rode the bike back. To make it interesting, I rode the bike all-out, barely beating them home. (I blocked the one-lane road to our complex, but a win's a win!)	5.1
Mon.	7/12/10	Hit the gym at 2p for some light lifting (mostly legs, with some upper-body). At 5:30, I ran 4 miles to Weymouth High for drills. I accelerated each mile, clocking 7:45, 7:25, 6:40, and 6:13. Still, I felt flat, which is how I've felt since resuming training after the foot injury. I did the drills at moderate intensity because the New Balance workout is tomorrow.	4.8
Tues.	7/13/10	Had my first track workout with New Balance Boston. Only two guys showed (Jeff Caronand Stephen Stewart[71]), but with the caliber of talent on this team, that's all it takes. The warm-up was 3.5 miles with stretching; the workout was 8 x 800m in 2:26 with 1 min rest (with the option to bail at 600m). I made 4 reps laboring a little bit. The pace was fine, but 1 min rest was not enough. I crashed on the 5th rep, struggling through 400m in 84 sec. I jumped back in for the 6th rep and completed 600m then did the same for the 7th rep. I could not run the 8th. We warmed down for 3 miles and thankfully it rained to alleviate the heat.	10.4
Weds.	7/14/10	Sore and tired. Strained something between my right ankle and calf. Perhaps wearing spikes yesterday wasn't the best idea. I'll be fine, but it slowed me down today. Yesterday's workout was the alarm bell I needed to get back into training mode. In the evening, I plodded through a 6-mile recovery run (46:00). My body needs to be reacclimatized to the rigors of hardcore training.	6.0
Total		Averaged 6:59 per mile for the week	**39.3**

---

71 Jeff Caron, University of Maine '06, trained under coach Mark Lech (formerly head coach at Northeastern University). His PRs range from 3:54 in the 1,500m to 30:39 for 10K, cross country. Stephen Stewart was an 800-meter specialist at Amherst College.

Dietary Research and Findings

Creatine: Creatine is a well-publicized supplement that I researched multiple times, and like caffeine, I found contradictory findings. Initially, I decided against incorporating it into my supplement stack. Creatine's reported side effects include water retention, weight gain, muscle tears, and similar injuries. Additionally, there was no clear-cut consensus on how much to take and at what times in relation to my workouts.

Another determinant against creatine came from a friend from my high school days, Karim-Ben Saunders[72] Saunders was a standout sprinter from Cambridge, Mass., who went to be an All-American at Auburn University. He recommended against Creatine, citing many of the side effects I listed above. He also theorized the change in body mass would likely alter my running form (which I had worked diligently to optimize). Instead of Creatine, Saunders suggested building speed and power via better plyometric and weight-training. He also recommended whey protein *with* glutamine to assist with recovery.

In Hindsight – *Nine months after my talk with Saunders, I experimented with creatine anyway. After more research I learned two things: creatine is a key contributor to ATP reproduction, and it acts as a lactic acid buffer… two benefits in one supplement. After trying it for a few weeks, I concluded it was one of the most important supplements in my stack! At first, I gained weight (mostly water retention – I increased my daily water intake to about 1.5 gallons on creatine, per instruction), but after a few weeks I returned to normal. Also I later learned Kre-Alkalyn, a specific type of creatine, supposedly results in very little weight gain and thus may be a better option for runners.*

Training Log Week 76

Day	Date	Notes	Mileage
Thurs.	7/15/10	Still sore from the workout with New Balance Boston. Julie and Jamie hit the track, so I biked out to meet them. I kept a moderate pace but focused on loosening up my lower right leg. I joined Jamie for the last 2.7 miles of her first-ever 3-mile run, then biked home, a 6.7 mile training equivalent. Later, I hit the roads for 6 miles – same course as yesterday -- still slow but 2:00 quicker. My leg is sore but not apparently injured.	12.7
Fri.	7/16/10	I biked to Weymouth High to coach Julie and Jamie through drills, but I didn't participate. Between sets I stretched and did pushups. After, I biked home. Total ride was 8 miles in 28:17 (17 mph). Later, I jogged to Cousin Christina's house: 4.8 miles uphill, hot and humid (34:42; 7:11 pace) – still not great, but considering the conditions and leg, it's progress. I capped the session by working on my lung capacity.	8.8
Sat.	7/17/10	After two days of doubles, it was time for a break. I slept in, then hit the pool for some resistance drills. At 7p I ran 4 miles at moderate effort (27:25; 6:51 pace), the fastest I've gone since the New Balance workout.	4.0
Sun.	7/18/10	Drove to Weymouth High School and ran 3.1 miles with Jamie, her longest run to date. She fought through the last mile and was proud of her accomplishment. (I was too.) She even had the strength to do some strides after! After the strides, she took the car and I completed a 4-mile jog home (7:00 pace).	7.2
Mon.	7/19/10	In the afternoon, Jamie went to visit her dad. She called 1 hr later, very upset. I hoped Jack was ok. As it turned out, *Jamie* had checked herself into the ER. She was feeling dizzy and out of sorts, possibly from her run yesterday. I wasn't about to let her drive home, so I biked to Norwood Hospital, 17.7 miles with a wrong turn. (Definitely the furthest I've ridden on a bike!) When I got there, Jamie was a little out of it, but ok.	8.8
Tues.	7/20/10	A bad day at work, plus some miscommunication with the New Balance team. Web site said to meet in Coolidge Corner, but if you know Boston, that's a vague instruction. I knew the workout was repeat Heartbreak Hill, so I went there instead, alone. Luckily, as I finished my warm-up, a few obvious runner-types appeared. Coach Curtain assigned us 8-12 x 60 sec on the Hill, with active rest. I hung at the back of the group, moving up during the final 2 reps. I did a 2-mile warm-down, partly with the group, which was headed back to Cleveland Circle. (That's right, Cleveland Circle, not Coolidge Corner!)	7.2
Weds.	7/21/10	After a night and day of icing, stretching, foam rolling, and "Recovery Socking" – and proper nutrition – the calf felt a lot better than after last week's hard workout. In the late afternoon, I drove to Braintree High School to jog around the fields and pond. The calf didn't feel great, but it was much better than I expected. I ran 5.4 miles at 7:36 pace.	5.4
Total		Averaged 7:32 per mile for the week	54.1

---

72 Karim-Ben Saunders' Auburn University 4 x 400-meter relay teams earned numerous podium finishes at the NCAA indoor and outdoor championships. His PRs include a 10.2 100 meters, 20.5 200 meters, and 45.1 400 meters (relay split).

Race Reports, Records, and Results

2010 Bay State Games Trials: The Bay State Games Trials are held in four different regions across Massachusetts to determine who will race at the Bay State Games Finals later in the summer. The top four finishers in each event were invited to the finals at the University of Lowell.

As an experiment, I decided to go into the June 19th race completely aloof and completely mentally unprepared. I anticipated little competition, so it seemed like a good time to study how attitude affects race performance. It also allowed me to take it easy on my injured foot.

While registering, I spied Ryan O'Connell and some of his old teammates from Coyle & Cassidy High School. Ryan planned on running the 5,000 meters. O'Connell and I would race in the same heat, because at the Bay State Games Trials the 5,000 meters doubles as the qualifying event for the Finals' 3,000-meter steeplechase.

(They do this because many facilities in Massachusetts aren't equipped with steeples and a water pit. Why they don't use the 3000-meter run as the qualifier for the 3,000-meter steeplechase is beyond me...)

As I suspected, there was little competition for the steeplechase. In fact, there was none! There were five other entrants in the 5,000-meters, so all but one of them were assured to advance to the finals. If that wasn't enough, O'Connell decided to declare himself a steeplechaser at the last minute – so everyone was sure to qualify and no one needed to race hard. All we had to do was finish and not be disqualified.

Only O'Connell gave any effort, treating the race like a solid workout. He ran somewhere around 16:30 and lapped everyone in the field, except me. Between my bum foot and not having run on roads in more than three weeks, I treated the race like a brisk jog, clocking just under 6:00 per mile.

As for my experiment with my pre-race attitude, I think it definitely impacted how I performed. Without focus, intensity, and competitive spirit, my body didn't feel the same as it did during most races. I don't know if it was a lack of adrenaline, but it was noticeable. The intensity was even a step down from the sensation I'd get from doing the same distance and time during a well-prepped training run. The experiment was unscientific, but I am convinced that being focused and serious is a no small advantage when getting ready to race.

2010 Bay State Games Finals: I ran the steeplechase at the Bay State Games Finals on July 10th. The weather was *awful*. Coach Dave, Ryan O'Connell, my mom, and I drove to UMass Lowell together. The second we got to the track, the skies opened up. O'Connell and I spent most of that time under the bleachers, trying to stay dry and trying to loosen up in the confined space. When the rain passed, we had only 25 minutes to prepare. We were able to do a couple laps and a few strides before being called to the line. Adding to the adversity, the steeplechase water pit was as full as it could be from the rain. The temperature was hot and ridiculously humid.

O'Connell led for most of the race. By the final lap, he had a 30-meter lead. Strategically, it was in my best interests to let him have it and try to sneak by him in the final 200 meters. He had better endurance than me, but I had better steeple form, especially over the water pit. I almost pulled it off... I cleared the entire pit on the last lap (seven for seven on the day). That alone cut his 30-meter lead in half. I caught him as we hit the final barrier. My form was weak and cost me some, but I don't think it mattered. He kicked and beat me by over a second (which is a lot, considering we were neck and neck with 50 meters to go).

Despite the exciting finish, our times both *sucked*: 10:34 and 10:35. In fact, I ran a second slower than last year. I could only take solace in the fact that there wasn't a good time all day. The mile was won in a pedestrian 4:35 and the 800-meters was won in an equally bad 2:05. The weather was just too much for anyone to overcome.

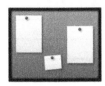

Bulletin Board Material – *In USATF Masters action, Ivan Ivanov literally ran away with the 2010 national steeplechase title. His 9:32.1 clocking was over a minute faster than the next competitor and a minute faster than my performance at the Bay State Games Finals. Nick Berra took nationals gold in the 800 meters again (1:56.1). His time beat my Hurricane Invitational performance (1:57.5) by a decent margin, from a half-miler's perspective. Then he went on to win the 1,500 meters (4:04.3) the following day. No matter which event I focused on, there was no shortage of talent standing between me and a Masters gold medal.*

Two additional names made their way onto my watch list: Blair DeSio, 39 years old like I was, won the 800 meters for his age group (1:59.4), and Jaime Heilpern finished second to Berra in the 40-year-old category with a 1:58.6.

Training Log Week 77

Day	Date	Notes	Mileage
Thurs.	7/22/10	Calf was still sore, but it's recovering a lot faster than last week. Ice and the Recovery Sock is likely doing the trick. I hopped on a mountain bike and cruised around town. I had some steam to blow off due to a bad day at work, so I went for over 40 min (17 mph).	6.1
Fri.	7/23/10	It was rainy, and I was busy with the stock market. By the time I finished, there wasn't much time left to work out, so I ran my Grove Street 4-mile loop. Mile 1 was 7:05 (uphill). Mile 2 was around 6:55 and the final 2 miles were 6:30 each. Total was 27:21 (6:41 pace) – 10 sec per mile faster than I ran 6 days ago. I'm starting to get my conditioning back. In other news, the 2010 USA Masters Outdoor Nationals got underway in Sacramento, CA.	4.1
Sat.	7/24/10	I rolled out of bed and ran a hard 4 miles (25:34; 6:23 pace). It was notably faster than yesterday and felt like it. I ran early because we were hosting our annual Polo Tailgate Party. (See Aug 11 2009 for details.) As is tradition, I wore my cow outfit for the kids and made my traditional lap around the polo grounds. I've become something of a mascot for the event! The field is about 800m around and the horses keep a brisk pace. After running around all day, that final lap can be tough. Thankfully, it felt a lot easier this year!	5.0
Sun.	7/25/10	Jamie, her brother, and I headed to Jack's place for lunch. He's finally to the point where he can take care of himself, and he asked that we bring his car back – a big step! I put a bike in the trunk of my car to ride home. The ride went as expected. I knew how to navigate the hilly roads through Stoughton, Canton, and Randolph, eventually popping out at the "Five Corners" in Braintree. From there, it was only 3 miles home, almost all downhill. I finished with 22.8 miles in 1:16:29 (17.9 mph). I logged it as 10.7 running miles. (instead of 50% of the biking distance) because I noticed that the last 15 min of a 75-min ride is a lot easier than the last 15 min of a 75-min run. I calculated that 10.7 miles would translate into 7:09 per mile. That felt about right.	10.7
Mon.	7/26/10	Limited to a brisk run on the same 4-mile course I did Saturday. I ran with less effort but still completed the run 10 sec faster than Saturday, possibly because I wore flats or because I was on the bike yesterday.	4.0
Tues.	7/27/10	Workout day with the New Balance crew. No drama and I had little trouble finding them in Cleveland Circle this time. We did a 20-min warm-up and some strides around the Cleveland Circle reservoir. The workout was two sets of 3-min/2-min/1-min with half rest. Between sets, we got 5 min rest. It was a tough workout, but I breezed through it. The calf was 100% for the workout and 2-mile warm-down.	8.5
Weds.	7/28/10	Easy bike "recovery ride" to Weymouth High. I met Jamie and helped her through drills. I did pushups instead of drills; however, I ran the 70yd strides with her. Julie showed up with a fractured foot and wanted to do a core workout, so we did 15 min of core exercises. It was tough. I hadn't done a core workout in a long time. After, I biked home and had my normal protein drink and lunch (chicken, rice, and an apple and a banana); all while icing my legs. In the evening, I went for an easy 4-miler, but I got antsy and started pushing the pace. The day turned into an example of how you can turn an "off" day into an "on" day. This is how I get hurt.	8.3
Total		Averaged 6:54 per mile for the week	**46.7**

Training Log Week 78			
<u>Day</u>	<u>Date</u>	<u>Notes</u>	<u>Mileage</u>
Thurs.	7/29/10	Slowed it way down today, but did a high volume of work (especially from a time standpoint) on soft trails.	9.8
Fri.	7/30/10	Did 8 x 100m almost all out; total time: 1:51.5. May 7th, I did a similar workout and ran 2:00. My warm-up and warm-down was a 4-mile bike ride to and from Weymouth High.	5.0
Sat.	7/31/10	Trip to Mohegan Sun casino with the Cambridge Boys. We started the trip walking 9 holes of golf. Afterward, I went out for a "recovery" run. It's hard to recover in that area of Connecticut though. Everything's a steep hill. Did 4.1 miles in 29:00 (6:59 pace). It was an effort, but I didn't mind getting the hill work in.	4.1
Sun.	8/1/10	After 23 years knowing Jamalh Prince, we went on our first run together. He weighs 180lbs now, but you wouldn't know it. He's getting in shape and handled the hills well. Still, we took the hills slow to go easy on our knees. Totaled 6.5 miles just under 8:00 pace.	6.4
Mon.	8/2/10	Easy day. Jamie and I headed to Weymouth High. She did drills. I did pushups (120 total) but joined her for the 70m strides (5 total). After, I did an 8-mile mountain bike ride at an easy pace.	4.8
Tues.	8/3/10	New Balance workout day. I was still sore from Friday's 8 x 100m workout, but not too bad. We hit Heartbreak Hill again for 8 x 1 min. Totaled 6.6 miles for the day. My knees were sore on the warm-down, so I'll do a lot of icing and hit the bike tomorrow.	6.6
Weds.	8/4/10	Recovery day included drills in the pool and an 8-mile bike ride.	4.9
Total		Averaged 7:30 per mile for the week	41.6

Miscellaneous Research and Notes

<u>Lung Capacity:</u> I added lung capacity work to some of my regular training sessions. For this, I did five sets of holding my breath and sitting at the bottom of a swimming pool for as long as possible. (Note: There are *obvious* inherent dangers to doing this, so do <u>not</u> try this alone and let people know exactly what you're doing and how to look for signs of trouble!)

This exercise was designed to acclimatize my lung sacs to hold air longer, thus stretching them out. I found a few great articles on the subject, including a Viewzone.com article[73] with quotes from the great Brazilian middle distance coach Luiz De Oliveira.

> *World-renown Brazilian track coach Luiz De Oliveira has trained champion runners like Mary Decker Slaney and Olympic gold and silver medalist, Joaquim Cruz. De Oliveira claims his breath-holding drill allows middle and long distance runners to improve their endurance by adapting to increased levels of lactic acid. "I have a breath-holding drill that I use once a week," says De Oliveira. "I try to drive the lactic acid up quicker than it would in a regular race. That way, my runners get used to it. What I have them do is take a running start, then inhale and hold their breath when they hit the starting line, then they run for 25 meters. They work on technique while holding their breath. When they reach the finish line, they exhale and breathe normally."*

> *De Oliveira then has them jog back and do the same drill for 30 meters, then 35 - all the way to 90 meters. "Everybody's capable of holding their breath for a very long time. But you've got to do three of these sets. By the final set, you're going to become very, very tired. It's hard to hold your breath at that point. But if you use my drill, you will see results."*

Some additional Web articles provided more information about lung capacity, so I incorporated these exercises into my routine on an occasional basis.[74]

---

73 Source: [Google: viewzone + breathing + luiz]

74 Sources: [Google: wikihow + increase + lung + capacity; Google: ehow + increase + lung + capacity + running]

Training Log Week 79			
Day	Date	Notes	Mileage
Thurs.	8/5/10	18-month anniversary of my training streak. To "celebrate" I joined Ryan O'Connell at the Blue Hills. The workout was 4 reps up a very steep 3/4-mile hill, and I was in over my head! Ryan's in for a great year. I hung with him for the first 4 min of the first rep then fell back. I actually had to stop before reaching the top. Ryan got there between 6:30 and 7:00. For the final 3 reps, my goal was to hang with Ryan as long as possible, which was about 3:00 each time. After letting him go on the final set, I did three hard 30-sec reps just to feel a little better about myself. I biked the 10 miles home. Unfortunately I was surprised to discover Google Maps guided me right over the Blue Hills. Needless to say it was a tough ride. At home I iced for about an hr.	9.1
Fri.	8/6/10	Jamie and I visited our friends, the Chesky's, in Haverhill, MA. We golfed 9 holes. After, I ran 4 miles in the Chesky's backyard. The circumference of the field behind their house measures close to 3/4-mile. The run brought me back to high school — the last time I won a cross country race. The memories made me run faster with each lap, starting at 7:00 pace and finishing at 6:00 pace. I completed 4.1 miles in 26:35 (6:31 pace), iced, and enjoyed a Friday-night Chesky BBQ, featuring steak and boar (which Vito killed on a hunting trip).	4.1
Sat.	8/7/10	With a long run looming tomorrow, I did 8 miles on the mountain bike. Considering my effort level felt normal, the faster time was encouraging (28:42; 16.7 mph).	4.0
Sun.	8/8/10	Was hoping for 10 miles, but it wasn't meant to be. I felt sluggish in the morning and when I finally hit the roads, I felt the same. I decided not to fight it – just run to get the mileage in. Aerobically, I felt fine, but my knees starting hurting. At 50 min I decided to pack it in. I jogged home, completing 7.8 miles in 63:00 (about 8:00 pace). Tough day.	7.8
Mon.	8/9/10	Sluggish again. I needed a nap in the afternoon. At 6:30p, I went for a 4-mile jog on the trails. My knees felt better, possibly from shortening my stride and striking closer to my mid-foot. Halfway through I was able to pick it up, but only closed with a 6:59 mile. Totaled 4 miles (30:17; 7:34 pace). Another disappointing day. I plan to cut back my anaerobic work a bit. Lydiard said too much anaerobic work can retard development. He claims only 4-5 wks are needed to develop optimal anaerobic capacity.	4.0
Tues.	8/10/10	Somewhat back on track for New Balance day: a repeat of the reservoir workout from 2 wks ago (2 sets of 3 min/2 min/1 min, with half rest). Everyone ran well, making me look less impressive; however, my workout improved from last time. I averaged 6:39 pace for over 7 miles; 2 wks ago, I ran 7:05 for 8.5 miles. I may be snapping out of my recent funk. Also, my knees didn't flare up until the warm-down.	7.0
Weds.	8/11/10	Flew to Illinois to visit Jamie's family. It was blistering hot at midday, and by 9p the heat index was still 95 degrees. My college rival Mike Atwood[75] posted on Facebook that he ran 9 miles in 62 min. That brought out the competitor in me, but by 4 miles I knew it wasn't going to happen. The heat was still too much, so I headed home: 58:30 for 8 miles. Given the conditions and yesterday's workout, I was satisfied just to finish.	8.0
Total		Averaged 7:22 per mile for the week	**44.0**

Heat Training: Heart rate training improves the cardiovascular system by pushing one's heart rate to a target level for a period of time (regardless of running pace). During a late-summer visit to Jamie's family in southern Illinois, I found myself running in 90-degree heat for most of trip. My heart rate and breathing were accelerated for most of the runs, despite that I was running shorter distances. I wondered if the hot, humid weather had a heart rate effect. A quote from an article by Mark Higginbotham on the Web site howtobefit.com seemed to confirm my suspicions:[76]

> *"The two best training environments in which to maximize aerobic fitness are training at high altitudes or working out in the heat and humidity."*

If this logic is true, high heat and humidity can enable a runner to build a strong cardiovascular base with fewer miles of pounding on the body. All things being equal, heat and humidity will create a faster heart rate at a slower pace. Additional sources suggested adding 30 seconds per mile for every five-degree temperature increase above 60 degrees. The sources also advised making adjustments for humidity.

Initially I thought 30 seconds slower per mile was too drastic a compensation, but when I checked my log it held up. Considering the difference in heat index in southern Illinois versus in Boston, I was running about 30 seconds slower per mile for each five-degree increase.

---

75 Mike Atwood ran track and cross country for Boston College. As a freshman, he qualified for the U.S. National Junior Championships by running 8:28 for 3,000 meters, and he went on to run PRs of 14:47 for 5,000 meters and 24:50 for 5 miles.

76 Source: [Google: howtobefit.com + "running in heat"]

This realization prompted me to buy a heart-rate monitor and train at a target heart rate – not at a target pace. My heart rate fluctuates at different temperatures, altitudes, and humidity levels, but for base training it is the heart rate zone that matters most to me.

The Web site Run The Planet posted several articles on heat training, as it pertains to marathoning and long, slow distance running.[77]

Double Sessions: My young Miami protégé, Matt Kiss, sent a *Runner's World* article about running twice a day, written by Ed Eyestone.[78] Eyestone was a 10-time NCAA All-American and two-time Olympian when I was in high school and college, so I read it with rapt attention. A key quote:

> *I definitely felt the advantages of running twice a day. My morning run was easy enough that I wasn't exhausted in the afternoon. But I wasn't fresh either, so it got me used to training through fatigue. I always rehydrated, rested, and refueled before the afternoon run, so I had a much better chance of hitting a quality pace than if I'd tried to grind out those same miles on the end of one long run.*

Because of my work schedule, travel schedule, and occasionally the elements (like on really hot days), I would employ double sessions, so Eyestone's positive opinion of them made me feel good about my work.

Some training schedules we researched (including Lydiard) felt there was greater benefit to conducting all training during one elongated session, but my experience was different. If I adhered to the hard-day/easy-day principle, I was fine. I felt like I experienced an additional benefit: a very easy morning workout seemed to circulate nourishing blood to the muscles, enabling a stronger afternoon workout. The fatigue Eyestone cites above is the tradeoff. However, if my morning workout was moderate and performed on a machine to save wear and tear, my body experienced accelerated recovery with very little fatigue.

Food Tip: *I looked into ginseng as an additional supplement to add to my arsenal. Ginseng is claimed to increase energy levels, relieve stress, enhance athletic performance, enhance immune system function, control blood sugar, improve mental function, and promote general well-being. That's a lot of benefit from one supplement. However, when I researched it further, I found ginseng is a difficult supplement to use accurately.* The American Journal of Clinical Nutrition *published a study that took 25 commercial ginseng supplements and compared the actual content of the supplements to what was labeled. The amount of active ingredient significantly varied from the label – as much as 15-36 fold.*[79] *Energy drinks like Red Bull list ginseng as an ingredient, but do not provide the quantity.*

While many studies tout ginseng's benefits, a number rebutted the positive findings – and part of the problem may be the difficulty in finding standardized measures of the supplement. Accurate measures aside, I found variations in the recommended daily dose for ginseng. Some studies indicated performance enhancement with 200 milligrams per day; other studies provided 8-15 times that much to the subjects. Ultimately I opted against using it; however, there seem to be very few reported downsides to ginseng. You could probably experiment on your own safely.

77 Sources: [Google: runtheplanet + marathon + tempextreme; Google: runtheplanet + safety + heat]

78 Source: [Google: "twice a day" + "ed eyestone"]

79 Source: Beginner Triathlete [Google: ginseng + performance + beginner triathlete]

Training Log Week 80

Day	Date	Notes	Mileage
Thurs.	8/12/10	Started with a short midday run around a golf course and park. Running fast isn't an option in this heat, so I found grass to give my knees a break. I was breathing heavy but settled in after 800m – but after 1.5 miles, the heat got the best of me. I totaled 2.5 miles in 19:23 (7:45 pace). That's some killer heat! About 45 min before sunset, I laced 'em up again. I felt a lot better than earlier, but this was a fleeting sensation. I found myself walking soon after 2 miles. I resumed running but had to stop a few more times. I kept my heart rate above 120 bpm, but each time I had to stop it took longer for my heart rate to come back to 120. I completed 6.5 miles of running in 49:58 (7:41 pace), not including my time walking.	9.0
Fri.	8/13/10	Surprisingly sore today. I had to wonder if this is a side effect of heat and humidity. I decided a recovery day was in order: 4 miles in 29:11 (7:18 pace) – faster than yesterday. because of the shorter distance and the fact that a rain storm cooled me down.	4.0
Sat.	8/14/10	Ran 8 miles very slow, mostly on grass: 63+ min. After, I immediately hopped in a cold shower, iced my knees, had a protein bar and milk, and took in as much fluid as my stomach could hold. It took 1 hr to recover.	8.0
Sun.	8/15/10	Cooler temps: "only" 84 degrees. I could feel the difference. I stayed on grass as much as possible (90% of the run). I went out cautiously then loosened up finished 8 miles comfortably in 58:25 (7:18 pace).	8.0
Mon.	8/16/10	Weather and workout a repeat of yesterday, with a moderately faster time and easier effort level: 8 miles in 57:16 (7:09 pace). I recovered with a cold shower, ice, and elevated legs (to aid with venous pooling).[80]	8.0
Tues.	8/17/10	A cooler and faster day (heat index ~ 80 degrees). Ran 8 miles in 56:11 (7:01 pace). I didn't want to overdo it just to get under 56 min; however, my last mile was the quickest (6:41).	8.0
Weds.	8/18/10	About 10-degrees warmer, but I had planned to take it easy anyway… I went out in 8:30 then settled into 7:30 pace until 6 miles. I ran Mile 7 in 7:10 and closed in 6:27 to finish in 59:37 (7:27 pace). No cross training this week. I definitely feel tired, but I think running on grass made a difference. My injuries remained completely under control and I worked a number of supporting muscles on the soft, bumpier terrain.	8.0
Total		Averaged 7:25 per mile for the week	**53.0**

Training Log Week 81

Day	Date	Notes	Mileage
Thurs.	8/19/10	Travel day. We hung out at Jeff Baker's place in Chicago until it was time to leave for the airport. I hit the jogging path along Lake Michigan for 6 miles (43:25; 7:14 pace).	6.0
Fri.	8/20/10	After wks of training cautiously – often in hot/humid conditions – I received another affirmation for the "Train Smart" philosophy. On a 70-degree night (with a slight breeze), I cranked out 7 miles in 45:27 (6:30 pace). It was almost effortless; totally in control.	7.0
Sat.	8/21/10	Took it easy: 8 miles on grass in 56 min (7:01 pace). After a 7:25 first mile, most of the run was 7:10 pace. The last two miles were quicker, especially the last one, when I closed in 6:09. My knees were a little sore, no doubt from yesterday. My right foot still hurts, but nothing worrisome. It's exactly as the podiatrist said it would be on June 28.	8.0
Sun.	8/22/10	Another easy 8 miler. Braintree doesn't have much grass, so I hit the roads. I was careful to tread softly for the sake of my knees. Everything went well (57:09; 7:03 pace).	8.1
Mon.	8/23/10	Rainy evening. I didn't feel like running and neither did my knees. I suspect they were barking because of the weather. I begrudgingly jogged 7 miles, but took my time about it (52:50; 7:33 pace). I should be rested for tomorrow's New Balance workout.	7.0
Tues.	8/24/10	Rainy day at the BC reservoir. We did a 15-min warm-up and warm-down; workout was a 5K tempo run, followed by 8 x 30 sec. I did the 5K in 16:58. By the halfway point, it was hard staying in contact with the younger distance runners. I wanted to stop, but held on for the final 1.5 miles. I felt good on the 30-sec repeats. Health-wise I feel good. My knees still ache, but Kevin Curtin thinks I could have tight IT bands or glutes. That makes sense and serves as a big relief. Tight muscles are easier to deal with than bad knees.	8.4
Weds.	8/25/10	I was sore from yesterday's workout and thought I'd be running slowly. It started out that way (7:32 first mile). After that, I picked up the pace and felt fine doing so. My last 3 miles were in 18:41, giving me a total of 7 miles in 46:41 (6:38 pace).	7.0
Total		Averaged 6:56 per mile for the week	**51.5**

80 Venous pooling is the normal tendency for blood to remain in the lower extremities due to gravity. A leg drain is a pose in which you lie on the floor with your legs vertical for three to four minutes (usually supported by a wall or other object). This drains the blood from your legs so fresh, clean blood is pumped back into them when you stand.

Chapter 10
Jenny, Jenny, Who Can I Turn To?

Weeks 82-91

Following the 2010 Bay State Games Finals, and my subsequent decision to re-focus on the 800-meter event, I went into aerobic limbo with a prolonged base-building phase (as evidenced by many of the log entries in the previous chapter). In the meantime, I researched what the all-time greatest 800-meter runners did during their base-building phases. The best information I found was from Tony Wilson, who presented consolidated base-training philosophies from some of the greatest 800-meter runners of all time.[81]

The key takeaway was that long, slow distance is very important. The only counter to this came from Sebastian Coe who, along with Wilson Kipketer, piqued my interest most significantly with regard to training tactics. There are conflicting reports on Coe's mileage. Most of the controversy comes from Coe and his father/coach, Peter, who claims that Seb did very low mileage. However, I found plenty of evidence to suggest that they were either lying or had a funny way of counting mileage.

To make a long story short, my research leads me to believe that lots of mileage at the right point in the season is important for 800-meter success.

Frequent lactic threshold workouts and races (as I had done for the better part of the previous year) take longer to recover from and will actually break the body down over time. Instead, continuous easy runs are advised. But just because long, slow distance and base building are important, they clearly aren't the end-all, be-all to running a fast two-lapper. Long slow distance, aerobic threshold runs, tempo runs, and speed work are all important. Sebastian Coe used to train at five different speeds.

Example of Five-Pace Training (Used by Sebastian Coe in the Pre-Competition Phase)	
Day 1	3 x 2,000m or (2 x 1,200m) + (1 x 800m) + (2 x 400m) **5000m pace**
Day 2	Fartlek Run
Day 3	6 to 8 x 800m **3000m pace**
Day 4	Distance Running
Day 5	16 to 30 x 200m alternating with 10 x 400m **1500m pace**
Day 6	Rest day if race the next day, or fartlek if not
Day 7	Race or time trial
Day 8	4 to 6 x 400m or 9 x 300m **800m pace**
Day 9	Distance running on roads
Day 10	1 x 300m + 2 x 200m + 4 x 100m + 8 x 60m **400m pace**

As I thought more about focusing on the 800-meter event at Nationals instead of the steeplechase, I researched legendary half-miler Johnny Gray's training techniques – something I should have done years ago. Gray holds the U.S. indoor and outdoor 800-meter records; his outdoor record has stood since 1985. Gray's approach was different than most training regimens I had seen.

---

81 http://tonywilson.wordpress.com/2010/05/05/base-training-for-the-800-m-runner/

In the weeks/months leading up to racing season, Gray logged 60-mile weeks, but two consecutive days would be on the track. The first day would consist of six easy miles, followed by a set of 16 x 200 meters (going fast every fourth rep), then followed by a set of 6 x 150 meters (fast), followed by a set of 10 x 100 meters (easy). The second day would also start with six easy miles, but the track workout would consist of longer intervals: 8 x 400 meters with 200 meters rest in between (again, going fast on every fourth rep), followed by 4 x 200 meters (fast), followed by 10 x 100 meters (easy). The remainder of these weeks was pure distance running. One day would he would run easy distance; the next day he would alternate a slower mile with a quicker mile (or two easy miles and two quicker miles). During this phase of his training, his longest easy run would be 12 miles.

During racing season, he was on the track almost every day, doing all kinds of crazy stuff. Each workout started with a warm-up jog – the harder the workout, the shorter the warm-up – and 12 x 100 meters, alternating between a quick rep and an easy rep. The workouts all ended with 10 x 100 meters (easy). As for the actual workouts, Monday and Tuesday appeared to be the hardest days:

- ➢ Monday = 8 x 400 meters and 8 x 200 meters (alternating hard/easy reps), followed by a couple of easy miles before ending the meat of the workout with 2 x 600 meters (fast).
- ➢ Tuesday = 4 x 800 meters (hard), 3 x 400 meters (easy), and 15 x 150 meters (alternating hard/easy).

Wednesday was reportedly a road day, in which Gray would run an easy seven miles, followed by 1 x 800 meters on the track in 1:49. Yes, 1:49 is *very* fast for almost anyone, but this was seven seconds off of Gray's PR. Keep that in perspective when considering how you might incorporate his regimen into your own. For an athlete like Gray this was likely an easy day of distance with a moderate 800-meter rep just to get some leg turnover.

Thursday appeared to be a "quickness" day, loaded with 100-, 150-, and 200-meter reps. Friday was an easy pre-race day: six easy miles. Saturday was race day, and Sunday was a day of pure rest.

All in all, there are varied accounts of *exactly* what Gray did, but the principles seem to be pretty clear. The pre-season was focused on building a strong endurance base, with some light track work mixed in for leg turnover. This base would give him the strength to make it through racing season, when distance gave way to track work. It appears he wouldn't do more than seven consecutive miles during track season (although I calculated that his toughest track workouts added up to 12 miles).

A key to Johnny Gray's training was his long-time coach, Mihaly Igloi. Igloi is a legendary Hungarian coach who came to the U.S. in the 1950s. To say he was big on interval work would be a monumental understatement. That said, I don't think you'll find many detractors to his methods. The number of medals won and records established by his pupils is staggering.

Igloi's methods loosely map with the University of Oregon's, but seem to take things to an extreme. An Oregon coach once said that if you give one runner nothing but distance and another runner nothing but track workouts, the one doing nothing but track workouts would run the fastest PR, but the one doing nothing but distance would be able to sustain his peak for a longer period of time.

Most track programs focus on base-building then *mixing in* a track regimen. Igloi's regimen seemed to incorporate the best of both worlds more aggressively by building the base first and then switching almost solely to track workouts. Obviously, not everyone is an 800-meter runner, but I believe Igloi's approach for Gray can work for shorter and longer events. The mileage and track workouts would simply be altered to fit the chosen event.

For more on Igloi and the history of U.S. training, I highly recommend a piece written by Ben Raphelson, which is essentially his thesis from his work at Grinnell College: *Peaks And Valleys: The History of Competitive Distance Running in the U.S. Since 1954.*[82]

---

82 Source: [Google letsrun.com + history of us running 1954]

Training Log Week 82

Day	Date	Notes	Mileage
Thurs.	8/26/10	Comfortable 1-hr run: 8.8 miles (6:48 pace).	8.8
Fri.	8/27/10	Ran 4 miles to Weymouth High and jogged 800m with Jamie, who was already there. Did a handful of 50m strides, then headed home. Grand total: 8.77 miles in 1:01:22 (7:00 pace). Weighed in at 144lbs.	8.8
Sat.	8/28/10	7 miles in 48:17 (6:54 pace). 80-degree weather and tired legs kept it slow. Opened in 7:34; closed in 6:17.	7.0
Sun.	8/29/10	Biked to Jack's place in Foxboro; 90-degree weather. A few wks ago, I averaged 17.9 mph, but today I averaged 16.1 mph and I'm in better shape now. It was almost 1.5 hrs of constant pedaling. (Later, we had a Stoughton High School cross country reunion at Town Spa with Coach Dave.)	11.3
Mon.	8/30/10	Needed to take it easy, so went 4 miles at a moderate pace (normal loop). First 2 miles in 14:00 (7:00 pace); second 2 miles in 12:30 (6:15 pace).	4.0
Tues.	8/31/10	Hell of a workout on 4 hrs sleep. 6 x Heartbreak Hill (about 1:40 per rep). Andrea Sorgato and Jeff Caron weren't there, but a couple of new guys showed up. Paul Rupprecht,[83] a tall middle-distance runner, made the hills look easy. His stride was long and powerful but looked slow and effortless. He led all but the sixth rep (which I led, but to be fair, Paul added a rep after). Overall, I'd say that I was the #2 guy out there today. The final tally was 63 min (8.5 miles; 7:20 pace) Afterward, I weighed in under 145lb. Progress continues.	8.6
Weds.	9/1/10	Recovery run. Julie biked while I ran. 8.3 miles in 1:03 (7:37 pace).	8.3
Total		Averaged 7:09 per mile for the week	**56.8**

Training Log Week 83

Day	Date	Notes	Mileage
Thurs.	9/2/10	Standard run. 7 miles in 48:28 (6:55 pace).	7.0
Fri.	9/3/10	Standard 7-mile run, but a coming hurricane made for extremely muggy conditions. When combined with 80-degree temps, I felt like I was back in Springfield, IL. Had to stop at Mile 4 for a min before continuing. I struggled through the last 3 miles at 8:00 pace instead 6:40 pace. I definitely got more cardio benefit for the distance (50:48; 7:15 pace).	7.0
Sat.	9/4/10	Ran 4 miles, accelerating, to Weymouth High School (7:22, 6:40, 6:28, 6:10). With elevated heart rate, I did barefoot 4 x 200m (32.5-sec avg), then took a solid rest and did a 60-sec 400m (smooth and easy). Finished with 6 x 65m strides, totaling 1 mile of speed work. Ran home at accelerating pace (7:30, 7:20, 7:10, 6:09).	9.0
Sun.	9/5/10	Standard 7 miles in 48:34 (6:56 pace).	7.0
Mon.	9/6/10	Easy pre-workout day run: 7.7 miles in 57:16 (7:25 pace).	7.7
Tues.	9/7/10	Tough day with the New Balance team. We started with a 5K warm-up at about 7:00 pace. The workout was two sets of 3 min/2 min/1 min, with 1 min rest. After the second interval, I could tell it wasn't going to end well. Sure enough, my third rep was flat, and I lagged for the rest of the workout. We finished with about 1.2 miles to warm down. Afterward, my knees and hips were sore. I think I need rest.	7.8
Weds.	9/8/10	After a few wks of sore knees and a mediocre workout, I decided that taking it easy is smarter than trying to push through. I hit the exercise bike for 30 min.	4.0
Total		Averaged 6:59 per mile for the week	**49.5**

Injury Reports and Medical Findings

Chondromalacia: Not long after I addressed my foot issues, my knees started to hurt. I kept them under control by icing and wearing braces when I ran. However, the problem grew more and more difficult to mitigate with ice and braces. Some research uncovered a few things:

Striking the ground with your heel creates a lot of impact on the knees. It's like trying to come to a halt with every step. Mid-foot striking is easier on the knees. Shortening your stride also alleviates some impact. I'm closer to being

---

83 Paul Rupprecht is a Mark Lech-trained runner from University of Maine. He recorded PRs of 1:51 in the 800 meters, 3:49 in the 1,500 meters, and went on to win the Penn Relays Men's Open Steeplechase in 2011.

a toe-striker, so heel-striking wasn't a big problem – but I have a longer stride, so I tinkered around with shortening it. Even toe-strikers do a lot more heel-striking on long slow runs, and considering the slower pace of some of my runs at the time I noticed trouble, that may have been a contributor.

Chondromalacia, also known as runner's knee, tends to be most painful after hill running. I was doing a *lot* of hill work when my knees started to hurt. Beyond hill work, the most common causes of chondromalacia include over-pronation (which I have in spades), tight hamstrings/IT band (also one of my problems), and weak quads (not a problem for me). The recommended remedies for each symptom are pretty logical: proper shoes for over-pronation, stretching for tight muscles/tendons, and strengthening exercises for weak quads... and of course, icing the knees after workouts.

Knee and hip injuries are very common among bikers, and I was biking a fair amount when my knees flared up. Hip injuries are usually the result of a tight IT band, which is often a side effect of biking. Proper seat position can be a quick fix for the problem. The knee should have about 30 degrees of flexion when the pedal is in the down position. Several other adjustments might help (e.g., better cleat position, orthotics for pronation, lower gear choice, gluteus stretches, optimal handlebar height, and proper tire inflation). In other words, if you plan to do a lot of biking, you probably need a professional to tailor-fit you to a bike.

Dietary Research and Findings

Iron Consumption: In late summer 2010, my September 7th workout with the New Balance team was the exclamation point on a couple of disappointing weeks of work. I knew from my college days that fatigue is often associated with an iron deficiency. I realized I hadn't been eating as much of the foods that serve as my key sources of iron (e.g., lentils). That said, I had assumed that my daily "mega-vitamin" would pick up the slack.

Surprise... I looked at the bottle to see how much iron I was getting from the mega. Nothing. That's right – *zero* iron in my daily vitamin supplement. I figured I was on to something, so I went to the grocery store and bought a bottle of iron supplements. Note: To optimize absorption, take vitamin C with the iron and avoid dairy products (which hinder absorption).

I was even more convinced of the importance of iron after talking to New Balance Boston teammate Paul Rupprecht. He has a near-chronic iron deficiency. For some reason, his system doesn't absorb iron well on a consistent basis. He has to get tested often to figure out how much iron to take, to avoid taking too much (which is dangerous) or too little.

Before a recent iron test, he ran a workout where he was only able to complete a few reps of 800 meters at his assigned pace. Not surprisingly, the subsequent iron test revealed that his iron levels were low. He increased his iron intake, and shortly thereafter he ran a similar workout and managed to complete twice as many 800-meter reps at the same pace... with less rest in between.

This is a dramatic result and shows that proper iron levels are important to performance. Iron is a critical component in the transport of oxygen to the muscles. I often remarked that my training sessions were stronger 24-48 hours after a steak dinner (a meal I didn't often eat). Paul's experience and my results reinforce numerous research sources I found on the topic.[84] Make sure your iron levels are strong – but not too strong. Overcompensating can cause significant problems... both in long-term health and in some very acute, more immediate terms (as I found out the hard way).

One Saturday morning later in the season, the New Balance guys gathered at a field in Lexington that is bordered by a 1,000-meter path. We warmed up with an easy 5K and planned a workout of 3 x 3 minutes, 3 x 2 minutes, and 4 x 1 minute, with varied rest of a minute or two. The pace was expected to be around 5K race pace for the 3 x 3s, a bit faster for the 2 x 2s, and even faster for the 4 x 1s. In short, it played to my strengths.

84 Sources: [Google: rice + jenky + iron; Google: parenting science + iron absorption]

I started the workout in the back of the pack. Each of the guys were faster 5K runners than I was, so I simply stayed tight with the group. I felt fine after the first three-minute interval and recovered quickly, so I moved up in the pack for the second and third intervals. During each of the 3 x 2s, I hung with Paul Rupprecht longer and pulled further from the rest of the crew. Once those were done, it was time for the home stretch. At the start of the first one-minute rep, I finished right where I wanted to – close behind my measuring stick, Rupprecht. By the last few reps it was just me chasing Paul; the rest of the pack had fallen off. It wasn't like I won a race, but it was a great workout... and then I learned my lesson about iron overload.

Early in our three-mile warm-down, I had to stop and double over – nearly sick to my stomach. The workout was challenging, but at this point it felt like I ran a really nasty race. I gathered myself for the rest of the warm-down. On the drive home, the violently nauseous feeling hit me again. When I got home, it worsened. I was supposed to attend a family dinner, but that did not look promising as of 1 p.m. I decided to take a nap. When I awoke, I felt better at first but soon doubled over again... and then again. I felt food poisoned, but I hadn't eaten anything that Jamie hadn't, and she was fine – and her stomach is far more sensitive than mine. I suspected something else and quickly started researching.

Coming into the workout, I had taken iron supplements for three days straight, as opposed to my typical every-other-day routine. Sure enough, my symptoms fit the iron-overload description caused by unabsorbed iron in the gastrointestinal tract. "Unabsorbed" seemed to be the key word. After reading several Web sites, I concluded that my condition was due to the unwise combining of iron supplements with calcium-magnesium and Tums (which I took for better lactic acid tolerance). Calcium inhibits the absorption of iron. Thus, there was probably a decent amount of it sitting in my stomach, wreaking havoc.

Adding insult to injury, when I first got home I downed a bunch of Tums to quell my sour stomach, which only prolonging my ordeal! The better treatment was the exact opposite of what one would expect - orange juice and red meat. Yes... an acidic fluid and an iron-rich, hard-to-digest solid. Intuitively, I was afraid to follow though, but the logic was actually sound. The best iron-absorption enablers are Vitamin C and red meat. Unfortunately, I had neither in the fridge at the time, so I settled for the next best things... chicken breast and lemon juice, which I combined into a grilled lemon-chicken dish.

Sure enough, the symptoms start to ease soon after. The contractions continued into the evening, but became less frequent. I was able to attend the family dinner (with no ill-effect on my appetite), and was 100 percent by Sunday morning.

Going forward, I took my iron supplements with vitamin C and well in advance of any races or critical workouts. (Iron is not noted to be an immediate performance enhancer – nor do its benefits fade quickly). That allowed me to focus on lactic-acid buffers closer to the races and workouts, which provided significant benefit.

Researching the iron topic further, I found the National Institute of Health (NIH) published some basic-but-important findings on iron.[85] Among the findings is vitamin A's important role in activating iron stores within the body. After reading that, I researched good sources of Vitamin A to help activate my iron stores. A simple search on Wikipedia reveals the common sources of Vitamin A. To maximize the benefits of iron, I took an occasional iron pill with nothing but fruit and followed it with some raw carrots a few hours later to aid with iron activation. I had no further problems, and I believe solving the "iron problem" can provide a distinct competitive advantage.

---

85 Source: [Google: NIH.gov + Iron]

Training Log Week 84

Day	Date	Notes	Mileage
Thurs.	9/9/10	Hit the weights for upper- and lower-body lifting. Later, I hit the elliptical for about 30 min.	4.2
Fri.	9/10/10	Planned on 7 miles, but my knees hurt so I cut it to about 5 miles. I'd like to see an expert and figure this out. Incidentally, Chris Simpson has the same issue, stemming from the same origin (a near-plantar experience, followed by orthotics, followed by a knee problem). With any luck, one of us will figure out a solution soon.	5.2
Sat.	9/11/10	To keep the pressure off my knees. I did 8 miles (30 min) on a mountain bike. The bike I use is a loaner from the condo complex; it's rusty and the tires are half flat. I don't mind, but I should note that 8 miles in 30:00 is actually a pretty good workout on that bike! After the bike, I did a fairly continuous 30-min lower-body weight workout (calves, hamstrings, and quads).	4.0
Sun.	9/12/10	Did 65 min elliptical... felt ridiculously easy. Maybe I just needed a few easy days and the iron supplements I started yesterday. After, I did a 20-min upper/lower-body weight workout: body-weight squats and 10-sec squat-&-holds (a.k.a. isometric squats). The squat-&-holds are supposed to be good for my knees' supporting muscles. Also did standard lunges, and step-back lunges. I'm paying more attention to the total time I spend working out: 6-6.5 hrs/wk, plus lifting, seems to be my sweet spot.	8.5
Mon.	9/13/10	The NFL can make 2 hrs fly by. I spent 1:45 and 13.5 miles on the elliptical happily watching the Jets lose. From April until December last year, most of my workouts were on the elliptical. My road/track running didn't suffer. I broke 50:00 for 8 miles and ran several strong track workouts during that time. The only thing that suffered was my quad strength. After my elliptical workout tonight, I spent 15 min doing leg lifts to work my quads and strengthen my knees' supporting muscles. My knees are feeling better. As long as my feet don't feel strained again from the elliptical, I'll have to balance it with road work.	13.5
Tues.	9/14/10	After yesterday's long session on the elliptical, I returned to the roads for a short run (4 miles). I wanted to test my knees and my conditioning, after starting iron supplementation last week. The results were pretty good: 6:32 pace. Not awesome, but a step up from last week.	4.0
Weds.	9/15/10	Back to the elliptical today: 63 min, plus a strong 5-10 min ab workout.	8.0
Total		Averaged 7:36 per mile for the week	**47.4**

Training Log Week 85

Day	Date	Notes	Mileage
Thurs.	9/16/10	70-min elliptical, plus extensive leg-weight work.	9.0
Fri.	9/17/10	62-min elliptical. Slightly fatigued from yesterday. This weekend marks my 5th anniversary with Jamie, so I'll be running around the streets on Kennebunkport the next few days.	8.0
Sat.	9/18/10	Some delayed soreness from the previous long ellipticals, so I kept it short today: 5.2 miles in Kennebunkport at a quick 6:22 pace. The elliptical and/or iron supplements seem to be making a difference. Meanwhile, Ryan O'Connell ran a great cross country race, covering 5 miles in 25:10. Barring injury, he'll run some great mile and 800m PRs later this year.	5.2
Sun.	9/19/10	Another quick run in Kennebunkport. I did an extra half-mile (5.7 total), kept the same pace (6:22), and felt better afterward. Not feeling fatigued anymore.	5.7
Mon.	9/20/10	Jamie and I got back from Maine today. I have a New Balance workout tomorrow, so I hit the elliptical for an easy 45-min session.	6.0
Tues.	9/21/10	Back to Heartbreak Hill for strength work. The workout was called 90/60/30: run up Heartbreak for 90 sec, jog down quickly, then up for 60 sec, down quickly again, etc. Wash, rinse and repeat. I was assigned 4 sets. We warmed up for 2.9 miles at 7:00 pace. In the workout I felt good from the get-go. I didn't push the first 90 sec. I worked the 60 sec a little harder, finishing among the leaders. The 30-sec rep was tailor-made for me. I led it. I settled into a pattern of struggling on the 90s, running mid-pack for the 60s, and leading the 30s. I still felt good, so I joined some of the top guys for an extra 60 and two extra 30s. We finished with a 2.6-mile warm-down. My knees were sore, but overall I felt good.	10.1
Weds.	9/22/10	1-hr recovery session on the elliptical.	8.6
Total		Averaged 7:08 per mile for the week	**52.5**

Common Sources of Vitamin A, Including Microgram Count and RDA Percentage	
Most meat and fish (6,500 µg; 722%)	Cheddar cheese (265 µg; 29%)
Carrots (835 µg; 93%)	Cantaloupe melon (169 µg; 19%)
Broccoli leaf (800 µg; 89%)	Egg (140 µg; 16%)
Sweet potato (709 µg; 79%)	Apricot (96 µg; 11%)
Butter (684 µg; 76%)	Papaya (55 µg; 6%)
Kale (681 µg; 76%)	Mango (38 µg; 4%)
Spinach (469 µg; 52%)	Peas (38 µg; 4%)
Pumpkin (400 µg; 41%)	Broccoli florets (31 µg; 3%)
Collard greens (333 µg; 37%)	Milk (28 µg; 3%)

Source: Wikipedia

Training Log Week 86

Day	Date	Notes	Mileage
Thurs.	9/23/10	1 hr on the elliptical; 15 min on leg lifts. Good workout.	8.7
Fri.	9/24/10	52-min shortened session on the elliptical. Had to rush to catch a flight to Chicago.	7.5
Sat.	9/25/10	31 min along the lake in Chicago. Spent some time running in the sand, slowing to near 10-min pace. It'll be interesting to try longer runs in the sand in Miami. Later, at Rick Miller's birthday party, I spent 2 hrs dancing. With my recouped leg strength, I had some old moves back: which is good news and bad news; I'll be sore tomorrow.	4.8
Sun.	9/26/10	An arduous day... but not of training. After celebrating Miller's birthday in Chicago, I went straight from the festivities (4a Chicago time) to the Patriots' game at Gillette Stadium. It was a hell of an all-nighter, with planes, cabs, cars, friends and favors. (Thanks Terry!) By game's end, I was beyond exhausted and sore from last night. I got home around 6p and took a nap. I woke up around 8p and hit the elliptical for an hr during the late game (Miami versus the Jets).	8.7
Mon.	9/27/10	Today was Day 600 of my training streak. For a milestone, it was uneventful. I slept in and did an easy 30-min elliptical session. Tomorrow is New Balance workout day.	4.4
Tues.	9/28/10	Back to the BC reservoir. Workout was 23 min of continuous running, alternating 5 min hard, 1 min easy. This is not my kind of workout. Plus, my legs were still sore and tired from the Chicago dance-fest. My only goal was to keep up for the first 5-min set. After a 3-mile warm-up (in which I ran with the slowest group) we got started. The top guys quickly separated themselves. I hung back, waiting for everyone to settle in. After that, I just tried to run efficiently and stay relaxed. At about 3 min, I felt surprisingly comfortable. My breathing picked up, but that was it. The next 2 min were more of the same, and I finished in the middle of the 2nd pack. After 1 min rest, I was ready to go. The entire workout continued this way. The last couple of min were tough, but I actually led my group to the finish. I was shocked. Our pace was under 5:30 per mile for the entire workout, which isn't blistering, but it's solid – I couldn't have done that a few wks ago. I believe those iron pills made a difference.	9.3
Weds.	9/29/10	My left leg has a line of pain running down the side. Hoping it's not my IT band. 1 hr on the elliptical to avoid pounding my body. That tactic has worked well in the past (barring trouble with plantar strain).	8.7
Total		Averaged 6:49 per mile for the week	52.1

Training Log Week 87			
Day	Date	Notes	Mileage
Thurs.	9/30/10	1-hr elliptical.	8.7
Fri.	10/1/10	1-hr elliptical.	8.7
Sat.	10/2/10	Ran to my grandmother's house (4.3 miles), visited for 20 min, then ran back. I took it fairly easy: 6:48 pace for each leg of the run. It's a hilly trek, so the performance is notable.	8.6
Sun.	10/3/10	Played flag football; first time in nearly two years. I was rusty, but fast. Definitely got a workout out of the deal. After, I hit the elliptical for a *long* session: 1:45:00. Thank God for the NFL. I'll be sore tomorrow… and probably Tuesday too.	16.5
Mon.	10/4/10	Sore all over. Couldn't lift my legs past 90 degrees. Hit the elliptical for 30 min. New Balance tomorrow. Considering how I felt today, I'm worried about my performance.	4.4
Tues.	10/5/10	I was officially added to the New Balance Boston roster, entitling me to 40% off their gear. I bought some shorts, trainers and flats. I shamefully had been wearing my Brooks flats to practice. I wasn't feeling competitive though. Jamie was sick and I was fighting it. Plus I was aching from Sunday. I strongly considering skipping. Adding insult to injury, I got there late, so I missed most of the warm-up. I did a mile on my own. The workout: a 5K tempo run around the BC Reservoir. Great… my weakness. When it started, I actually felt good. I went out with the first group before coming to my senses and dropping back to my usual pack. Still, the pace felt pretty easy. I hoped to get around the rez once with the boys and not look like a fool as we passed Coach Curtin. I made it through the first lap and felt pretty good. Now, if I imploded, I could do it out of Coach's sight, but oddly I felt good and focused on catching some guys. With about 800m to go, I felt fatigue set in. Nonetheless, I finished the 5K in 17:20. A good time, considering. If it were a race, I could have run faster. After, I did some 30-sec strides. My new flats were chafing my Achilles, so I skipped the warm-down.	5.3
Weds.	10/6/10	35-min recovery session on the elliptical.	5.2
Total		Averaged 6:51 per mile for the week	**57.4**

Race Reports, Records and Results

<u>2010 Mayor's Cup</u>: On a whim, I decided to run Boston's Mayor's Cup cross country championship, an annual mid-autumn meet, held on the specifically designed Franklin Park course. As an 800-meter specialist, I wasn't a fan of a 5K over grassy, rolling hills – but Mayor's Cup is a unique experience, and the occasional 5K is good for conditioning (and mental toughness).

Coach Dave picked me up in his old pickup truck and we carpooled to the race. Heading to Franklin Park felt like old times… except Coach Dave has a son now!

The weather was dreary (overcast and breezy) but well-suited for a cross country race. I ran fairly well for that time of the year: 17:05 for the 5K, finishing 19th out of more than 350 harriers. I managed to fend off all the women (including some elites) and was only beaten by one guy older than me. I keyed off of my New Balance Boston teammates, which made a big difference, and ran a pretty evenly-paced race.

Miscellaneous Research and Notes

<u>Racing Weight</u>: *Peak Performance* and other publications make a strong argument for targeting a goal weight based on a formula provided by the legendary Dr. George Sheehan.[86]

The ideal weight for an average man of my height (5' 7 1/2") is considered to be 151 pounds. I was intentionally maintaining my weight at 150 pounds. However, for middle-distance runners of my height, the ideal weight is supposedly 12 percent less than that of the average man. This works out to 133 pounds for me. It was outlandish to think I could get to that weight. Body fat tests placed me somewhere in the 10-15 percent range. I would have had to lose every ounce of fat to reach Sheehan's "ideal weight," which was obviously impossible and likely counterproductive.

---

86 Source: [Google: "peak performance" + "george sheehan" + "lose some weight"]

That said, I thought my 10-15 percent body fat content might have been too much. In maintaining my 150 pounds, I ate carefully most days, but splurged heavily on Wednesdays (date night), Fridays and Saturdays. By implementing stricter dietary controls, I felt I could reasonably drop to somewhere between 135 and 142.5 pounds.

Based on Sheehan's research, 400-meter runners were lumped in with sprinters, which are said to be ideal when weighing in only 2.5 percent lighter than the average man. One could argue that the ideal weight should be different for each event. As such, an 800-meter runner (more similar to a 400-meter runner than a 10K guy) could very well have an ideal weight at something closer to 8-10 percent under the norm. That would make my ideal weight 136-139 pounds.

The *Peak Performance* article went on to say that dense bone structure could account for about 6 pounds of additional weight. Assuming that my bone structure qualifies, my ideal weight might actually be 142-145 pounds.

Thus, my ideal weight ranged between 133 pounds at the low-end and 145 pounds at the high-end. The mid-point of that range is 139 pounds, which is one pound more than I weighed when I entered Northeastern University as a freshman. When I set the school record in the 1,000 meters a little over a year later, I weighed 153lbs, but I was a lot more muscular by that point.

Netting it all out, I got the sense that I could safely shed up to 10 pounds of body fat by cutting out my Wednesday/Friday/Saturday eat-fests. This sounded reasonable. When I imagined running 800 meters with a 5-pound barbell in each hand, I could easily envision that adding 3.5 seconds to my time.

Shedding 10 pounds would drop my total weight to 140 pounds. All else being equal, that would surely make me faster – assuming it didn't also make me sickly or weak. The article cited an example where an athlete dropped two stone (28 pounds) and was rewarded with a 16-second PR in the mile. Simple math would suggest that a 10-pound drop would knock 2.5-seconds from my 800-meter time. Based on my earlier 1:57.5, I'd be running 1:55-flat, which was one second faster than Nick Berra, the reigning American Masters champ.

In the first week I eased back on my binging, I lost one pound. I felt hungrier, but not any weaker. I was trying to trim 500 calories per day (about 14 percent of my intake), and because I usually took in 300 percent of the RDA of all nutrients, I didn't think I'd suffer nutritionally.

In Hindsight: *A few months after finding this research, by mid-December 2010, I was weighing in at 142 pounds – only two pounds away from my championship goal weight. I was happy and frankly surprised by how easy it was to shed the weight. I lost an average of two pounds per week, despite my annual road trip to Miami and weight I would gain on vacation in St. Lucia.*

Logging an extra 20 miles of work per week certainly helped. (That accounted for roughly 2,500 calories, or 0.7 pounds per week of weight loss). However, it became clear that proper diet trumps exercise if the primary goal is shedding weight. Portion control was the cornerstone of my success. Pulling way back on what I ate on Wednesdays, combined with exercising a little bit of prudence on Fridays and Saturdays, made all the difference. I dropped weight fast without sacrificing much in the way of nutrition or health – but I would soon learn the hard way that weight charts and formulae are good guidelines, but everyone's physiology functions very, very differently.

Training Log Week 88

Day	Date	Notes	Mileage
Thurs.	10/7/10	60-min elliptical plus weights.	8.7
Fri.	10/8/10	60-min elliptical	8.8
Sat.	10/9/10	30-min elliptical.	4.5
Sun.	10/10/10	I tried my hand at flag football again and got another good workout. After, I hit the elliptical for 90 min during the early NFL games. I found I could easily handle elliptical work after a tough workout. I think I can do more workouts/weights each wk without sacrificing distance work. I could increase my volume *and* train more efficiently without risking injury. Reviewing my training log, I see a pattern of endurance and good health during periods when I've done a lot of elliptical work.	14.7
Mon.	10/11/10	Not as sore as last week. I focused on recovery this wk (ice, protein, etc.) and did a noon recovery session on the elliptical to go with my regular 30-min session in the evening. I think the noon session helped. Tomorrow's New Balance workout will be the test.	8.9
Tues.	10/12/10	Back to Heartbreak Hill. This is my favorite New Balance workout, as I've become proficient at it. Distance runners were assigned 8-10x the full hill (about 1:40 to the top). Middle-distance runners (my group) ran 8 x 1 min and then 8 x 30 sec, with a brisk downhill rest. I felt a *lot* better this wk than last week, so I'll probably continue flag football or do sprints on Sundays. With 5 months until Indoor Nationals, I think it's time to reacclimatize myself to moving quickly. As for the workout, I felt fluid and powerful. Could have gone harder, but Coach Curtain didn't want that level of effort.	9.5
Weds.	10/13/10	Jogged with Jamie for a bit at the Braintree track. I felt yesterday's workout more than I expected; probably the 16 reps more than the pace. Later, I hit the elliptical for 40 min.	6.8
Total		Averaged 6:55 per mile for the week	**61.9**

Training Log Week 89

Day	Date	Notes	Mileage
Thurs.	10/14/10	Moderate 60-min elliptical and weights.	8.7
Fri.	10/15/10	Easy 35-min elliptical, then drove to Hartford CT to see Roger Waters in concert. Even if you aren't a big Pink Floyd fan, this is something to see.	5.0
Sat.	10/16/10	Got in late from Hartford last night, which made this morning's New Balance workout a challenge. Distance guys did a 2-lap tempo around Fresh Pond in Cambridge (1 lap = 2.4 miles); middle distance guys did 2 miles, then jogged the remaining 0.4, then did another 2 miles at tempo pace. My first 2-miler was 10:56; the second was 11:00. It was tough.	9.0
Sun.	10/17/10	Another late night and another early morning. I awoke on 6 hrs sleep for another round of flag football. It allows me to get out there, run fast, and catch a few balls without worrying too much about getting hurt; quite useful for getting my speed back. Today, I felt faster and stronger for a longer span. When the game was done, I ran a few extra sprints. Later, I hopped on the elliptical for 100 min of cardio. Tough, but I felt better than the previous two Sundays. I have a feeling that I'll be 100% for my Tuesday workout.	15.5
Mon.	10/18/10	A little tired and sore, but not too bad. I felt great about my weekend of work and rewarded myself with an easy 40-min recovery session on the elliptical.	5.8
Tues.	10/19/10	New Balance day. I felt good, ate well, took my iron, and got to the BC Reservoir ready to work. It was chilly, so I wore jogging sweats and an old gray long-sleeve with holes I poked in the sleeves to put my thumbs through to help keep my hands warm. Kinda ghetto, but it works. The workout was 6 x 3 min @ 5K pace, with 2 min recovery jog for the elite distance guys; 4 x 3 min @ 5K pace, with 2 min recovery jog, plus 4 x 1 min with a 1-min jog for the middle distance guys. We started together, as usual, then the two groups separated – but this time I stayed with the elites. The 4:45 mile pace felt fine; I fell off pace slightly on the third rep, but caught up during recovery. I finished the fourth rep with the elite group, but my reward was to run my 4 x 1-min intervals alone. However, when I finished, Coach Curtain alerted me that New Balance left some gear for the team and I got first dibs. I picked a sweet blue long sleeve – with holes in the sleeves, pre-cut!	10.9
Weds.	10/20/10	40 min on the elliptical. This mode of training has worked well. I plan to increase the volume to get more out of it because I feel almost no risk of injury.	5.8
Total		Averaged 6:53 per mile for the week	**60.7**

Training Log Week 90

Day	Date	Notes	Mileage
Thurs.	10/21/10	60-min elliptical.	8.7
Fri.	10/22/10	60-min elliptical.	8.7
Sat.	10/23/10	40-min elliptical.	5.8
Sun.	10/24/10	Decided to run the Mayor's Cup cross country meet. I ran fairly well for this time of the year: 17:05 for 5K, finishing 19th out of 350. Solid day's work.	7.2
Mon.	10/25/10	110 min on the elliptical. I logged it as an equivalent of 15 road miles.	15.0
Tues.	10/26/10	40-min elliptical.	5.9
Weds.	10/27/10	New Balance workout was held today to give extra rest from Mayor's Cup. Warmed up with 5K at 7:00 pace. Workout was a tempo run: 3 x 7 min at 5K pace, with 3 min rest at 40 sec above 5K pace. Hard to be exact using GPS, but I think I ran 5:33 per mile for the intervals and 6:11 per mile for the rest. This compares to the 5:30 pace I averaged in the race and the 6:10 target pace for my rest… so I was close to goal pace. I led my group again – odd because two of them beat me Sunday. They must be able to hold pace longer while I'm better at shorter intervals. Most importantly, I feel fresh (mentally and physically), which prepares me to up my workload for Indoor Nationals, which are 4 months away.	10.6
Total		Averaged 6:53 per mile for the week	61.9

Technical Tip – *Sebastian Coe's coach and father, Peter Coe, called 5K pace "the golden pace" and claimed it eradicates the need for big mileage. Workouts at 5K pace take the athlete to 95 percent of VO_2 max and, according to leading physiologists, are the greatest improver of oxygen uptake. Seb Coe's VO_2 max was measured at 82mls/kg/min, one of the highest ever recorded. His workouts included:*

➢ *7 x 800 meters at 5K pace with 45 seconds rest.*
➢ *3 x 1.5 miles at 5K pace (the Roger Bannister workout)*
➢ *5 x 1,000 meters at 5K pace with 60 seconds rest (claimed by some physiologists to be the "ideal" workout)*

Training Log Week 91

Day	Date	Notes	Mileage
Thurs.	10/28/10	60-min elliptical, plus weights. Decided to increase my workout volume to test my low-impact cardio theory. I hope to follow a hard workout like yesterday's with a workout like this, instead of needing a "recovery day".	8.7
Fri.	10/29/10	40-min elliptical in preparation for the Saturday New Balance workout.	5.8
Sat.	10/30/10	Hard waking up because my brother visited last night, and we scarfed BBQ until 2a. Not helpful before a 9a workout, but I made this bed… Workout was 2 x 4 min, 2 x 2 min, and 4 x 1 min at faster than tempo pace, with 1 min rest. I did the 4-min reps at 5:25 pace the 2-min reps at 5:00 pace, and the 1-min reps at 4:40 pace. It felt hard enough. At home I crashed for a 90-min nap, which is rare. That's my kind of workout. A little less pain during and a little more pain after…	10.2
Sun.	10/31/10	Jamie and I attended a wild Halloween party last night and didn't get home until after 2a. I was up early to meet my buddy Dolan to tailgate before the Patriot's game. It was a late game and long tailgate, followed by a long trek home. Then, it was time for my long workout. I dragged my butt onto the elliptical for two full hours. Can't let drunken shenanigans get in the way of training. I logged it as a 16-mile running equivalent.	16.3
Mon.	11/1/10	40-min elliptical on top of our prep work for our move back to Miami for the winter.	5.8
Tues.	11/2/10	Tough day at Heartbreak Hill. I felt tight and sore all morning, so I expected trouble. I felt heavy during most of the 12 x 1-min reps. I lagged guys I normally beat. Days like this happen, but it may be time for some rest. I've averaged 60+ training-equivalent miles each wk for the past month. That hasn't happened since April… and ended with an injury.	8.9
Weds.	11/3/10	Easy 30 min on the elliptical (my shortest workout in wks).	4.4
Total		Averaged 6:53 per mile for the week	60.1

Chapter 11
I Don't Know Where I Am, but I Know I Don't Like It

Weeks 92-102

It was summer, 2004. Through blurry eyes, I saw a bear-like figure looming overhead. I was fully clothed in a bathtub of lukewarm water with a waterlogged pillow holding my head upright. I had just regained consciousness. I was disoriented and confused... and in that instant I found the whole scene amusing.

"Dude, you okay?" the bear-like figure, a close friend named John Burke, asked me.

"Where are we?" I replied.

"Newport, Rhode Island."

"How'd we get here?"

"Um, you drove here."

The scene was becoming less amusing considering I didn't remember driving. I didn't remember much of the preceding 12 hours.

Burkie continued, "You decided to see at which speed your BMW's governor kicks in..."

Ugh.

"...as you were driving over the Newport Bridge."

Every hole has a bottom. That was mine.

A decade removed from Northeastern University, I was divorced and living with my brother in downtown Boston. I had just started my business and was working about 100 hours per week. Most of my spare time was spent eating or sleeping. My bed was about five feet from my desk. My kitchen wasn't much further away. You couldn't name a presweetened cereal that didn't exist in my cupboard, and my typical dinner consisted of a large store-bought steak fried in butter, with a package of Lipton butter noodles on the side.

In the summers, I would break from work late on Fridays and speed from Boston to Newport to spend the weekend in a beach house with a bunch of single guys, living the single guy life. I had gained more than 30 pounds since graduation – maybe closer to 40 pounds – and I could breeze through half a case of beer with no effort at all.

One Sunday morning in Newport, a few of us decided to grab a ferry to nearby Block Island, a party spot halfway between the coast of Rhode Island and the tip of New York's Long Island. The ferry left from Port Judith, 20-25 minutes away by car. It was a common day trip for locals and weekend warriors alike. After a few full summers vacationing there, my friends and I had befriended many of the Rhode Island natives – an easygoing, quick-to-party, bunch – and on the way to the boat we were spotted by a few of them.

Before long we were sucking down cocktails on the ferry and gearing up to spend the day on the island drinking beer and watching a popular cover band play at Ballard's Beach Club. Before we even landed at Block Island we were four drinks deep. While the band played, we took turns buying rounds of beer, and like most things we did, it turned into a race. The moment your bottle was empty, you called the waitress for the next go-around. Falling behind wasn't an option, and we were keeping receipts as proof. By sunset I had receipts for 35 beers in my pocket, a chipped tooth, and a fickle grip on reality.

A few hours later, I was racing my BMW over the Newport Bridge at 136 mph. In the wee hours of the morning, I awoke fully clothed in the bathtub.

Burke, satisfied I hadn't drowned, headed toward the kitchen. I lingered in the tub for a minute, my initial amusement fading into disgust. Consuming 35 beers in a day was bad enough. Piloting my sports car at high rates of speed over country roads and ocean-spanning bridges was inexcusable. Getting back to the summer house without killing someone was an act of God; Passing out in a bathtub three-fourths-filled with water and not drowning... I wouldn't have blamed God if he had taken me then, considering my behavior.

But that was the bottom. I resolved to stop my self-destructive path even as I started to realize that many of the factors that had driven me to succeed as an athlete, as a professional, were the same factors that provoked me to drink 35 beers in an afternoon. I knew it wouldn't be easy. I needed to figure out the right balance of who I was. Some of the changes started small, but when I began my quest for a national championship five years later in 2009, I would frequently think back to that time in my life – perhaps even more frequently as I geared up for my first winter of hard racing in 20 years.

Training Log Week 92			
Day	Date	Notes	Mileage
Thurs.	11/4/10	A day of rest was all I needed to recover from Heartbreak Hill. Did a 1-hr elliptical, followed by leg weights, and felt strong. I also took a body fat test, which registered 10-15%.	8.7
Fri.	11/5/10	Starting elliptical double sessions. It causes no real wear and tear, so I think sneaking in an extra 30 min early in the day should do more good than harm. Today, I did 30 min in the morning and 34 min in the evening.	9.4
Sat.	11/6/10	60-min elliptical.	8.7
Sun.	11/7/10	The New Balance Boston team ran the USATF New England Cross Country Championships. My calf was acting up a bit, so I chose easy distance instead of racing. No sense risking insult *and* injury. I went to cheer on my old teammate Erik Nedeau, who was racing. I joined him for a 3-mile warm-up. During the race, I ran from spot to spot, to cheer, getting some decent short sprints in. Ned finished in 32:04, and a few of us joined him for a warm-down. I ended up running 7 miles, then at home later in the day I logged 1 hr on the elliptical and some weight work. Being at the race got me pretty motivated.	19.2
Mon.	11/8/10	Woke up sore. For me, soreness peaks about 24 hrs after hard work, so I figured on a tough day. Nonetheless, I did a morning elliptical session, knowing I could take the afternoon easy (or off). Opened with a 30-min session in the morning and felt good. At night I hit the gym for a 1-hr elliptical, plus weights, drills, stretching, and foam rolling. I may be sore tomorrow from the lunges...	13.0
Tues.	11/9/10	Took it easy. I was a little sore from yesterday's work (only in my hamstrings though, which is typical after I do lunges). Did 40 min on the elliptical and iced during the day.	5.8
Weds.	11/10/10	Today's New Balance workout was tempo/hills/tempo. Started with 2 miles at faster-than-5K pace, then 3 min rest, followed by 8 x 30-sec sprints up Heartbreak Hill. After 3 min rest, we added another 2 miles at 5K pace for good measure. With a 3-mile warm-up and warm-down, we logged some distance.	11.3
Total		Averaged 6:53 per mile for the week	76.1

Training Log Week 93

Day	Date	Notes	Mileage
Thurs.	11/11/10	Jamie kicked me out of the house for a morning recovery session on the elliptical (30:00; 4.3 equivalent miles). Later I did a 6-mile elliptical session at 7:00 pace. I felt yesterday's workout, but overall, I was fine. With New Balance workouts on Wednesdays and Saturdays now, the trick is to recover by Saturday morning.	10.3
Fri.	11/12/10	Took it easy: 30-min elliptical at 7:00 pace.	5.8
Sat.	11/13/10	My last New Balance workout before I leave for Miami. The workout was 3 x 3 min, 3 x 2 min, and 4 x 1 min – with 2 min rest after the longer reps and 1 min rest after the 1-min reps. In the last rep, I held off Paul Rupprecht and was clearly the #2 guy on this day. However, I ran into problems related to iron consumption (see Chapter 10).	11.7
Sun.	11/14/10	Miami moving day. My cousins helped pack our stuff in my new Boston-to-Miami transport: a 2007 Infiniti Qx56! The move went smoothly. After, I snuck in a 30 min elliptical before starting the 20-hr drive to Miami.	4.4
Mon.	11/15/10	Ran 4.7 miles on grass in 31:36 (6:45 pace), then drove until we reached a hotel in South Carolina with a Life Fitness elliptical machine. I logged 91 min during Monday Night Football, giving me 17.7 miles for the day. The hot tub had strong water jets. Well needed!	17.7
Tues.	11/16/10	Hopped on the elliptical for 30 min before the drive. Made Florida that night by driving straight through. Only did one training session today, but I did a lot of work yesterday.	4.4
Weds.	11/17/10	First day in Miami brought a sunny, 80-degree run on thick grass. The surface slowed me, but this run was about heat/heart-rate training, not speed. After, I stretched and did 6 x 70m strides. That evening, my back was sore but didn't impact my night run. I ran a dirt path around a golf course for about 6 miles. My overall pace was 6:51, but I started slow (over 7:30 pace). I have a great base but very little speed. I'll work on that.	10.5
Total		Averaged 6:54 per mile for the week	64.8

Training Log Week 94

Day	Date	Notes	Mileage
Thurs.	11/18/10	Did 4.3 miles through thick grass in 30:15 (6:58 pace) – 14 sec faster pace than yesterday. Later, we moved into our new place in South Beach. The complex has a great gym, pool, and hot tub. Am I wrong to find it funny that our condo has a bidet? At 7p, I had my first Nike tempo run. Started with a 2.3-mile warm-up (6:41 pace), then the 2.9-mile tempo. After a slow start with the group (as usual), I finished in 17:06 (5:50 pace). The final 2 miles were probably 10:40. Bryan Huberty and I warmed-down with a 3.5-mile jog	13.1
Fri.	11/19/10	Easy day on the legs: 30 min morning elliptical and 30 min in the evening. Matt Kiss and I did some upper-body lifting, runners' curls, and breath-holding exercises. Per earlier research, breath-holding supposedly increases lung capacity. We did 3 sets. Matt did 0:54, 1:02, and 1:24. I surprised myself by going 1:46, 1:55, and 2:19. My all-time best is 2:45.	8.6
Sat.	11/20/10	Started with an easy 7-miler in the morning, immediately followed by a core workout. An hr later, I led an easy drill workout (5 sets, with 50m strides, and 15 pushups). Later, I did 30 min on the elliptical.	14.4
Sun.	11/21/10	Met Bryan and Matt for a 12-mile run on the grass at Tropical Park – where I won my first 1-mile race in 13 years last winter. We finished in 1:26:47 (7:14 pace). Later, the gang gathered at my place for a Sunday Night Football elliptical session. I did 60 min, giving me a total of 20.5 miles for the day. After a big weekend of work, there wasn't much left of me.	20.5
Mon.	11/22/10	Took it fairly easy: 30 min elliptical in the morning and another 45 min during Monday Night Football. I also did some light foam roller exercises and 3 sets of breath-holding.	10.7
Tues.	11/23/10	Important day: my first track workout in preparation for the Masters Indoor Nationals. Started the day with a 30-min elliptical at noon. Did a lot of stretching and icing in preparation for the evening workout at FIU. We started with a 3-mile warm-up in 21:00, then some stretching and strides. My workout was 6 x 800m at 5K pace with 600m active rest. Physically, the workout wasn't much different than the New Balance Boston workouts. The first couple of sets felt easy (2:35 and 2:32). The second 2 sets were tougher, but my times remained solid -- 2:33 and 2:30. The final 2 sets took a lot of toughness to get through. I finished strong in 2:31 and 2:29. It was 76 degrees and humid, so I had a hell of a sweat going. After a protein drink and some water, we did 6 x 50m strides and a 3-mile warm-down.	15.5
Weds.	11/24/10	Woke up sore but no worse than expected. I hit the elliptical for 30 min before my first session of the season with Alex at Miami Flexibility Trainers. Alex went relatively easy on me but noted that I had regressed quite a bit since seeing him last. I agreed. After an hr of work, I felt a lot better. Later, I hit the elliptical for 30 min.	8.6
Total		Averaged 7:01 per mile for the week	91.4

Injury Reports and Medical Findings

Psychological and Physiological Stress: Excluding my recent Masters-era coaches (Mike Ward and Kevin Curtin) I had only two 800-meter coaches in my career: Dave Barbato in high school and Mark Lech in college. I was in regular contact with Coach Dave, but I didn't want to leave any stone unturned, so I reached out to Lech.

I wasn't looking for advice on any one specific topic, but a number of topics that seemed related were puzzling me. I was seeking general observations from my time under him at Northeastern that I could compare to present day. He didn't disappoint. In fact, most everything he wrote was unique, additive, and insightful relative to the things I was focusing on during my comeback:

Gomser,

I have been taking a couple of weeks to think about your situation (trying to set the wayback machine a decade or so) and getting your most recent email [I] have come to some conclusions that I hope help. First of all see if you can get a sports psych person to help you keep things in perspective and help keep you relaxed, deal with stress etc. Second if you have disposable income you might want to either get a blood lactate meter or find someone/someplace that can do it for you on a regular basis. This is what I used to do by educated guess after I got to know your idiosyncrasies. The blood lactate test will give you a more scientific indication of the level of lactic acid in your system to tell you if you have recovered enough from the last workout to do the next one.

To use one, you just need to get a reading when your body is in equilibrium or recovery. Then, when you do a hard workout and lactase (the new word for lactic acid) is increased you want to make sure that your body has recovered enough (gone back to normal level) for the next hard workout. Another clue to over-training is taking your pulse first thing in the morning after you wake but before you get up. Take it when you feel normal then you can monitor it when you feel lousy. As a rule of thumb, if it is 10 beats/minute more than usual, your body needs more rest... or you might be getting sick.

The last thing you want to do now is beat your head against the wall working hard and run yourself into the ground. It's great to think you have to be tough on yourself but at the same time you have to listen to your body. Knowing when to back off and recover is the supreme sign of a pro. You don't want to do all of this work for months on end and get sick or hurt just before the big race. Like Bowerman said, it's better to be a bit undertrained and make it to the starting line than to try and balance on that tightrope between highly fine-tuned and being over-trained. Remember to keep the recovery days recovery pace, don't dig a hole for yourself. You have to ask yourself how long you can hold the level of work you are doing. Physiologically you should only need 6 weeks of specific training before your race and a week or so to rest/peak if you think you need it.

As for workouts make lactate threshold work a big part of your training (every 10th day or so) and do workouts that are specific to what you want to accomplish. It's not that complicated, like Roger Bannister did, just take the components of the race and break them down for your workouts. How much work/distance do you have to do to race 800 meters? For the latest kid I had that broke 4 minutes in the mile, I gave 4 x 400 meters under 60 seconds with 20 seconds rest in-between. Once he could accomplish that, he knew he was ready to run sub-4... Let me know if you have any questions.

Good luck,

Mark Lech

One thing that was different during my comeback was the level of stress I felt when compared with high school and college – so I didn't take Lech's suggestion about the sports psych expert. Make no mistake about it, I still put myself through intense torture every race day – and still felt an ominous pit in my stomach before races or even hard workouts – but I didn't feel that the stress obviated good performances. Truth be told, in hindsight I don't think I ran a bad race as a Master. Some races were closer to perfect than others, but none of them were clunkers. You might blame that on maturity/perspective; I think some of it was due to my process. On race days – and really almost every day – I had a specific order with which I approached my time leading up to races or workouts. I also played around with my pre-race playlist on my iPod – which probably sounds trivial, but given that I'm such a music-oriented person, I think it had a real effect.

I became pretty good at tricking myself that I wouldn't have to suffer much through rationalization. I would tell myself, "Well, the first 400 meters of an 800 shouldn't feel like much at all if I'm running the race right, then the next 200 meters is controlled intensity, so it's really only the last 200 meters that is bad... and that should be less than 30 seconds."

I was never able to get my hands on a blood-lactate meter either, but Lech's advice here cemented my theories around supercompensation – which I continued to research and attempted to perfect until the end of my mission. To this day, it's one of my guiding principles behind any training program.

Training Log Week 95

Day	Date	Notes	Mileage
Thurs.	11/25/10	Turkey Trot 5K today. Despite being late and cutting short my warm-up, I went out at a very controlled pace (5:20). I remained steady through Mile 2 (another 5:20) but I started feeling it. The last mile required a lot of toughness. I only ran 5:40, but that was enough. The last 0.2 miles were on the track where I ran the 4:29 mile last year. That was enough inspiration to kick and finish in 16:50. Did a 4-mile warm-down at 7:15-7:30 pace.	10.0
Fri.	11/26/10	Jamie and I left Miami for St. Lucia. I turn 40 in a few days, so some friends are meeting us to celebrate. I did 30 min on the elliptical before we left and hoped to do more in the evening, but it took longer to get to the resort than expected and hitting the roads didn't seem so smart. I did some plyometrics at the resort (lateral lunges and step-ups). It wasn't much, but it was solid for what I had to work with.	4.3
Sat.	11/27/10	After a night of partying, I woke up with the St. Lucia sun. Considering the revelry I expected later, I decided to get my morning run out of the way. There was only one problem: the compound was 500 ft above sea level, and the only direction to run was toward the sea about a mile away – steep! Later I did 40 min of high-knee running in the pool and some step-ups.	10.9
Sun.	11/28/10	Woke up early again. Today my friends Ian and Jeremi turned 40, so I expected the partying would reach a fever pitch. Thus, I hit the roads for 60 min to ensure a full day's work. St. Lucia's hills gave me another lesson in humility. The down-hills were too steep to run fast. The up-hills were too steep to run fast. I logged my mileage based on effort, rather than the actual pace, which was a laughable 9+ min per mile.	8.3
Mon.	11/29/10	33 min on St. Lucia's ridiculous hills. The Garmin estimates that some of my route was at 50% grade, and that's probably right. At points I could reach out and touch the road in front of me with my hand. Rick Miller and Jeff Baker couldn't believe I could run these routes at all. At midnight I am officially a Masters athlete!	4.7
Tues.	11/30/10	To celebrate my birthday, Miller and Baker joined me in a fool's errand: we decided to hike the Gros Piton. It's 3,000ft straight up – not a rolling 3,000ft mountain you'd find in the States. The guides didn't tell us until we finished, but most tourists can't finish the climb. *No one* had climbed it since a recent hurricane. Halfway up, my climb turned into a race with one of the guides; Miller and Baker hung back. It took us 3 hrs round-trip. The guides gave us props, revealing that those who make it typically take 5 hrs and start from a higher elevation. However a hike doesn't qualify as a "training day" for me. I had to hit the pool for 30 min of cardio.	14.3
Weds.	12/1/10	Jamie and I headed home to Miami. I suited up for an 11:30p elliptical session – just enough time to keep my training streak alive. I learned the hard way our gym closes at 11:00. I scrambled upstairs to grab my watch and ran 4 miles in 26:50 (6:42 pace).	4.0
Total		Averaged 7:30 per mile for the week	56.4

Dietary Research and Findings

Endurolytes: Bryan Huberty recommended Hammer Nutrition's Endurolytes product. Eudurolytes is supposed to replenish an athlete's full complement of electrolytes. Based on my research, I believe it is a legitimate product. It's a specially formulated mix of nutrients, primarily vitamin B-6 and manganese. That said, my diet was already rich in B-6, manganese, and the other nutrients found in Endurolytes. After a hard workout, I gravitated toward a protein shake followed by a meal shortly after that. Combing these whole foods with Endurolytes seemed at best redundant and at worst counter-effective, so I did not include it in my regular diet. However, it might be good for athletes with different eating habits.

SportLegs: Bryan Huberty also resurfaced the topic of SportLegs. I first researched SportLegs when I was exploring lactic buffers, but I didn't explore too deeply. SportLegs is a direct competitor to generic cal-mag pills, but it is specifically formulated for athletes. It uses calcium lactate monohydrate and magnesium lactate dihydrate. (Calcium and magnesium have a variety of suffixes, like carbonate, citrate, gluconate, oxide, and phosphate. Each of these forms acts differently. The most notable difference tends to be the speed and volume with which the calcium or magnesium gets absorbed by your system.)

SportLegs explains this in great depth on their Web site:[87]

> *Lactate, commonly called lactic acid, is turning out to be seriously amazing stuff. Science no longer regards it as a waste product of anaerobic exercise, as was thought for most of the 20th century. Lactate is now recognized as a key carbohydrate muscle fuel source which muscles produce, exchange and consume both at rest and during exercise... At rest and during light exercise, your muscles balance lactate production and consumption, producing just as much lactate as they consume. But kicking up the pace upsets the balance:*

> *When you start serious exercise, muscles produce more lactate than they consume, particularly at altitude, which is why skiers and mountain bike racers suffer more "burn" than most. This continues until the concentration of lactate in your blood rises enough to signal muscles to stop producing excess lactate. Until this happens, a domino effect begins which limits your subsequent performance: Lactate accumulates in muscles; limbs "pump up" and feel heavier. The harder you exercise, the more lactate accumulates. Lactate accumulated from flow imbalance quickly becomes acidic and even less mobile, further exacerbating accumulation. This "Lactic Acidosis" is classically associated with reduced Lactate Threshold, reaching the "burn point" at a lower level of exertion. Muscular strength plummets as well...*

> *SportLegs uses lactate, your body's primary high-exertion muscle fuel, to signal muscles not to overproduce lactate before you even begin exercise. Muscles switch from lactate overproduction to net lactate consumption in response to a rise in blood lactate concentration, regardless of whether blood lactate is raised naturally or from exogenous infusion.*

Based on what I learned about lactate, lactic acid, and calcium/magnesium, SportLegs claims sounded valid. Just to be sure, I did a little research on the key ingredients: calcium lactate monohydrate and magnesium lactate dehydrate. I determined that these ingredients are indeed superior for absorption:

➤ The solubility and bioavailability of magnesium L-lactate dihydrate are higher than those of other magnesium formulations, and the low incidence of side effects and a bid dosing schedule may provide the additional benefit of patient compliance.[88]
➤ According to Cathy Carlson-Rink, MD, a doctor of naturopathic medicine and member of the Canadian Naturopathic Association, calcium lactate and calcium gluconate have the highest levels of solubility in the

---

87 www.SportLegs.com/how/how.asp

88 Source: [Google: geriatric times + improving magnesium absorption]

body, making it easier for calcium to be absorbed in the intestines. As a result, calcium lactate is sometimes prescribed to prevent or treat calcium deficiencies.[89]

I wished the calcium lactate monohydrate and magnesium lactate dehydrate were in separate pills, to minimize the calcium and magnesium competing for absorption – but when an athlete is within a couple hours of competition, there's no choice but to take them together.

Technical Tip – *Magnesium is extremely vital to athletes, and unless you really overdo it, it's hard to over-supplement (although you can; I learned the hard way). That said, magnesium and calcium compete with one another for absorption. As such, it's best to consume them at different times of the day to maximize the absorption of each. calcium citrate and magnesium citrate are superior alternatives to cal-mag pills. The calcium citrate can be taken first in the day. The magnesium citrate can be taken later. Rice bran is a great low-calcium source of magnesium. It also contains a healthy dose of potassium.*

Training Log Week 96			
<u>Day</u>	<u>Date</u>	<u>Notes</u>	<u>Mileage</u>
Thurs.	12/2/10	Woke up *sore*. St. Lucia's hills and Grand Piton hike had a delayed effect; my quads felt shredded to the bone. But the show must go on: 30-min elliptical in the morning, then the Nike 5K tempo run at night – with a 5K warm-up and 4.5-mile warm-down. The tempo run started slow as usual but quickly accelerated to sub-6:00 pace. Strong first day back.	15.0
Fri.	12/3/10	Much needed recovery day. 30-min elliptical sessions in the morning and evening.	8.6
Sat.	12/4/10	Started the day with drills. John Cormier and I did 6 sets of 30-sec drills, with 100m sprints. John kicked my ass on 5 of the 6 sprints. He's fast! His goal is to run a sub 18:00 5K, but I think he could place at the Masters' Indoor Nationals in the 400m. That night I put in a 30-min elliptical session.	11.7
Sun.	12/5/10	Woke "early" at 10a. Jamie and I were out until 4a and I had wanted a full 8 hrs sleep, so I strapped on some ice packs, swallowed a tablespoon of honey,[90] and went back to bed. When I got up for real, I hit the elliptical for 10 miles. Then, I put in 4 miles on the roads (6:20 pace). I hopped in the ocean to cool my legs (good for recovery) and did four 20-sec sprints while I was waist deep, plus some recovery jogging. Long day.	18.3
Mon.	12/6/10	Opened the wk at 145.5lbs – 7 or 8lbs less than I was opening the wk a month ago. More importantly, I feel 100% healthy. I think I'll hit 140lbs and settle at that weight until Indoor Nationals. Training-wise, I did my standard recovery routine: 30-min elliptical sessions in the morning and evening.	8.6
Tues.	12/7/10	Jogged to Alex's office for a 30-min flexibility session. I usually see him on Wednesdays (*after* speed work), but he was booked. He loosened me up and applied some Kinesio tape to my calf (just as a precaution). The evening's workout was listed as 800/200, 600/200, 400/200 at 70% of goal pace. "800/200" meant that we had to run a strong 800m, then "float" for 100m, then go right into a fast 200m. After, we'd get 200m rest. The concept applied to all the reps. Using a chart provided by Brian "Jackson" Moore and my peak target of 1:55 for 800m, I estimated my goals to be: 2:29, 1:49, and 65, respectively, and 31.5 for the 200s. The 800m rep went smoothly in 2:28; I floated the 100m in 28 sec and went straight into a 32-sec 200m. The rest of the workout got progressively harder. I ran a 1:48/30 and a 64/31, all faster than the prescribed times. The whole workout only took 11 min, but it felt as bad as a longer workout. I added 4 x 200m in 28-30 sec after taking plenty of rest. Immediately after, I gulped down a protein drink, did some strides, stretching, and drills. I didn't feel like warming down on the unlit track, so at home I did a 2.5-mile equivalent on the elliptical.	13.2
Weds.	12/8/10	Recovery day: 30-min elliptical with Bryan in the morning; 30-min elliptical with Matt in the evening, plus hamstring stretches, runners' curls and 10 min of upper-body work.	8.6
Total		Averaged 6:51 per mile for the week	**84.0**

---

89 Source: [Google: livestrong + calcium lactate + 22077]

90 Honey is great for recovery due to its high fructose content and anti-inflammatory properties; Source: [Google:"outside online" + honey + recovery]

Training Log Week 97			
Day	Date	Notes	Mileage
Thurs.	12/9/10	30-min elliptical in the morning, then my usual 5K warm-up/5K tempo run with the Nike crew. Ran 18:00 – a slow-ish first mile (6:21), then 2 miles in 5:32 each and a fast finish. Jamie and I had an event to attend that night, so I had no time to warm-down. I hit the elliptical for 30 min after the event. This is the strongest, freshest I've felt since my 1:57 800m, despite averaging about 75 miles per wk for the past month.	14.8
Fri.	12/10/10	Recovery day. I felt strong, so I hit the packed sand of South Beach with Bryan Huberty in the morning. We covered 4 miles in 30 min (7:16 pace), solid work considering the surface. Later I added some elliptical.	8.4
Sat.	12/11/10	Drill day. We were able to work out on the Flamingo Track infield, which is usually closed to the public – it's a soft surface, as opposed to the hard asphalt of the track. We took our time warming up and did 6 sets of 30-sec drills, with 100m sprints. It was pretty easy for me. In fact, I felt so unfulfilled that I decided to head out with Bryan for an evening 7-mile run. I felt more fulfilled after that. After both workouts, I engaged in standard recovery activities (protein drink, stretching, icing).	15.1
Sun.	12/12/10	Bryan and I ran 14 miles in 75-degree heat around South Beach and Miami, averaging a steady 7:09 per mile. It may have been the easiest 14-miler of my life. With the water loss, I weighed in at 138lbs, my lightest since I was a freshman at NU! I took an ice bath, stretched, and downed a protein drink, a low-cal Gatorade, and a banana. Next, I took a hot shower, slapped on some ice bags, and had a balanced lunch. Later, I did 30 min on the elliptical while watching Sunday Night Football.	18.3
Mon.	12/13/10	Opened the wk at exactly 142lbs, 2lbs shy of my goal weight for Indoor Nationals. I did 30 min of elliptical work in the morning and evening. I also spent 20 min stretching, working abs and doing runners' curls.	8.6
Tues.	12/14/10	Put in a 30-min elliptical session in the early afternoon before a chilly (45 degrees) evening track workout, which was 4 x 600m/100m float/200m with 200 rest between reps. Similar to last week, but done at 75% of goal pace. The goal-paces for a 1:55 800m at 75% effort were 1:45.4 for 600m and 30.3 for 200m. After the second set, I worried that I bit off more than I could chew. I told myself to treat the 3rd set like it was the last and hope for the best on the final set. My recent spike in mileage must have kicked in, because my final set was 1:42.4 for 600m and 30.9 for 200m – my best of the night. My average was 1:44.9 for the 600s, better than goal pace, but this was offset by my 200s: a 31.8-sec average. Strange -- I thought I was doing the 200s right. We cooled down with a very easy 3 miles.	13.0
Weds.	12/15/10	Recovery day. I had a flexibility session with Alex, which included a 1.25 mile warm-up and warm-down. As usual, the flexibility session was a light workout unto itself. Today, Alex did some work on my sore hammy, but everything else feels 100%.	7.9
Total		Averaged 6:51 per mile for the week	84.0

Mapping Diet to Race Weight: Based on Dr. George Sheehan's research on race weight (see Chapter 10), I took steps to drop from a steady 150 pounds into the low 140s. I felt this would have me in peak condition in time for my first attempt at a national Masters title – in March of 2011 at the USATF Masters Indoor Track Championships, in Albuquerque. This meant another visit to the Web site FItDay.com.

According to FitDay, I was taking in 2,800 calories per day, versus 3,200 earlier in my training. I had cut my portion sizes by about 15 percent. Meanwhile, my caloric output increased from 3,200 to 3,400 (via more mileage). With 2,800 calories in and 3,400 out, I was losing a little over one pound per week on average; 3,500 calories = one pound. After eight weeks, I was close to 140 pounds, lean, and ripped.

One way I cut calories while training heavily – and not feeling like I was fasting – was to focus on foods with a very low calories-to-gram ratio. By keeping the calorie/gram count low, I could eat plenty of food without packing in calories. I tried to stick to foods that have less than 3 calories per gram, but I made a few exceptions in moderation (most notably raisins and nuts). Pure fat has nine calories per gram; pure protein has four calories per gram, as do carbohydrates – but the non fat/protein/carb content of foods can get the calories-to-gram ratio under three if you make the right choices. Many foods with low calorie/gram ratios are rich in protein, which can ease the mental burden of sticking to a diet. Obviously protein is essential to building the muscle for athletic performance, as well.

As the table below shows, canned tuna is a calories-per-gram and protein powerhouse, offering a 28-to-1 ratio of protein to other nutrients. By adding tuna to my daily diet, I increased my daily protein intake significantly while still dropping weight in preparation for the 2011 Indoor Nationals.

Calorie and Protein Ratios in Common Foods

Food	Cals	Fat (g)	Carbs (g)	Protein (g)	Protein-to-Other Nutrients Ratio	Cals-per-Protein Gram
Tuna, canned, water packed	39	0.3	0.0	8.5	28.3x	4.6 cals
GNC Whey Protein	120	1.0	3.0	24.0	6.0x	5.0 cals
Salmon, cooked	30	0.9	0.0	5.0	5.6x	6.0 cal
Chicken, roasted/broiled/baked, no skin	422	16.5	0.0	64.3	3.9x	6.6 cals
Beef steak	71	4.3	0.0	7.7	1.8x	9.2 cals
Egg, whole, cooked	33	2.4	0.3	2.5	0.9x	13.2 cals
Spinach, raw	7	0.1	1.1	0.9	0.8x	7.8 cals

Training Log Week 98

Day	Date	Notes	Mileage
Thurs.	12/16/10	Due to a change in plans, I made today an easy day: two 30-min sessions on the elliptical. The change is, I'll be working out with Mike Ward's guys at FIU tomorrow – essentially a try-out. The former long-time University of Miami coach has guided multiple middle-distance runners to the Olympics and/or NCAA championships.	8.6
Fri.	12/17/10	Met Coach Ward and his team at 9a. The assignment was 2 x 400m at goal pace with 2 min rest. It sounded easy, but it was designed to simulate an 800m race, so clearly it was not. We started with a different warm-up than I had ever done. Rather than an easy run, we did a series of drills on grass, involving skipping, hopping, and something that was like a lateral-moving jumping jack. Then, we moved to the track for some more familiar drills, like butt kicks, high knees, A-skips, and B-skips. Finally, we did 4 x 150m accelerating strides, the first two in flats and the second two in spikes. By the end of the 150s, I had felt some lactic acid buildup. At the starting line, Coach Ward told us to focus on running even splits. The pace seemed fast, but I didn't question it. I passed 200m in 27.5 sec, started feeling the lactic acid kick in around 300m, and struggled to keep up on the final straightaway. I finished in 55.9 sec. After 2 min, we lined up again. Coach Ward advised us to relax and maintain form, then sent us off. By the 200m, I was toast. I finished in 61 sec. Clearly, I wasn't ready for this kind of workout. I needed more speed and lactic-acid tolerance. We did a 3-mile warm-down, then Coach Ward had us do circuit drills. Later, I rounded out the day with 30 min on the elliptical.	13.7
Sat.	12/18/10	Coach Ward gave me the green light to train with his 800m runners; I'm pretty excited. Bryan and I ran 10 miles (7:00 pace), mostly on pavement but on grass where possible.	10.0
Sun.	12/19/10	Did 50 min on the elliptical around 1pm and massaged my legs with The Stick before bed.	7.2
Mon.	12/20/10	Hit the track with Coach Ward's guys. Same warm-up as Friday's, sans the 150m strides. The workout was 8 x 400m in 74 sec with 74 sec rest. The pace was easy for me and the rest period was much more than I needed. But Coach picked the pace and rest for a reason, so I tried to hold myself in check. Still, I finished most of the 400s in under 70 sec, including a 65 at the end. After, I asked Coach Ward if I pushed it too hard. He said, "A little." Usually, I would have kept myself under control, but there was a little chip on my shoulder from Friday. I think I needed to show that I was legit. It was selfish, but I'll be good from now on. After the workout, we cooled down with 2.5 miles, followed by 2 x 20-sec circuit drills.	12.0
Tues.	12/21/10	Recovery Day. Jogged to and from Alex's office for 1 hr flexibility training. In the p.m., I did a 30-min elliptical.	6.5
Weds.	12/22/10	Workout day: We did the standard Coach Ward warm-up drills, plus 3 x 150m strides to prepare for 8 x 150m at 19 sec each. We ran the first 4 sets in flats to acclimate our muscles to the speed, then we laced up the spikes. I was able to hit the time, but it was 100% effort. After, we did a 3-mile cool-down, then a set of 20-sec circuits. At home, I went heavy on recovery activities. I did some runners' curls, worked with the foam roller, and hit the elliptical for a 35-min easy session.	9.5
Total		Averaged 6:49 per mile for the week	63.1

Training Log Week 99			
Day	Date	Notes	Mileage
Thurs.	12/23/10	Woke up sore, but not really worse for wear. I started tracking my resting heart rate, which was 58, identical to yesterday. I didn't feel any strains, even in my calves. I did my standard recovery-day 30-min elliptical sessions in the morning and evening.	7.2
Fri.	12/24/10	With the Christmas weekend pending, I decided to do my long run early. I met John, Bryan, Jason Miller, and Dan Potter for an easy run on the beach. We found a new grassy field and a nearby golf course to take some of the strain off our legs, and we finished with 10.8 miles in 1:21:08 (7:31 pace). I barely broke a sweat. Later, Bryan, John, and I hit the gym for 20 min on the elliptical, plus stretching, ab and upper-body work, and some light quad lifts.	10.3
Sat.	12/25/10	Started my Christmas with drills. John and I were joined by Alex, who is new to Track Club Miami. He is training for a sprint triathlon and the Miami Marathon. I warmed up for 1.5 miles (6:00 pace) and added a slow mile with the group. Next we did 8 x 30-sec drills with 100m strides and 15 pushups. I cooled down for 2 miles and later hit the elliptical for 32 min prior to a great Christmas dinner with Jamie.	12.0
Sun.	12/26/10	Recovery day: 30-min elliptical, plus stretching and "The Stick."	7.2
Mon.	12/27/10	Workout day with Coach Ward's guys. Standard drill-based warm-up, then intervals: 2 x 1,000m; 2 x 800m; 1 x 400m – all run at 5-min mile pace. Rest time matched the interval time. I achieved or exceeded the goals: 3:10, 3:06, 2:28, 2:28, and 69 sec. After, we did 2 slow miles to warm down. That night I logged a 45-min elliptical and several weight circuits, focusing on hamstrings, calves, quads, abs and runners' curls.	10.4
Tues.	12/28/10	Recovery day. I did 50 min on the elliptical at a decent pace. Later, I hit the gym for stretching and work with the foam roller.	4.8
Weds.	12/29/10	Another Coach Ward workout: 18 x 200m at 32 sec per, with 60 sec rest. Endurance-wise, this was an easy workout. I was very comfortable and below 32 sec on all but the 3rd rep. I had no trouble with the rest. I could feel the intervals getting to me after the 12th, but not enough to slow me or affect my perfect form. However, if I had to go all-out for one rep, I wouldn't have run well. My calves started to strain after the 10th rep. I adjusted my form, which helped. After the intervals, we did a slow 2.2-mile warm down, followed by 2 sets of circuit drills. When I got home, I iced thoroughly and took a hot shower, which left just enough time to put on a fresh running clothes and head to see Alex. I was still loose from the workout, so the jog to Alex's was fairly brisk (6:09 pace). The session itself was the most painful part of the day. My calves were pretty troubled after that workout. Alex advised me to walk home and then ice the calves again. I complied. Later, I hit the elliptical for 30 min of aerobic/recovery work.	12.1
Total		Averaged 6:41 per mile for the week	63.9

In presenting data on diet, I feel it is important to note another key component to my training philosophy: Diet is but a tool in your workshop, and you should wield this tool in *different ways* depending on where you are in your training cycle and what your physiological needs may be at the time. I utilized a low-calorie, high-protein diet to accomplish two things simultaneously – shed weight and build muscle for the 800 meters, which is arguably a power event. Most Kenyans, who specialize in long distance events, maintain high-carb diets with high nitrate contents (see Chapter 7). Consuming 1,400 grams of protein each week, like I was during my pre-indoor nationals training phase, probably wouldn't help them prepare for world-class marathons.

An extreme example of wielding diet as a training tool was evidenced by my co-author, Rick Miller. After struggling with a severe foot injury for more than a year – and packing on some serious weight due to missed training and general malaise – Miller underwent invasive surgery that had him in a cast for months. Unable to train in any capacity, he focused aggressively on diet, adopting Tim Ferriss' "Slow Carb" approach. He shed more than 20 pounds from diet alone, and when he resumed training got up to speed quickly and mostly injury-free – then shed almost 20lbs more.

Researching and planning your diet can seem daunting because there are many sources that advise what a "proper" diet is. The International Sports Sciences Association (ISSA) advises athletes to follow a 1-2-3 Nutritional Rule-of-Thumb. In short, 1-2-3 means that for every 1 gram of fat you take in, you should take in two grams of protein and three grams of carbs. On a percentage basis, the right mix would be 50 percent carbs, 33 percent protein, and 16 percent fat.[91] But that probably wouldn't work for a Kenyan marathoner.

---

91 www.criticalbench.com/nutrient_ratios.htm

The American Heart Association's Nutrition Committee presents somewhat different guidelines for healthy Americans, at least around fat consumption – where they allow fat to comprise 25-35 percent of total intake, but suggest these additional practices:

➢ Limit *saturated* fat intake to less than 7 percent of total daily calories
➢ Limit *trans* fat intake to less than 1 percent of total daily calories
➢ Remaining fat should come from sources of monounsaturated and polyunsaturated fats such as nuts, seeds, fish and vegetable oils
➢ Limit cholesterol intake to less than 300mg per day, but if you have coronary heart disease or your LDL cholesterol level is 100 mg/dL or greater, limit your cholesterol intake to less than 200mg per day."

Those guidelines are certainly useful to members of the general public aiming to live healthy; they weren't completely useful to me when I was trying to shed weight.

Training Log Week 100

Day	Date	Notes	Mileage
Thurs.	12/30/10	Recovery day. I started with some icing and stretching at dawn. After a nap, I did 50 min on the elliptical.	7.2
Fri.	12/31/10	As is Coach Ward's norm, his final speed workout of the wk was the toughest: standard warm-up, 3 x 150m strides, then 2 sets of 4 x 200m at 26- to 27-sec pace, with 90 sec rest between reps and 5 min rest between sets. At this point in the season, 27-sec 200s were a 90%+ effort for me. It got harder for everyone as the workout wore on; I felt lactic acid build-up at the end of the 3rd rep. The 5-min break between sets wasn't enough. My times slipped, despite my best efforts to push and maintain good form, but I put in a good effort and will benefit from it. My average time was under 28 sec until the last rep. We finished the workout with a slow 3-mile cool-down, followed by 1 set of circuits. At home, I performed my typical recovery activities. I hit the gym in the afternoon for a 30-min elliptical, runners' curls and a few sets on the ab machine. I rallied in time for Jamie and I to enjoy a great New Year's dinner at Indomania!	10.3
Sat.	1/1/11	I started 2011 by hitting the track for a light drill workout. I did a slow 1-mile warm-up and some stretching beforehand. Then I did a handful of drills, 60m strides, and pushups, but kept the effort very easy. Next Bryan and I went out for some easy distance; I went 10 miles, picking it up sharply the final 2. When I finished, I guzzled a Mix 1 recovery drink and went into full recovery mode. Later, I hit the gym for a weight workout.	12.0
Sun.	1/2/11	Recovery day: 50-min elliptical session and plenty of stretching throughout the day. I felt good, considering the weekend I had. I think a month of double sessions is paying dividends.	7.2
Mon.	1/3/11	Track workout: 8 x 400m in 73 sec with 73 sec rest. We started with 71 sec and steadily picked it up. After the 7th rep (67 sec), Coach Ward reprimanded us. I nodded apologetically and dropped to the back of the pack. We came through in 70 sec to finish the workout – not a 73, but not a 67 either. Immediately after, I drank a banana/whey-protein mix, did a 3-mile cool-down, and asked Coach Ward the optimal time/days to lift. He said I should lift right after our workouts, leaving the maximum amount of time for between-workout recovery. Later I did 6 x 60m sprints in the thick grass behind our building, then 45 min of lifting. I focused on leg exercises, mixing dynamic reps with static (lift and hold) reps and a 90-degree bend at the knee. After that, I hit the elliptical for 30 min and headed home for recovery (banana/whey-protein drink/ice bath/hot Jacuzzi).	10.4
Tues.	1/4/11	Recovery day: stretching, a few drills, a few strides, and 32:30 on the elliptical.	4.8
Weds.	1/5/11	Speed work with Coach Ward: standard warm-up, followed by 2 sets, 4 x 100m w/rest of 100m walk back to the starting line. The first set was in flats; the second in spikes. Coach Ward sought 13-sec 100s for the first set and 12.5-sec 100s for the second set. For me, every rep of every set was all-out. Coach Ward clocked most of my reps in the low- to mid-13s, with 12.9s for the 5th and 6th reps. I fatigued on the 7th and 8th sets, but aerobically I recovered quickly. We did a 4-mile warm-down and a set of circuits. I had a flexibility session with Alex. The sprints did a number on my calves, tightening them up like rocks. Alex did a number on them, loosening them back up. (I jogged there at 6:51 pace, but Alex advised me to walk home.) I hit the gym at 6p, for a weight workout and 35 min on the elliptical. Date Night was a 2-hr Salsa class with Jamie!	12.1
Total		Averaged 6:59 per mile for the week	63.9

Race Reports, Records and Results

<u>**2010 Run Miami Turkey Trot:**</u> I went to bed at 10:30 the night before Thanksgiving in anticipation of the Turkey Trot. Unfortunately, my body didn't like the idea. I awoke just after midnight. After a lot of tossing, turning, and some reading, I finally fell back asleep around 2:45. My alarm went off three hours later.

I was tired and still sore from a workout I did two days prior and from a flexibility session with Alex. I suited up and called my building's valet to pull my car around. Unfortunately, the valet couldn't find my car. *Great...* they actually found a way to lose my gigantic SUV.

"So much for the Turkey Trot," I thought. The day was not starting well.

Luckily, the vehicle turned up after 10 minutes of the valets scrambling around. I was off to the race, but now I was late. By the time I got there, I had two choices. Warm up or register for the race. That was a no brainer. I headed out for a 2.85-mile warm-up and did a few strides.

I got to the starting line with a couple minutes to spare. I started at a very controlled pace, going out in a 5:20 first mile. Along the course, I endured a few "bandito" calls, referring to my lack of a race number. No worries. I remained steady through Mile 2 with another 5:20. The last mile was hard and required a lot of toughness. My third mile was only 5:40, but that was good enough. The finish was on the same track where I ran the 4:29 mile earlier that year. That was enough inspiration to muster up a kick and finish in 16:50.

I was very happy with that performance. It was faster than I ran at the Tropical 5K 10 months earlier and 15 seconds faster than what I ran at the Mayor's Cup in Boston. Considering the situation and the intense training coming into the race, this was a much stronger performance than the small improvement implied on paper.

Miscellaneous Research and Notes

<u>**Racing at Altitude:**</u> Knowing that I'd be racing at altitude when I visited Albuquerque for the USATF Masters Indoor Nationals, I sought the advice a pair of former world-class athletes who had dealt with altitude in their travels. I asked them about the benefits of devices like altitude tents to prepare. Here is what they said:

➢ **Erik Nedeau:** Altitude is a funny, tricky thing, with mixed results for different people. I have been at it on two occasions... three if you count NCAAs in Boise my senior year, which was [roughly] 3,000 feet. I did not feel like altitude affected me in Boise. In my first run there I felt a little heavier, and the run was a little harder than it should have been for an easy day, but the actual racing did not feel any different.

  I was in Utah two years ago for two weeks, and I was in Colorado *and* Utah this year for two weeks, and I certainly noticed a difference because the altitude was between 6,500 and 10,000 feet. I expended more effort and the runs definitely were tougher than they should have been, but I seemed to figure things out after a week. My biggest problem was hydration. I am not the best at drinking water, and I really suffered in the first few days. The runs were not *too* bad, but shortly after I was on the crapper constantly because of dehydration. Until I got a good handle on that, it was not all that enjoyable.

  I have heard two things about altitude: Get in the night before and race the next day, *or* get in more than a week before and take the time to adjust. The middle ground is the toughest– coming in Wednesday or Thursday for a Saturday race.

Training Log Week 101

Day	Date	Notes	Mileage
Thurs.	1/6/11	Woke up very sore. Yesterday's 100s wrecked my hamstrings and the weight work wrecked everything else. And tomorrow I have a critical race simulation with Coach Ward. I spent the day in heavy recovery mode and only did 35 min on the elliptical to loosen the legs.	5.0
Fri.	1/7/11	Very evident that I worked too hard on Wednesday. We did our standard warm-up, and I felt ok until we did strides. My hamstrings were sore, and on the second stride, I felt a pop in my left quad. It was a slight twinge, but I knew it was trouble for the workout: 3 x 300m in 42 sec. Coach Ward decided a race simulation was too risky. I did 18 x 200m at 32-sec pace with 1 min rest. Fortunately it went smoothly. We jogged 3 miles at 7:15 pace and did two sets of circuit drills. At home, I focused on recovery and skipped my evening elliptical.	6.2
Sat.	1/8/11	Went to the track to lead drills, but I took it easy. *Leading* the workout isn't the same as *doing* it! I warmed up for a few miles, and did a few drills and all the pushups with the group. After, John Cormier joined me for a long jog; neither of us wanted to push. At 8 miles, he dropped off at his house and I continued to mine. Totaled 9.6 miles (8:09 pace) – easy but a lot of sun time. Back to recovery, starting with a long ice bath.	12.2
Sun.	1/9/11	*Still* not 100% healthy (hamstrings). I opted for a 30-min elliptical and a leisurely walk on Lincoln Road with Jamie, my sister Tammy, nephew Austin, niece Karina, and Karina's baby daughter, Avah.	4.3
Mon.	1/10/11	Recovered and legs felt ready for today's workout. I made good progress since my first track workout of the season, back in November, when I did 6 x 800m with about 3 min rest. (I averaged 2:32 per rep.) Today, we did 5 x 800m with 2:30 rest. My adjusted times were 2:23, 2:19, 2:17, 2:23, and 2:16 – under 2:20 average. After the workout, I drank a banana/milk/protein-powder mix, then we did a 2-mile warm-down at 7:06 pace. Later, I worked the foam roller and weights. I need to shore up my strength/power. I did upper- and lower-body, but I moderated my effort, aiming for the right balance between effort and recovery.	5.6
Tues.	1/11/11	Easy day: I jogged to a PT/flexibility session with Alex at 1p. Later, I hit the gym for 35 min on the elliptical.	6.1
Weds.	1/12/11	Coach Ward changed our workout from a speed session to something more strength-related: 2 sets of 8 x 200m – the first set at 32-sec pace (in flats), with 1:00 rest per rep; then a break to change into spikes, followed by the second set at 30-sec pace. With the exception of the 14th rep, I fared well, averaging 29.8 sec in the first set and 29.7 sec in the second set. Later I hit the elliptical for a 30-min recovery session.	10.2
Total		Averaged 6:53 per mile for the week	**49.6**

Training Log Week 102

Day	Date	Notes	Mileage
Thurs.	1/13/11	With my first meet of the season in two days, I did a 60-min elliptical and called it a day.	8.6
Fri.	1/14/11	Pre-race day: hit the elliptical for the minimum (30 min) and spent the day relaxing and eating easy-to-digest foods (more carbs; less protein). I didn't get nearly as much sleep as I prefer two nights before a meet (8-10 hrs). We'll see if that impacts my performance. After yesterday's workout, my hamstrings felt mildly strained, and my right calf was back to its old tricks. I called Alex for an emergency visit, and he was able to work me in.	4.3
Sat.	1/´5/11	Pros and cons in a debacle of a track meet. We got a late start, drove 3 hrs, and dealt with typical Florida meet mismanagement. I won the 800m in a disappointing 2:02.6, but there was no one near me the entire race. I did run a 53-sec 400m leg on the relay – surprisingly fast. (See this chapter's Race Results section.)	3.2
Sun.	1/16/11	Long, easy day. My aerobic base is off the charts for an 800m runner, so more than 10 miles now is likely a waste and maybe even a hindrance. I hit the elliptical for 70 min.	10.0
Mon.	1/17/11	Coach Ward's guys did distance today, so I worked separately. Rain prevented drills, so John Cormier and I did stairs: 3 x 45 sec hard (double-steps), then 4 x 22 sec hard (single steps). It was difficult; we had to adjust downward mid-session. Next, we hit the gym for plyometric drills and lower body lifting exercises. Later, we reconvened at the gym for a recovery elliptical session and upper-body workout.	6.6
Tues.	1/18/11	Sore from yesterday. Planned an easy day, plus an Alex session. Did elliptical work (40 min) then jogged to his office. Alex worked his magic, but I was still sore. I focused on recovery, alternating ice baths and the hot tub.	5.8
Weds.	1/19/11	Still not recovered from Monday. I should have incorporated weight work on my legs earlier in my training cycle. I'm paying for it with poor recovery times. Today's workout was 2 sets of 4 x 400m – the first set at 70 sec; the second set at 65 sec. Rest was 90 sec per rep, with 4-min active rest between sets. I was under the goal times on each rep, but it hurt. After the 8th rep, I dropped to the track. I was wiped out and definitely felt worse than I did after my races last weekend. I drank half of a Muscle Milk Light for recovery then headed out on a 2.5-mile recovery jog. After, I worked the foam roller, incorporating dumbbells as handles to make it a simultaneous core/arm/leg-recovery session. After my recovery routine, I hit the elliptical (50 min), did some rowing and 20 min of upper-body weights. I'm adapting to the upper-body workouts and building muscle without gaining any weight.	13.6
Total		Averaged 6:48 per mile for the week	**52.0**

> **Kevin Curtin:** I wouldn't get an altitude tent. Being at altitude makes you ill-equipped to deal with humidity. My concern is that sleeping in the tent to prepare for Indoor Nationals would sacrifice your training in Miami.
>
> Bob Sevene[92] used to feel there were a lot of similarities between altitude and humidity training. At altitude your body learns to deal with less oxygen and thus gets more efficient, so when you go to sea level you spend less energy and can do more. In high humidity, your body devotes more blood to help keep you cool, so you get more efficient due to decreased blood volumes. So when you go somewhere without humidity, you have more blood to help you with oxygen uptake. Similar principles, different systems... Hydration is huge, especially if your travel to the race involves flying."

In my additional research, I found some notable data on altitude from one of the all-time pioneers of running research, Jack Daniels. Daniels reported that performance starts to be affected at about 3,000 feet, and the effect is not linear. A runner who is not acclimated will lose 10 to 12 percent in VO2 max at an altitude of about 6,500 feet and 12 to 15 percent at 7,500 feet. However, performance will not degrade to the same degree because running economy is better at altitude (because of the less dense air). Daniels' research at 6,500 feet indicated a 12 percent loss of VO2 max, but 6 percent improvement in running economy, resulting in 6 percent total loss in performance. The duration of a race is also a factor. A 1,500-meter race may be six to 10 seconds slower for an acclimated runner (but perhaps 20 seconds slower for an unacclimated runner). The longer the race, the more performance degradation.

Here is what *I* concluded about altitude – especially as it pertains to the 800-meter run. Although the 800-meters is *mostly* anaerobic, it's still at least 33 percent aerobic. I graphed the meters-per-second rate of world records at every distance and found that aerobic capacity *begins* to be a factor around 300 meters, so aerobic capacity in the 800-meters is important, despite its relatively short duration. (No third-party study I could find indicates aerobic capacity contributes to less than 33 percent of an 800-meter performance.) Thus, while the effect of altitude is small and largely offset by lower wind resistance, I asked, "Why not acclimate and let wind resistance become a positive, instead of merely an offset?"

The time-loss due to altitude appears linear at increasing distances, so one could surmise that the loss at 800 meters could be three to five seconds for the acclimated runner and 10 seconds for the unacclimated. If I only counted the 33 percent of the 800-meter run that is aerobic, that still equated to 1.7 seconds of performance. In a championship-level 800-meter run, that's a lot of time.

My plan was to get to Albuquerque in time to watch the USATF Open Indoor Nationals, which would give me nine or 10 days before the Masters Indoor Nationals to acclimate. I figured most of my competition would show up the Friday night before the Sunday race. Therein lay an advantage for me.

Canned Oxygen: I researched the potential benefits of canned oxygen. It is no longer banned by the World Anti-Doping Agency (WADA), but I gathered that it's probably not very useful. Some letsrun.com commenters refuted canned oxygen with some basic physiological data:

> *At rest, at sea level, your arterial blood will be between 98 percent and 99 percent saturated with oxygen. At extreme levels of exercise your arterial blood will still be at the same saturation.*
> *Getting oxygen into your body is not the limiting factor of exercise. You breathe hard when running a mile, not because you need more oxygen, but because you need to get rid of CO_2, which is a by-product of acid buffering.*

The debate on Let's Run started because someone inquired about performance mouthpieces that supposedly improve the efficiency of breathing – lessening the energy consumed through that aspect of athletic activity. In other words, let's say that breathing represents 3 percent of the energy consumption in a race. If a mouthpiece can

---

92 Bob Sevene is the legendary distance coach who trained Joan Benoit Samuelson to victory in the first-ever women's Olympic marathon in 1984. He coached many elite and sub-elite runners in New England for years, including my co-author Rick Miller.

make you 10 percent more efficient at breathing, the total performance optimization would be 0.3 percent. However, does the weight (and perhaps discomfort) of the mouthpiece have an opposite effect, thus rendering it less effective – or perhaps even counterproductive? I decided that the product was too niche to research deeper.

Although I decided *against* using canned oxygen, the research yielded some useful science on athletic performance. It became clearer to me how oxygen affects performance. ATP is what the cells in your muscles use for energy. Oxygen is needed to breakdown glucose and create ATP.

Glucose + O_2 = CO_2 + H_2O + ATP + heat

When your muscles use up the readily available oxygen, they go into "oxygen debt," where they begin to convert glucose to lactic acid and start to fatigue. If the muscles have sufficient amounts of oxygen, they will not produce lactic acid and therefore will not fatigue as quickly. Muscles store oxygen using a protein called myoglobin. It is this storage capacity that limits performance. After researching this, my question was, "How can I increase my myoglobin levels?"

David Holt, author of *10K & 5K Running, Training & Racing: The Running Pyramid*, reports that running at 80 percent of VO2 max "improves your aerobic pathways at the cellular level, stimulates more and larger mitochondria, red blood cells and myoglobin." Running up to 80 miles per week can improve fitness by as much as 12 percent. Holt claims that anything above 80 miles per week provides a lower per-mile benefit.

Other ways to increase myogloblin levels generally involve starving the muscles of blood:[93]

➤ High-angle isometric exercise – High angle means bending the limb to at least 90 degrees. In that position, blood flow to the muscles is constricted. Isometric basically means that you don't move. A good example of this would be a "wall sit" or getting into a squatted position (with knees bent about 90 degrees) and just holding it (basically, a wall-sit without the wall).
➤ Swimming in cold water – The cold would result in constricted blood vessels, thus starving the muscles.

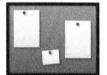

Bulletin Board Material – *Right after New Years, I received some exciting news from Chris Simpson. He had contacted Steve Vaitones, the Managing Director of USATF's New England chapter, and inquired about taking a shot at the Masters 4 x 800-meter indoor world record. Vaitones was going see if one of the upcoming indoor meets would feature a race for us to go for it.*

The logistics behind a record attempt are not as simple as one might think. For example, Harvard University's track would have made a great venue, but it was a 220 yard track, not 200 meters. The baton exchange zones were not in the right places to make a 4 x 800-meter record legitimate. After a few weeks, Chris Simpson researched a better opportunity. A meet at Tufts University would feature a 4 x 800 relay. Soon, my goals would not only include a U.S. title; they'd include a world record and a place in the sport's history books.

---

93 Source: [Google: deeperblue.com + seals + myoglobin]

Chapter 12
You're the Fastest Runner, But You're Not Allowed to Win

Weeks 103-109

My first memory of Scott Cody is from the 1987 Massachusetts State Finals in the one-mile run – my junior year. To that point, my best mile time was 4:27. Cody was several seconds faster. His Cambridge Rindge & Latin teammate, Jamahl Prince, was even faster and also in the race… In fact Prince was the best miler in the state. (Along with Cody and Prince, about 10 other guys were running comfortably under 4:30. It was a pretty deep year for the mile by Massachusetts standards.)

Luckily, my time got me into the seeded heat, which went out very fast – under 63 seconds at 400 meters, if I remember correctly. As we approached the bell lap, I found myself still in contention, feeling okay, and passing the 1,200-meter mark in 3:17. My brain said, "That's way too fast." But my body said, "That's about right." I started my kick, passed a couple kids and started chasing down Prince, who had the lead.

With 100 meters to go, Prince turned on the jets… just as mine were fizzling out. With 50 meters to go, I looked back and saw a comfortable gap between me and the next runner. I was disappointed to lose to Prince but excited to be comfortably in second place. Runner-up at the state meet was not too shabby. I pushed forward but not with 100-percent effort.

I'm sure you see what's coming…

Sure enough, just as I was taking my final step to the line, I saw something in my periphery. It was Scott Cody… and it looked like he might have out-leaned me. The officials couldn't tell. While they went for the cameras, I went for the ground.

I remember being in abject pain and begging Coach Dave to never ask me to run again. At that moment, I didn't care that I had closed the final lap in 63 seconds, giving me a huge PR. Nor did I care that I had just finished top-two or top-three in one of the hottest races of the year. All I cared about was not feeling any more pain. Of course, 20 minutes later the pain passed, and suddenly I cared about all of the above very much. Most of all, I cared about whether or not Cody had caught me. An official turned on the PA system to announce the results.

He counted down the sixth-, fifth-, and fourth-place finishers. Blah, blah, and blah. Then…

"In third place, in a time of 4:20.69, Mark Gomes from Stoughton."

Ugh.

"In second place, in a time of 4:20.66, Scott Cody from Cambridge R&L."

Ugh!! Three one-hundredths of a second!

The newspaper headline the next day read, "Cambridge Phenoms Take Top Honors in State Mile."

It could have read "Stoughton Junior Breaks Up Cambridge Phenoms," but I didn't sprint through the finish line. In hindsight, it was one of the biggest disappointments in my racing career. Sure, I was psyched to have crushed my previous PR. Finishing third in such a stacked race also felt great. But to this day, getting out-leaned by Cody is the overwhelming memory, overshadowing all the good.

It turned out to be a good lesson though. After that day, I never gave anyone the chance to catch me at less than 100-percent effort. The lesson came in handy my freshman year at Northeastern, when I outkicked Prince (who was racing for Boston College) to win the 1,000-meters at the New England Championships. On a separate occasion, Prince and I raced to an indistinguishable photo finish and were crowned Greater Boston co-champions.

At least he didn't out-lean me.

These days, Cody and Prince coach and teach in the Cambridge school system. They're both married with children and far from having run their last steps – and we are close friends.

Training Log Week 103			
Day	Date	Notes	Mileage
Thurs.	1/20/11	Post-workout recovery day. I've started to adjust these slightly. I've modestly increased the duration of my elliptical sessions to maintain my endurance and started seeing Alex more often to further my recovery. Last spring, as I peaked, my body almost fell to pieces. Preparing differently this year.	6.9
Fri.	1/21/11	The extra visits to Alex are paying dividends. I went into today's speed workout feeling healthier than I have in some time. I even felt largely recovered from the weight work I did on Wednesday. The workout consisted of fast-paced 100m, 200m, and 300m reps designed to acclimatize our bodies to getting out fast, holding a strong pace, and enduring the lactic rush down the final straightaway. In other words, I was going to be taken to task by the young guns... and it was going to hurt. Each set added up to 800m total (2 sets). My adjusted totals were 1:49.3 and 1:54.8. Later I hit the elliptical for 30 min. I weighed in at 140lbs exactly.	7.8
Sat.	1/22/11	Started my day with 30 min upper and lower body weights. Later, Matt Kiss came over to test his endurance. He'd been running 10 miles a day, but only at 8:00-8:30 pace. Today he was to stay with me for as long as possible at 7:00 pace. His 5K pace is in the low 6-min range. By training at 8:00-8:30 pace he's been putting the *slow* in long, slow distance. This workout would determine if *slow* can be too slow. My guess was yes. It didn't take long to confirm my suspicions. One mile into the run, he was breathing heavy. A half-mile later, he was 5m behind. He surged to my shoulder, but soon fell back. I demanded that he shoulder-up again. This continued until the futility was palpable. At that point, we hit the elliptical. That way, I could give Matt advice and encouragement while we worked at our own pace. I did 70 min faster than usual.	13.2
Sun.	1/23/11	Easy day of elliptical work (30 min) and strides.	5.2
Mon.	1/24/11	Twisted my ankle. It wasn't a bad twist, but it cut my warm-down short. Workout was 2 x 1,000m (sub 3:00), 2 x 800m (sub 2:20), 2 x 400m (65.6 sec and 67.5 sec). I hit lactic threshold hard on the final rep and found myself scouring my mind's collection of Happy Places. "The Bear" typically jumps on my back with 100m to go. When it kicks in earlier, it's a bitch. Clearly dazed, I scuffled awkwardly on a root during the warm-down. I caught myself in time to minimize the damage, but it was bad enough to end my session. After an afternoon of alternating ice and heat, it felt a lot better. I went out to test it. It was a little tender, but it loosened up quickly and I found myself at Flamingo Track, exactly one mile from my flat. My watch read 6:30. Not bad. I did some drills. Later Bryan came over for a 30-min elliptical session and some weight work (upper- and lower-body). I also did several 20-sec sets of plyometric jumps. After that, it was back to the ice and heat.	12.7
Tues.	1/25/11	Easy day on the elliptical (30 min), with lots of weight work, drills, and exercises (pushups, foam roller, etc).	4.3
Weds.	1/26/11	A "self-against-self" tempo run to celebrate nearly two full years of training. 6.8 miles with miles splits of 6:08, 6:03, 5:46, 5:46, 5:46 and 5:44, plus a 4:41 closer for the final 0.8-mile. The ankle held up fine; if I felt any give, I would have ended this indulgence immediately.	6.8
Total		Averaged 6:42 per mile for the week	56.9

Training Log Week 104			
Day	Date	Notes	Mileage
Thurs.	1/27/11	Happy to wake up with few ill-effects from yesterday's run. My twisted ankle was a little sore, but I think more from sleeping awkwardly. I immediately put it on ice, then applied some heat. 30 min later, it was fine. Did 23 min elliptical and light weights/plyos in the afternoon. Did Nike Run Club at night. The Nike Run Club sends groups out in reverse order of speed. The slower and recreational runners start first. It's meant to get everyone to the finish around the same time for social activities.	8.0
Fri.	1/28/11	Easy 30-min elliptical.	4.3
Sat.	1/29/11	I defended my title in the Miami Tropical 5K today in 15:55. (See Race Results section.) More interesting is that I ran negative mile splits for the first time ever: 5:12 for Mile 1, 5:08 for Mile 2, and 4:59 for Mile 3.	9.1
Sun.	1/30/11	Paced Bryan Huberty for 2.5 miles of the ING Half Marathon (5:30 pace). I was supposed to hang with him for 5 miles, but I was a mess from the past few days of hard work. I focused on recovery for the rest of the day and hit the elliptical in the p.m. for 30 min.	9.3
Mon.	1/31/11	Still a mess from killing it for 3 of the past 5 days. Saw Alex in the a.m., which helped a lot. In the p.m., I hit the gym for an elliptical session and some weight training.	4.3
Tues.	2/01/11	Saw Alex again this morning. In the p.m., I hit the elliptical again. I feel a *lot* better. Sometimes, rest and recovery are your best friends.	4.3
Weds.	2/02/11	Workout: 8 x 400m. Ran 63-66 sec per rep until the final rep (68.6). My pace for the early reps was clearly a little too fast. Overall good effort.	5.6
Total		Averaged 6:26 per mile for the week	44.9

Injury Reports and Medical Findings

Antibiotics: While researching my main competitor for a Masters title, Nick Berra, I learned he once won a race despite being diagnosed with a sinus/bronchitis-like infection a few days prior. His doctor prescribed antibiotics, and Berra went on to run his fastest 800-meter time as a Master: 1:56.3. That learned, I wondered if antibiotics aided performance in any way or were even legal to take before a race. I didn't doubt Berra's competitive ethics; but given the thousands of dietary and medical substances athletes (or humans in general) ingest on a regular basis, I wondered if the USATF or anyone else had scrutinized antibiotics.

According to the USATF, all antibiotics are acceptable for use in competition. Further, "all antihistamines are allowed and many decongestant containing products available by prescription or over-the-counter are permitted due to the fact that pseudoephedrine and phenylephrine are now permitted in and out of competition time. A similar decongestant ingredient, ephedrine, is available in very few products but would still be considered a prohibited substance in-competition time as a stimulant."[94]

In addition, according to the World Anti-Doping Agency (WADA), bupropion, caffeine, phenylephrine, phenylpropanolamine, pipradol, pseudoephedrine, and synephrine were included in WADA's 2008 Monitoring Program and therefore *not* considered prohibited substances.

Adrenaline associated with local anesthetic agents or by local administration (e.g. nasal, ophthalmologic) is not prohibited. Cathine (a type of amphetamine) is prohibited, but only when its concentration in urine is greater than 5 micrograms per milliliter. WADA confirms that ephedrine and methylephedrine are prohibited, but only when its concentration in urine is greater than 10 micrograms per milliliter.[95]

A 2006 study performed by researchers at the School of Sport and Exercise Sciences at the University of Birmingham examined the effect of 2.5 milligram/kilogram supplement (a little more than 1.0 milligram/pound) of pseudoephedrine ingested 90 minutes before a 1,500-meter run. The results showed a 2.1-percent improvement in

94 Source: [Google: USATF + Legal + antidoping]

95 Source: [Google: Wada + AMA + prohibited list]

times with no side effects. For me, that would entail taking about 150mg or five Sudafeds and knocking 2.5 seconds off of my 800-meter time.[96] That is huge!

Understanding what is fair to put in your body is one of the trickiest things about track and field. I spent hours researching the optimal diet and optimal mix of legal health-related supplements. I had to ask myself, "Should I be researching the optimal mix of legal *prescription drugs* to take before a race, as well?"

Dietary Research and Findings

The Gomes Weight Loss Method in Brief: I decided to summarize my dietary philosophy as concisely as possible. Many people asked about my diet – especially those who knew me before I started training, when I was a portly 185 pounds at 5′ 8″-ish. This inevitably led to long discussions, in which I ended up thinking, "Man, I'm getting tired of hearing myself go through that speech over and over." (My girlfriend was getting pretty sick of hearing it too.)

I was also sure that the person who asked ended up thinking, "Great info, but he talked forever, and I won't remember any of it!"

Here is a concise description of my weight-loss principles.

Healthy Versus Weight-Friendly

In my opinion, the biggest error people make is to confuse healthy foods with weight-friendly foods. Nuts are extremely healthy, but if you ate them all day, you could get extremely fat. Similarly, salads are great, but the high-fat dressing can eliminate 100 percent (or more) of the weight benefits. I feel bad for people who suffer through salad after salad, when they can be eating something tastier (e.g., some skinless chicken and steamed veggies) that contains half the calories.

Calories per Gram or Milliliter

The second biggest weight control mistake I think people make is to look at a food's calories per serving. Manufacturers choose the serving size, enabling them to manipulate the calories per serving. It's no coincidence that many snacks have "just 100 calories," but if you examine the serving sizes they are ridiculously small. For example, a serving of Tostitos has "just" 150 calories, but the serving size is literally six chips! To get that snack down to 100 calories, you have to stop eating after four chips. Who eats only four Tostitos? I don't.

CalorieKing.com is a great source to gain a better understanding of how various foods compare to one another in calorie content. It has a huge database of foods and a drop-down menu that allows you to see the calorie content *per gram* (or *per milliliter* for liquids). Obviously, if you can reduce the number of calories in your daily diet without lowering your caloric output (activity level), you will lose weight.

You can cut down your total food intake by volume, but a better strategy seems to be eating the same volume but ingesting fewer calories. If you eat less, your body tends to "go conservative" and reduce your metabolic rate to conserve your precious calories for unforeseen future events. Eating frequently – but still keeping caloric intake lower than your caloric output – appears to be the fastest, safest way to weight loss.[97]

Calculating calories per gram creates a virtual 10-point scale. For example, fresh basil has less than one calorie per gram, so it's score is close to a perfect zero. On the other end of the spectrum, animal fat can approach a cataclysmic 10 calories per gram. That's especially bad when you consider that any score greater than four is higher than sugar. Interestingly, pure protein also approaches a four on the scale. However, you can get protein in foods like lentils. Boiled lentils score near one on the calorie-per-gram scale, despite being high in protein.

---

96 Source: www.ncbi.nlm.nih.gov/pubmed/16531903

97 Source: Katherine Tallmadge, M.A, R.D.

Calorie King's database also contains drinks. Manufacturers measure liquids in units including liters, gallons, and fluid ounces. As such, they need to be treated a little differently than solid foods. As a baseline, one gram of water and one milliliter of water are equal. So, for liquids, look at the calories per milliliter.

As everyone knows, water scores a perfect zero. On the flip side, meat drippings score the same disastrous near-10 calories per milliliter as solid animal fat scores per gram. Oils score very poorly. This includes olive oil (a whopping eight), even though olive oil is considered very healthy, thus illustrating that healthy and weight-friendly are not one and the same.

Looking at the nutritional label, you can quickly calculate a score by dividing the calories per serving by the serving size (grams for foods and milliliters for liquids). If the manufacturer doesn't provide the serving size in grams or milliliters, you'll have to convert whatever measure they use. (But, you only have to calculate it once for each food to know which parts of your diet score high and which score low.)

One final note – if the item in question melts at a room temperature (e.g., ice cream), it's a liquid, not a solid.

Keeping Taste; Shedding Weight

During the week, I generally kept my calorie-per-gram scores under three. I did this by eating lots of chicken, fish, fruits, veggies, and legumes (e.g., lentils). I made a few exceptions. For example, I ate some rice bran every night for its high fiber and magnesium content. I also ate a few nuts (not to be confused with a handful) for their concentrated nutritional benefits. However, most nuts score above 5. I also ate my share of raisins. They score a 3.3 on the scale – not bad although still on the high side of my weekday diet. But it doesn't take many raisins to greatly enhance the flavor of a salad or chicken dish, so they serve a great role, in addition to being healthy. I also ate a decent amount of pasta. Most people are surprised to discover that pasta only scores a 1.7. It's not the pasta that kills you; it's the olive oil, sauce or meatballs!

Another key tactic in my diet was to avoid butter, cooking oils, store-bought sauces, etc. For example, instead of butter or oil, I used non-stick pans and very light coatings of Pam. Of course, butter and olive oil taste good! So, how do you get any flavor? I leaned heavily on spices. Fresh spices are the best because they tend to provide health benefits and have almost no calories (like the aforementioned basil). I also used my fair share of dry spices, like garlic salt, chicken bouillon, and cayenne pepper. Dry spices like these are also low in calories and can add a lot of flavor. You have to beware of their sodium content because sodium is a major contributor to high blood pressure, but…

…For active runners, sodium intake isn't usually an issue. Runners tend to have low blood pressure and literally "sweat it out." Most runners don't have *enough* key electrolytes for running (e.g., sodium, calcium, magnesium, and potassium). The Livestrong.com Web site published a very concise summary of the nutrients you lose while running that need to be replaced regularly.[98]

You'll notice that many of the key food sources they cite also score well on the calories-per-gram scale… a win-win! And you're not even limited to the foods on my calories-per-gram scale *all* the time, leading me to the next principle in my dietary philosophy…

You Can Cheat!

Despite what you might think, I am *not* a diet fanatic. I merely act like one because I'm serious about my athletic goals. I'd prefer to eat steak, burgers, fries, pizza, onion rings, ice cream, soda, milk shakes, waffles, chips, etc., etc… and I do!

Every week, I made sure to give myself some "cheat time." One time was Wednesday night date nights with Jamie. The other time was from Friday evening until I went to sleep on Saturday night. During these times, I was known to

---

98 [Google: livestrong.com + important minerals for running]

put on epic displays of consumption. It was not uncommon for me to gain seven or eight pounds in a single sitting. Of course, much of that was water weight, but when you're eating burgers, fries, shakes, and chocolate, the calories pile up! However, when taken as a whole, my total weekly calorie consumption remained low enough to maintain my training weight. The great thing about it was that if I found myself getting out of line, losing an extra pound or two was as simple as skipping a few cheat meals.

You can even cheat your cheat meals!

If you know you're going to have a "bad" meal, eat a few stalks of celery or other low-calorie/high-fiber foods one hour or so beforehand. (Celery only has only one calorie per 10 grams.) Now you'll eat less before getting full – so what could have been a 4,000-calorie pig-out, might end up as only a 3,000-calorie pig-out.

I also found some research that implied celery provided an additional benefit – although I found some sources that refuted this as well: Celery strings are insoluble, they don't get absorbed in the digestive process. Some studies suggested celery impedes the absorption of what you eat until you've passed all of the celery fiber. As a result, you may only absorb 2,000 calories of that 3,000 calorie meal. In this example, your net savings would be 2,000 calories... and since 3,500 calories equals one pound, if you went through this scenario once a week, you could theoretically save 104,000 calories per year... almost 30 pounds!

As with many things I researched, I couldn't prove fact from fiction – but celery seemed to work wonders for me. Just be careful about this tactic. If the pro-celery research is right, calories wouldn't be the only thing you cheat. If that high-calorie steak dinner passes right through you, you miss out on critical iron and other valuable nutrients in addition to the calories.

Training Log Week 105			
Day	Date	Notes	Mileage
Thurs.	2/03/11	Easy day (30 min elliptical).	4.3
Fri.	2/04/11	Tough session with Coach Ward. We started with a sub-27 sec 200m. (I ran 26.5 sec.) After, we took 8 min rest before an 800m simulation: 500m at race pace, followed by 200m in 40 sec, followed by a final 100m at race pace (or whatever we had left). My 500m was 1:08.9. (I went through the 400m in 55.0 sec – too fast.) Not surprisingly, the 200m rest was a little slow and the final 100m was barely at race pace (14.8 sec).	4.9
Sat.	2/05/11	Recovery day: easy 47 min on the elliptical.	7.0
Sun.	2/06/11	Awoke to bad news. Chris Simpson strained his calf during the Master's Mile at the New Balance Indoor Grand Prix. We need him healthy for our Masters world record attempts over the next two wks. I hit the Booker T track with John Cormier. Did 1.5 miles warm-up and drills. I felt a slight quad strain during a kick-out, probably a remnant from the 800m simulation. I used The Stick and shook it out. It held up fine for the 6 x 200m workout: 28-29 sec with full rest between reps. The track closed and we did not get to warm down.	7.8
Mon.	2/07/11	Easy pace workout with John Cormier. We warmed up simulating race-day conditions (a mix of my routine from last year and the routine used by Coach Ward). I felt a slight strain in my quad during our first kick-out so I avoided further kick-outs and strides. I'm still not fully recovered from Friday's workout. I worked my quad with The Stick, then we got down to business: 6 x 200m @ 29 sec, with full rest. The goal was to practice getting out at the right pace. We were successful: 29.7, 30.7, 30.0, 29.9, 28.9, and 29.9 sec.	4.7
Tues.	2/08/11	Did a speed workout with John, as prescribed by Coach Ward. Two sets of 2 x 300m, 1 x 200m. Each rep was faster than Coach had set – which is both good and bad. I felt great, rested and fully recovered, but Coach Ward still chastised me over e-mail to leave some for the race. Times were 43.7, 42.1, and 28.8 sec for Set 1 and 41.5, 45.1, and 28.2 sec for Set 2.	4.3
Weds.	2/09/11	Did 30-min elliptical, plus stretching and foam roller exercises. I'm getting more sleep and gaining a little weight. I feel rested and strong and as if my testosterone levels are bouncing back. Tapering is fun!	4.3
Total		Averaged 6:30 per mile for the week	37.3

Training Log Week 106			
Day	Date	Notes	Mileage
Thurs.	2/10/11	Extended warm-up at the track: jogging laps, drills, and lots of dynamic stretching. My workout was 5 x 150m in 21-22 sec (1:57.2 avg 800m pace).	3.5
Fri.	2/11/11	Pre-race easy elliptical work in preparation for the Eliot Track Club 4 x 800m world record attempt in Boston.	4.3
Sat.	2/12/11	I ran 1:59.6 on my leg of the Eliot Track Club's 4 x 800m world record attempt. I ran hard enough to induce tunnel vision down the final 50m, but I could have run faster if I went out quicker. We failed to break the record of 8:07. The track proved too flat and slow to run a fast time. I drowned my disappointment in alcohol at the after-party with tons of friends, family, and old track colleagues. When I got back to my cousin's (where we were staying), I went out and did a hill workout. I also did drills and pushups until I was face-first in a snow drift. (I was not likely sober at the time.)	7.0
Sun.	2/13/11	Was a little sore from yesterday's race and drunken hill workout, but felt ok overall. Did 80 min elliptical and lots of stretching.	11.0
Mon.	2/14/11	Met Chris Simpson for a short run (3.65 miles). I did an additional 1.6 miles on my own and drove the brief distance from Harvard Square to Harvard's indoor track. There, I did dynamic stretching and drills, then 4 x 200m @ 28 sec, with 90 sec standing rest. After, I jogged about 0.75 mile to warm down.	7.0
Tues.	2/15/11	Hung out at Harvard Track with New Balance Boston and my Eliot Track Club teammates. I did a fair amount of jogging, drills, strides, and plank pushups. Since finishing *Born to Run*, I've been worrying less about exact distances/times and focusing more on fun and quality work. I have discovered that fun is... fun!	9.3
Weds.	2/16/11	Track workout at Harvard: 5-mile warm-up at 6:40 pace, then 4 x 400m in 64-67 sec with 67-82 sec rest between reps.	8.0
Total		Averaged 6:48 per mile for the week	50.1

Race Reports, Records and Results

January 2011 began my first intense period of racing in nearly 20 years. Although I ran a couple of challenging track races in winter/spring 2010, it was just that: a *couple*. In winter 2011, things got serious. I had two Masters world record attempts on the calendar and my first Masters Nationals competition. Not to mention I had the chance to defend my Miami Tropical 5K crown – and I was training for an event 2.5 miles shorter than 5K at the time.

2011 Miami Tropical 5K: January 9th – I was tired from a hard week of training and a busy week at work, so I wasn't certain to defend my title; I just wanted a hard workout. I decided to focus on running even mile splits, with 5:20 being the target. Those splits would give me the opportunity to break 16:30 if I felt good after Mile 2, without blowing my chance to better my Masters PR of 16:50 (5:26 pace) if I ran out of steam.

At the start of the race, Linkin Park's "Waiting for the End" blared over the PA system. Then the music faded, and the starter fired the gun. I took a quick lead, but only to establish position and avoid any scuffles with the pack; then I quickly settled in. "Waiting for the End" started an endless loop in the back of head, keeping me relaxed and occupied.

Three guys passed me and established a pace faster than 5:20. I let them go but stayed in contact. They pulled me through the first mile in 5:12. A truck on the side of the road blared Lady Gaga's "Bad Romance." I tried not to pay attention, but it was too late. Other than a lesser mental soundtrack, I felt fine though, so I kept contact with the leaders. They pulled me through Mile 2 in 10:20.

At that point, I was 80 meters behind the leader, with the second- and third-place runners about half the distance between the leader and me. I still felt pretty good. It occurred to me that I might have enough in the tank to close the gap. I gave chase.

I'm very familiar with the McArthur Causeway Bridge that leads into South Beach, the closing stretch of this race. I knew I could open up my stride on the downhill section of the bridge, thus increasing my pace while resting the muscles I used on the uphill. I worked the uphill extra hard, nearly catching the second- and third-place guys. I was tired, but when I opened my stride and leaned a little forward on the downhill, I accelerated quickly with no extra effort. I went past those two guys like they were standing still. This brought me within 40 meters of the leader. I took a quick peek at my GPS: 0.7 miles to go. "Plenty of time," I thought. This partially anesthetized the pain of racing.

The downhill momentum from the McArthur Causeway Bridge shot me onto Alton Road at a fast pace, which I fought to maintain on the flat. The narrowing space between me and the leader gave me the incentive to press on. Also playing into my favor was the ascending sun: my shadow would not give me away. As I closed in, I started to mirror the leader's stride and mute my breath.

Like any animal stalking its prey, I wanted my arrival to be a surprise. I figured he was already relaxing his intensity after breaking the only two other contenders. Finally, I pulled up close. He must have felt my presence because for the first time in the race, he glanced back.

I decided to sit tight. I was tired from the chase, but I also wanted to see how he would react. I was prepared for him to kick. If he did, I'd go with him. If he didn't, I'd know his fight was gone. That would enable me to catch my breath and think about how to approach the final stretch. To my delight, his reaction was nothing. He swiveled his head back toward the sun without a change in stride or pace.

I made a quick check of my GPS and saw that 800 meters remained. If he didn't make a move in the next 400 meters, I was confident that my kick would win. Soon, I could see the Mile 3 marker. It was time to go. I was eager but exhausted, so I decided to kick *hard*. I thought if I took off like a shot, he'd think, "My God, I can't do that. It's over." The race would be over before Mile 3.

It worked. I put in a 200-meter surge that left him 50 meters back. I hit three miles in 15:19 for a third mile in 4:59! For the first time in my life, I had run negative splits in a 5K. I was fading fast, but the race was won... or was it? A spectator noticed my fatigue and started to encourage my pursuer, "He's dead... get him!!"

"Shit!" I thought. I turned my head to see if he had reacted. "Please don't be coming," I thought. "Please don't be coming." He was coming.

Now *I* was the prey. I went with everything I had left. He was closing, but so was the finish line. The finish came first... barely. A photograph (posted on the Faster Than Forty Facebook page) captured the moment. I squeaked out a win, and the clock read 15:55. My previous time at this race was over a minute slower. It was a Masters PR!

Running negative splits (5:12, 5:08, 4:59) made all the difference. In doing so, I had the momentum going into the final mile. At the same time, my adversary – named Dustin Meeker – was already fatigued and mentally worn from battling two other competitors for most of the race. He confirmed my thoughts in a post-race interview:

"I heard the footsteps," said Meeker, a Baltimore resident, of Gomes passing him. "I'm a bit of a pessimist. I thought it was over. I was pretty much spent."

Masters World Record Attempt – 4 x 800 meters: Tufts University, February 12th – After weeks of searching for a venue, the Eliot Track Club finally received an invite to race a meet at Tufts University. Our goal: break the Masters 4 x 800-meter relay world record. The circumstances were not exactly ideal.

Old Man Winter had dumped several inches of snow in Boston, making the warm-up jog an adventure. Additionally, there was an issue with the competing 4 x 800-meter teams... there were none. We'd be running all alone if we couldn't find four able-bodied souls who could average about 2:02 per leg. There was a meet at Boston University scheduled the same day and most every 800 runner was competing there. (Luckily, we located four able bodies that fit the bill last-minute.) Worst of all, Tufts has a flat 200-meeter track. Unlike the banked ovals around town (Harvard, BU, Reggie Lewis Center), Tufts' track did not have a reputation for enabling speedy times.

Despite the obstacles, we walked into Tufts undeterred and ready to roll. It was a big event for us. Friends and family turned out to hopefully witness history. The serious expressions on my teammates' faces were unfamiliar to me. Chris Simpson, Doug Williams, and Andrew Darien are a jovial group of guys who usually laugh their way through their weekly track workouts until fatigue and lactic acid finally gets the better of them. When race time came, the enormity of the moment took center stage.

Doug Williams led off, followed by Andrew Darien. I'd love to provide lap-by-lap commentary, but I honestly don't remember much. The only thing I recall was being ushered onto the track as Andrew turned the final corner for home. I was fixated on the baton but couldn't ignore the anguished look on Darien's face. I didn't catch his split, but I was sure he had given it his all.

I took the baton in a close second, drafting my fellow New Balance Boston training mate, Brendan Collins. He ran a great leg too, hitting fairly even splits through 500 meters before yielding the first lane for my final kick.

Pushing down the home stretch, my vision started to go black around the periphery. For a moment, I worried that I'd pass out. Fortunately, that didn't happen. Chris Simpson took over after a smooth exchange. I thought for sure we were doing well, but when I looked up at the clock, something didn't seem quite right. Two minutes later I knew why.

We finished in 8:14, a full seven seconds off the record. As far as I could tell, everyone had done pretty well out there. It was disappointing, but before long everyone's attention turned to friends and family. We had pre-planned a celebration party. The celebration was for naught, but we weren't about to waste a good party. I chalked up our failure to the slow track and headed out for a pint of Guinness. We had another date with destiny a week later in the distance medley relay at one of Boston's finest facilities: Harvard University.

Masters World Record Attempt – Distance Medley Relay: Harvard University, February 20th – What should have been a great day (and redemption for last weekend's failed 4 x 800-meter World Record attempt) turned into an unmitigated disaster.

The Eliot Track Club and I hoped to rewrite age-group history in the distance medley relay: a 1,200-meter leg, followed by a 400-meter leg, followed by an 800-meter leg, then capped off with a one-mile leg as the anchor. Our attempt started well. Chris Simpson (1,200 meters) and Brian Moore (400 meters) ran great legs. That left Andrew 'Drew' Darien (800 meters) and me (one mile).

I watched Drew go through his first 400 meters. His time was quick and he looked strong. I thought, "This is it. It's on me now." It was time to go into my "unconscious zone" – a near-mindless state where I can run my fastest and withstand the most pain. When I'm in that zone, my coach (or a teammate) tells me what to do and I do it: Go faster. Pass that guy. *Sprint*. Whatever it is, I do it. In the zone, I only do two things well – follow directions and run. Everything else is a fog. Mind you, "the zone" is not an excuse when something goes wrong. We're all ultimately responsible for our performances. It's just how I, and a lot of runners, operate.

The first thing I remember is seeing a race official place the anchor for a competing team, the Greater Boston Track Club, on the track. I looked at the official and asked, "Now?"

He said, "Yes, now."

Something felt off, but in the zone, I just do what I'm told... I saw something in Drew's eyes as I reached for the baton. He looked confused, but in the zone, Drew just does what he's told and runs. We were chasing a world record and the fulfillment of a dream. This wasn't the time to think.

During my leg, I couldn't help but feel confused. It was hard to focus. In hindsight, I don't even remember the first lap. Come to think of it, I don't even know what happened to the GBTC guy. Did I pass him? Did he step off the track? I honestly had no idea. I just kept running, looked at Chris Simpson after each lap, listening for guidance.

I few laps later, I lost count of how many I had left. I never heard the bell lap. Nor do I recall anyone saying, "One to go." I remember passing our remaining competition and starting my final sprint. When I came around to the stands, I wasn't sure if I was done or had another lap to go... but I still had a lot left in the tank. Another lap or not, I knew I would finish the job: a world record!

I crossed the line, but I kept sprinting. I wasn't given any indication to stop. Back in 1988, an entire heat of 1,000-meter runners at The Eastern States Championships did the same thing. Twelve of the East Coast's finest high school runners ran an extra lap. Why? Because when in doubt, don't stop.

On the backstretch, I looked back and I noticed that my competitors were gone. It was only then that I knew for sure that the race was over. I finished the lap, raising the baton. Jubilance! World record!

...And then I got horrific news.

Apparently, my earlier confusion was justified. When the race official placed the GBTC anchor and me on the track, our teammates still had one lap to go. Thus, when that baton passed from Darien's hand to mine, we broke the rules... and in track & field, you don't lose 10-yards and a first down for breaking a rule. You get disqualified. You *lose*. And anything you did during the event gets wiped off the books. As far as the USATF was concerned, we didn't race. We weren't even there.

Training Log Week 107			
Day	Date	Notes	Mileage
Thurs.	2/17/11	Morning elliptical (65 min) with dynamic stretching, drills, and strides. Evening elliptical (35 min) with dynamic stretching and drills.	14.5
Fri.	2/18/11	Pre-race 4 x 200m workout at a very easy 27-28 sec per rep, w/2 min rest between reps.	5.8
Sat.	2/19/11	Easy elliptical (30 min) to prepare for tomorrow's world record attempt redux, this time in the distance medley event instead of the 4 x 800m.	4.3
Sun.	2/20/11	I ran something around 4:30 for the anchor leg of our distance medley relay world record attempt. (See Race Results section.) To run well and not get the world mark makes for a very disappointing and discouraging day.	4.0
Mon.	2/21/11	Flew to St. Louis/Springfield, IL to visit Jamie's family on the way to Albuquerque for the Masters Indoor National Championships. Yesterday's loss is not sitting well. Jogged 4 miles to the local YMCA to do a 1-hr elliptical session and drills.	15.5
Tues.	2/22/11	Finally watched the video of our DMR world record attempt. It was a sad sight, but confirmed almost everything I thought. I clearly see me questioning the official when he lined up the anchor legs. You can also see me ask, "Now?" just before the handoff. Oh, the humanity. Did a 45-min elliptical to try and eliminate the bad taste in my mouth.	6.5
Weds.	2/23/11	Reached New Mexico and UNM's outdoor track, where I planned a few workouts. I met the Lobos' sprint coach, Giles McDonnell, who entertained me for a bit and gave me the practice schedule for the indoor track – which proved useful later as the outdoor temp was low-50s. After an extended warm-up, my workout was 14 x 200m @ 33 sec w/1-min rest. I wanted to be cautious in my first workout at altitude. It was tough. After the 8th rep, I was uncertain if I would finish, but the times in the final reps were much faster than prescribed. I averaged 31.4 sec for the full workout.	4.5
Total		Averaged 6:53 per mile for the week	55.1

2011 USATF Masters Indoor Nationals: March 6th, Albuquerque, NM – The day before my race in the M40 800-meters, I went to the track to see Nick Berra and Lance Elliott battle in the one-mile run. Apparently, Berra had other plans. Like me, he scratched. In my case, the scratch was planned well in advance. In Berra's case, it was more illness-related, based on an entry I saw on his blog.[99]

I spotted Berra in the stands a couple sections from where Rick Miller, Dennis Shine, and John Cormier were sitting. I guess I wasn't the only one mining for competitive intelligence. Elliott clearly caught a huge break. Without Berra in the one-mile, he'd probably be able to coast to an easy victory. Rechecking the seeding sheet though, I discovered Andrew Duncan, a 43 year old seeded at 4:26.

---

[99] http://nickberra.wordpress.com/2011/03/05/no-mile-high-mile/

"That could be enough to push Elliott," I thought. This made happy because, I wanted the 800 meters to be a two-horse race between Berra and me. If nobody else was going to be there with 300 meters to go, I wouldn't have to worry about being boxed in for the final sprint.

Duncan lined up next to Elliott, who was granted the pole position. The gun went off, but that was about the only thing that did. The altitude must have psyched the boys out because they mustered only 35 or 36 seconds for the opening 200 meters, a pedestrian 4:40-ish mile pace. I cheered for Duncan to pick it up, but he didn't hear me... or didn't listen. I didn't see the half-mile split, but it was slow. This was clearly going to be little-more than a warm-up jog for Elliott... or was it?

With 500 meters to go, Duncan unleashed a serious surge. Elliott was slow to react but eventually gave chase. With 300 meters to go, he had closed much of the gap. With one lap to go, the gap was all but gone. Elliott was in striking distance. I was happy to see Elliott get pushed, but I knew it was over. I'd seen this movie before. The superior runner passes the spunky underdog and coasts to victory.

But the spunky underdog wasn't ready to go gently into that good night. Elliott tried to strike his killing blow, and Duncan responded with another gear. Duncan actually opened up a meter's length on Elliott... and then another. As they navigated the final turn, the improbable became a certainty. Duncan was going to take Elliott down.

And he did.

The time was slow (about 4:40), but Andrew Duncan won the 2011 U.S. Indoor Masters Mile. Despite the times, the last 500 meters was hard work for both runners. Not only was Elliott pushed, but I got to see his finishing kick (weak). The man likely runs a great 5K, but I figured the one-mile was his lower boundary. I was certain I would be the quickest guy in the field in the 800 meters the following day.

March 6th was proving day. After two years of training I was going to race the reigning Masters 800-meter world champion. I felt good. Getting to Albuquerque early was a smart move. Each workout felt easier than the last. I thought I had a good advantage going into the race. I got to the track early as usual and soaked in the environment. I started my warm-up at the usual time, about 70 minutes before my race. I headed outside and started with a slow quarter-mile jog (eight-minute mile pace). It winded me a bit. That was no surprise at altitude though. After a few minutes of stretching, I did another quarter-mile at six-minute pace. That felt no different than the slower quarter I had done a few minutes earlier. After a little more stretching, I did a half mile at six-minute-pace and that felt pretty good. It was time to head back to the track and do my drills.

The meet directors had sectioned off a large warm-up area. Berra was there and doing many of the same drills I was doing. He looked pretty good, but not particularly intimidating. As for me, with each rep, I felt looser and stronger. By the time I got around to doing my final strides I was feeling fantastic. I honestly felt that the race would be mine... but when you're dealing with a world champion you can never be too sure. Thus, I was prepared for a dogfight.

The time finally came, and we were ushered to the starting line. Not surprisingly, Berra's seed time earned him the pole position. I had not entered a seed time, so I was assigned Lane 6 at random. It was a single waterfall start – where everyone lines up on one curved starting line. The curve is designed such that each runner starts a little bit in front of the runner to his left. This helps to eliminate the advantage of being in an inside lane. In other words, being in Lane 6 wasn't a big deal. I would be allowed to cut into Lane 1 when I wanted (assuming I didn't interfere with another runner while doing so).

The stage was set. We were asked to approach the starting line. I dropped to a single knee as I usually do before race. Then I stood in a crouched starting position, balanced on one leg and ready to spring forward. Berra took a similar position.

Training Log Week 108			
Day	Date	Notes	Mileage
Thurs.	2/24/11	Eventful morning. I was researching stocks with one of my partners when Jamie appeared before me looking like death: nasty headache, short of breath, and lightheaded. It was clearly altitude sickness. I immediately started calling local hospitals while Googling remedies. After a few calls, it was clear the hospital would not help her cause. Instead, we focused on key prevention techniques: hydration, canned oxygen, aspirin and rest. She felt better after a bit, but she was going to need time to acclimate. My body seemed to have acclimated. I felt great and ran 4 miles on the indoor track comfortably in 6:08 pace.	4.0
Fri.	2/25/11	Massage therapy and ice bath in the morning, then speed work in the afternoon: 3 x 200m w/60 sec rest, 90 sec break, then 3 x 200m w/60 sec rest. Similar times to one year ago (27-28 sec), but this year was at altitude with a tougher morning session and tougher day-prior run. Altitude was the biggest difference. I felt comfortable with my opening 27-sec rep, but my breathing elevated very quickly. That said, I felt I was acclimating well.	4.0
Sat.	2/26/11	Started my day with a 1.5-mile warm-up (10:00), followed by stretching and ultrasound with a University of New Mexico trainer, followed by "massage therapy." It was not a traditional (enjoyable) massage, but it was therapeutic and should have me ready to run. Next I ran an easy 4 miles (30:00) with Dennis Shine, then we watched the USATF Indoor Nationals (open division). As an athlete, I could go everywhere! I met Galen Rupp and Bernard Lagat (easily one of the most gracious athletes and still dominant at 36 years old)! He said he can't wait to compete as a Master, and a number of world records are sure to fall when he does. Later Dennis and I had dinner with Erin Dromgoole, who runs with New Balance Boston.	5.5
Sun.	2/27/11	Dennis and I visited the University of New Mexico's outdoor track for drills: the typical Coach Ward warm-up, followed by 6 sets of 30-sec drills w/a 50m stride and 15 pushups. Solid work as I taper for the meet.	4.0
Mon.	2/28/11	Leisurely 4 miles with Dennis. My hamstrings were a little store from yesterday's sprints.	4.0
Tues.	3/1/11	Relaxing day: easy 30-min elliptical in the a.m. Later, Jamie, Dennis and I drove to Sante Fe. I got some good sun for the first time in a couple wks!	4.3
Weds.	3/2/11	Still sore from drills the other day. Decided to delay my track workout until early evening – disappointing because I wanted to acclimate to going fast at race time (11a). Workout: 4 x 200m w/2 min static rest (29, 28, 28, and 27 sec, respectively). Last year at this time, I did 4 x 300m, but I cut distance this year considering my sore hamstrings, the recovery time at altitude, and the fact that last year I wasn't fully recovered before my race. In massage later, the therapist reiterated the need for longer recovery.	4.0
Total		Averaged 6:43 per mile for the week	29.8

The starter gave his command, "On your marks…"

"This is it," I thought to myself. Time to win a national title.

"Set…"

Click.

"Click?"

The starter's gun had misfired. How anticlimactic. After some fiddling, he ordered us back to the line.

"On your marks… Set… Bang!" We were off!

Berra jumped to an early lead. I quickly moved from my position into the first lane behind him. The pace was comfortable; slow, in fact. Down the first backstretch, one of the other competitors, Jonathan Stone, rushed to the lead. He took us through the first lap in just over 30 seconds. I was chillin' behind Stone and Berra, relaxed and barely breathing.

As we came around the final turn of the second lap, Berra passed Stone to retake the lead. I gave chase. We passed the 400-meter mark in just over 60 seconds and pulled away from the rest of the field. It was just Berra and me now. The third lap was just a waiting game. My plan was to sit quietly behind him until there was one lap to go. Then, I would unleash with everything I had, hopefully catching him by surprise… and tired.

Down the back stretch of the third lap, I followed Nick step for step. I was a ghost. He clearly didn't know I was there. I wanted him to think he was alone until I was ready to strike. As we approached start of the bell lap, I still felt good. Then, I made my move.

I pushed past him with a hard surge and took the first lane before hitting the turn. I was now running with everything I had. I was a little surprised to hear Berra's footsteps right behind me. He had reacted instantaneously and was following me stride for stride. Despite that, I felt that the race was mine. I had never lost a race where I had taken the lead with 200 meters to go.

I continued to push hard down the back straightaway, and Berra's steps continued to echo behind me. For the first time, I started to feel a little worried. As we approached the final turn, I decided that I'd move to the outside of Lane 1, forcing Berra to go wide. And he did.

But the final surprise of the race was about to revealed. As Berra went wide, he pulled even with me. He came off the final turn – the finish line looming 50 meters ahead – then he powered by me. Two things happened at that moment. One, I was stunned. I hadn't lost a lead in this fashion since the Scott Cody incident in high school – and even then I was technically in second place, not leading. Two, a lactic tsunami swept over me with full force. I was incapable of accelerating any further. I was still moving at a good clip, but Berra was pulling away...

The race wasn't quite over, but it was finished.

I saw my boys near the finish line cheering me on, but it was no use. Berra crossed the finish line a half-second ahead of me, retaining his title as America's fastest Masters 800-meter runner. I still had a couple of steps to go, but I was already coming to grips with my silver-medal fate. Even as I urged my body across the finish line, I knew I had executed my plan to perfection. I came prepared and made every move at just the right time. Berra was just the stronger runner. There was no shame in that. There was disappointment, but no shame. The lessons learned from my high school days held true – he beat me, but I had given everything; I didn't coast.

I crossed the finish line and dropped to a knee. Catching my breath, I looked up at Rick Miller and shrugged my shoulders, "What can you do? The guy's a monster," I said.

I looked over at Berra, who was doubled over several meters away. He gathered himself, walked over to me, and said, "So, I guess I'll be seeing you around."

"Yup... You will."

Less than a minute later I was on my feet and quickly recovering from the ordeal... too quickly, in fact. As I had worried, I had done too much endurance training and not enough work on power and speed. Given a 30-minute rest, I could probably have run another 800 meters in 2:00, and maybe another after that. But I couldn't run a single one faster than Berra. "Adjustments are needed," I thought. Then I let it go.

What was done was done. A wave of relief rushed over my body. I actually felt happy. I bounced around the arena for a bit, posed for a couple of photos, and bought a few souvenirs. I chatted with Berra for a few minutes, which confirmed the impression he gives off via his blog... he's a great guy – unbeatable on that day, but not unbeatable.

A little while later John Cormier ran his final race of the competition – the 200-meter final. It was the strongest he looked all weekend. He was clearly getting the hang of competing at a high level. Cormier finished sixth, but he was clearly the most aerobically fit competitor. Like me, he had built up too much of a base and not enough power. We would have all spring to work on that.

Miscellaneous Research and Notes

Who is Lee Emanuel? While in Albuquerque I met the University of New Mexico's sprint coach, Giles McDonnell. The coaches' office is adjacent to the track, and I could see light and movement from within, so before my first workout there I walked in and introduced myself. Coach McDonnell is a good guy. He entertained me for a few minutes and photocopied the practice schedule for the indoor track – something I desperately needed at the time.

We talked about UNM's famous miler, Lee Emanuel, a two-time NCAA champion. Here are some of Emanuel's honors:

➢ Two-time NCAA Indoor Champion/All-American (Mile – 2009, 2010)
➢ Two-time NCAA Outdoor All-American (1,500 meters – 2009, 2010)
➢ Three-time MWC Indoor Champion (Mile/800 meters/DMR - 2010)

What I found most interesting about Emanuel came from an interview he did with the Web site preracejitters.com:

PRJ: You once said in an interview that your coach Joe Franklin, told you, "The stronger you are, the quicker you can finish." How has that influenced you?

LE: I did not believe him at first, the first time I raced a mile for him I got beat pretty badly. He asked me what I thought we should do next. I said speed work, he said the opposite. I thought he was wrong but he proved himself completely right, which was annoying! Last year I had my greatest year without once putting my spikes on for a training session and the fastest I ran all season in training was 28 seconds so it seems to work for me."

That harkened back to some research I received from Rick Miller regarding training paces and their role in lactic threshold training. I understood it, but I needed to reread it a few times to better understand how to adapt the principles to my training. Combining testimony from athletes like Lee Emanuel and additional research on lactic threshold training – plus the lessons learned from the beating Nick Berra gave me in Albuquerque – profoundly affected the way I trained leading up to the 2011 USATF Masters Outdoor Nationals in July.

Race Recovery for Old Men: Here's a short list of needs for all the old guys lacing up the spikes for the first time in a long time:

➢ Ice! Ice packs, ice baths, etc. Alternate ice/heat/ice.
➢ Recovery pays immediate benefits. When in doubt, rest.
➢ Protein receptors are most active within 30 minutes of a hard workout. Toss down a coconut-water drink with a Muscle Milk Light and you're replenishing most of what you need at a good calories-per-gram ratio.
➢ Ultrasound therapy is an old man's best friend. It was the number-one solution for my chronic calf issues.
➢ Enhanced blood flow is another best friend for recovery (and performance)...beet juice, Recovery Sock, compression gear, and area-specific heat/massage (obviously countering ice for anti-inflation).
➢ Spider (kinesio) tape supports the calves during training/races. My calves live in the stuff.

Training Log Week 109

Day	Date	Notes	Mileage
Thurs.	3/3/11	John Cormier and I hit an Albuquerque gym at 11a for a 30-min elliptical. The workout time synchs w/Sunday's race time, so I'm getting on schedule – but our team took a hit: Jamie's altitude sickness never improved. No amount of fluids, vitamins, or other supplements made her feel better, and she opted to go back to Miami – so I decided to dedicate Sunday's race to her.	4.3
Fri.	3/4/11	Did a 4 x 150m untimed workout. Started with an 800m jog and a full Coach-Ward-style warm-up. I warmed down with a 22-min elliptical session (3-mile equivalent). Two days until race day! Later I learned from Nick Berra's blog that he recently took ill. This bothered me for two reasons: 1) I wanted to race him on even ground; 2) he got sick before Indoor Nationals last year, took some antibiotics, and ended up running a Masters PR in the 800m: 1:56.3.	5.0
Sat.	3/5/11	Felt *awful* last night. Might have been the steak dinner, but I was wiped out. My stomach hurt, and I was congested. Right after dinner, I went to bed. I woke up at 6a to simulate tomorrow – giving my body plenty of time to be ready to race. To my surprise, the night's rest did me wonders. I felt as good as I have since arriving in Albuquerque. I had my pre-race day breakfast (a multi-vitamin, 4 oz of beet juice w/a teaspoon of peanut butter, Tropicana 50, a banana, some whole-wheat pasta w/steak sprinkled in, and a low-fat strawberry yogurt). Next, I loosened up lightly and went back to bed until 9:30a. At 10:30 I headed to the gym. There, I loosened up and did an easy 30-min elliptical, followed by a stretching session in the sauna. One day to go.	4.0
Sun.	3/6/11	Race day! 2011 USATF Masters Indoor 800-Meters runner up. (See Race Results section for details.)	2.0
Mon.	3/7/11	Back in Miami! A few days in the humidity will cure my nagging respiratory issues left over from Albuquerque's dry air, but for now, I'm pretty miserable. Reflecting on the season didn't make me feel any better. I hit exactly *none* of my goals. I believe the culprit was too much endurance training and not enough speed/power/lactic tolerance. I will be making changes. I jogged to Flamingo Track, did a few drills and ran a few reps with the group. After, I went for 4 miles alone.	6.0
Tues.	3/8/11	My nose, throat, and mind were still a mess. I felt a little better, but may take a few more days to get back to normal. Did close to 9 miles cardio, plus weights and a 30-min yoga class.	8.7
Weds.	3/9/11	Ramped up the intensity level today. 30-min elliptical in the morning, then later a stair workout with Matt Kiss. We started with a Coach Ward warm-up , then to make a game of it, I decided we would play "Chase Stairs." I gave Matt a head start and chased him up the stairs. If I caught him, I would get a point (but I also do 20 frog drills before the next rep). That made it impossible to catch him twice in a row. After a few reps we were both wiped out, but we had a lot more fun.	9.3
Total		Averaged 7:12 per mile for the week	**39.3**

Chapter 13
Police and Thieves In the Street

Weeks 110-120

Back in the day, not every disruption to a workout resulted in one of my teammates doing evil. Occasionally the disruptions resulted in acts of good.

One late-spring afternoon at Northeastern University, Erik Nedeau and Gwil Jones headed out for a recovery run, crossing campus and into the Fens park en route to the Charles River. As they crossed the footbridge over the pond (the same pond that was now home to Ken Kaczinski's former used car), they heard a girl screaming and saw her lying on the ground about 50 yards ahead of them along the path. A few feet away, a shadowy character was righting a fallen bike and trying to get his feet on the pedals in a hurry.

"Holy shit, he's robbing her!" yelled another student taking in the late afternoon sun from a blanket on the grass. Ned and Gwil needed no further instruction. They sprinted off the bridge after the would-be bicycle thief, who was pushing the bike along as fast as he could with one foot on a pedal, skateboard-style. He made it about 50 feet before he looked over his shoulder and, realizing the effort was fruitless, dropped the bike and ran on. Ned and Gwil let him go, happy enough to return the bike to its owner – to the cheers of their fellow students who had watched the whole scene unfold. One student was a writer for Northeastern's student newspaper, and the runners enjoyed some mini fame when the story ran a few days later.

Much more recently, Masters sprints standout John Cormier and I were involved in a similar event. After an easy Sunday afternoon elliptical session, we went outside the fitness center at Cormier's building in South Beach to run some wind sprints. We left our cell phones next to a walkway near his building and began our work. In between one of the reps we realized the phones were gone. We immediately assumed they were stolen (after all, this was South Beach), and we headed up to Cormier's apartment to try calling them. No answer.

Luckily, I had left my iPad at Cormier's apartment. Using the Find My iPhone app, I was able to see the phone on Google Maps. (The app even showed me which direction the phone was going.)

Not thinking much about whether they were "found" or stolen, we went into hot pursuit. As we ran up the road, the app refreshed, letting us know that the phone was on the move. As we sprinted towards the updated location, we saw a police car and decided to get the officer involved. He asked for the phone number of the phones and tried calling them. Again, no answer. He told us to hop into the back of his vehicle and we sped off.

Now we were really in hot pursuit!

The phones continued to move, but we were catching up. As this was happening, the officer called for backup. I remember thinking that this was probably overkill, but I was happy for the effort. Soon, we were in the vicinity of the phones. Cormier and I tried to identify the person with them, based on who was walking in the same direction that the iPad indicated. At this point, we wanted to get out of the car and finish the hunt on foot. The officer had other ideas. He asked me to show him where the phone was on the iPad. When I showed him, he took it, pulled the car over, and hopped out. Cormier and I tried to follow but quickly realized we were locked in.

From that point, we were relegated to witnessing everything through the back window of the police car. Two motorcycle cops and another squad car arrived on the scene. Blue lights were flashing everywhere. I figured if I were the thief, I'd be outta there fast. I feared we would never see our phones again. A minute later, another officer let us out of the vehicle. At the same time, the first officer was trying to call our phones again. Miraculously, this time someone picked up. It was a girl who said that someone had just dropped the phones on the sidewalk.

The officer asked for the girl's description and location. He then relayed the information to Cormier and me, so we could retrieve our phones. We found a girl (about 25 years old) accompanied by an older guy (about 55 years old). He had our phones in a plastic bag and handed them to us. We were in the middle of thanking him when he decided to admit that he had actually picked up the phones while we were doing our sprints, not from the sidewalk where the girl said she found them. He said he thought the phones were lost.

The whole situation turned fishy fast. I could tell by the look on Cormier's face that he was thinking the same thing. I didn't know if the guy had stolen our phones or if he legitimately "found" them and simply didn't want to get mixed up with the police. In the end, it didn't matter. We got our phones back and had one of the more interesting cool-downs in recent memory.

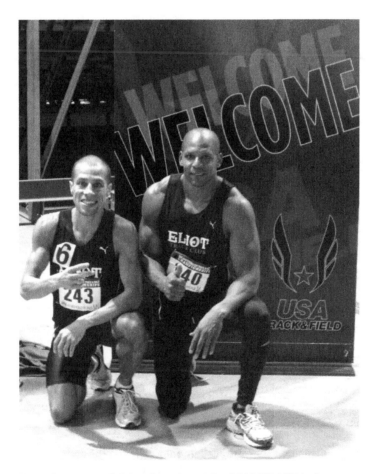

Mark Gomes and John Cormier at the 2011 USATF Indoor Nationals, Albuquerque, New Mexico.

Training Log Week 110			
Day	Date	Notes	Mileage
Thurs.	3/10/11	I'm getting angrier each passing day since Nationals. Stiff from yesterday's stairs, I waited until 1p for a 30-min elliptical. Later, I took a 45-min nap before heading to the Thursday Nike Run. I was still sore, but intent on a solid 3.5-mile tempo. Frank Green was game to go. We started at 6:00 pace. A few min in, I was disappointed to find myself laboring. Frank was unrelenting. We ran our second mile in 5:46. Frank started to fall back a bit, but I urged him on. Our third mile was 5:49, and our total run was 5:53 pace. After the tempo run, Bryan came by my place to use the gym. I added a combination rowing/elliptical workout while Bryan did his thing.	15.8
Fri.	3/11/11	Can't tell if I'm still angry about the race or just becoming more aggressive because I've added steak & eggs to my diet. Did two 30-min elliptical sessions (morning/early evening). Later Jeff Baker, visiting Miami for a medical conference, came by to use the gym. I lifted until I maxed out every muscle group.	8.6
Sat.	3/12/11	The torture continued today. I taught Matt pre-race tactics. We jogged 2 miles to the track, where we covered warm-up miles, stretching, and a series of 200m and 400m, followed by an 800m, with stretching between each rep. I ran the reps with Matt, but while he stretched, I did faster intervals – 200m and 400m reps. Later, I had dinner with Jamie and Jeff Baker. They went to a club; I headed home. I felt a little antsy, so I decided to do a stair workout. I started easy – 2 x 8 flrs, walking 2 stairs at a time. In total, I did 7 reps, pushing the last 4. After that I did weighted lunges. That wiped me out. I strapped on some ice packs and called it a night.	6.6
Sun.	3/13/11	Tired from last night's staircase and lunge workout. Sunday is my long day so I started with what was supposed to be an 8-miler. I decided to incorporate sand-based running to build strength and power. It was hot, which made the run tougher, but Outdoor Nationals will be held just outside Cleveland in late July. It will likely be very hot. I made about 45 min and had to call it. I was suffering. I went through my normal recovery routine, including a 20-min ice bath. After, I hit the beach to relax with Baker and some buddies visiting from Chicago. That evening I hit the gym for a 40-min elliptical and 15-20 min of weights (mostly upper body).	12.3
Mon.	3/14/11	Easy day. Afternoon elliptical session.	5.9
Tues.	3/15/11	John Cormier and I traveled to Curtis Track for a workout: full Coach Ward warm-up, then 3 x 300m with 5 min rest, followed by a 15-min break, followed by 3 x 150m at 90-95%. I was surprised to run the 300s in 40 to 41 sec and happy that I recovered quickly from each one. In the 150s, John *killed* me on the first one. I started faster, but he closed the gap after 20m and dusted me. On the second rep, I modified my arm motion. (In a video, I noticed that Berra's arms pump out to the side a bit, whereas mine pump straight. I also noticed that Berra's arms were bent at a 90-degree angle, whereas mine were bent more, so I copied his style.) Pumping my arms to the side generated more torso turn, which generated more speed. On the third 150m rep I got the hang of it and actually beat John. No warm-down, but later I ran 5 easy miles and did 30 min of yoga.	7.0
Weds.	3/16/11	Early afternoon weight workout with Matt Kiss. Evening elliptical, 11 miles (75:00), then 10 min rowing: 5 x 1 min w/1 min rest, felt easier than my previous rowing experiment. I added runners' curls, mimicking the arm motion I used in yesterday's interval workout – and I felt a big difference in my core. I finished with dynamic stretching and some strides, but I felt a tweak in my left quad during the strides and shut things down immediately to ice/heat/ice.	13.0
Total		Averaged 6:47 per mile for the week	69.1

Injury Reports and Medical Findings

Acupuncture: Acupuncture was one of the few remaining "mainstream" recovery techniques I hadn't tried. I rectified that with an appointment with Dr. Kasey Pryce. The first thing that surprised me was that Dr. Pryce attended four years of postgraduate school to earn a doctorate in Oriental medicine. When I got to her office, I went through similar process as I would at a traditional doctor's office – paperwork detailing my medical history, then a baseline physical exam.

When we began the session, she explained that the placement of the needles would be specific to my medical needs and the areas where I experienced pain. She believed I was generally healthy but suffered from inadequate hydration, a sub-optimal level of red blood cells, and possibly sub-optimal iron. I thought this diagnosis made sense in light of my heavy training regimen and poor attention to hydration. In theory, the needles would respond to my body to rectify the maladies and my areas of pain (although how they would fix apparent dietary conditions was beyond me).

I had no idea what to expect from the needles. I didn't think I would feel a thing when they went in – partly because they are very small needles and partly because I didn't think this form of therapy would have become popular if it was excruciating to the patients. The needles certainly were not excruciating but there was a tiny pinch as they went in. I could hardly describe the feeling as "pain," but some of the needles created a slight ache in my muscles. The doctor informed me that that was normal. Once all the needles were in, she manipulated them – rotating some, wiggling others, etc. When that process was complete, she situated a heat lamp over my back, shut off the lights, and left me in the treatment room for about 20 minutes. After that, she came back, removed the needles (a quicker process then inserting them), and the session was over.

I could still feel where the needles were placed and even felt some residual ache – nothing significant, and the doctor informed me that that was normal as well. I came away with insufficient evidence to call the session a success or failure. I learned a lot about acupuncture, but it remains to be seen whether this sort of treatment augments a training regimen.

Achilles Injuries and Injury Prevention: Based on some recurring tendinosis that cropped up during my spring training, I researched Achilles injuries and prevention.[100] Alternating ice, heat, and e-stim are good preventative measures. I also tried to limit my pounding to speed workouts and wear my short orthotics (which doubled as a heel-lift) when doing them. Running up hills was probably a major contributor to the tendonosis. I rounded out my strength training with rowing and stairs. (The flat stair surface is better than the tendon-stretching slope of hills.) I also added eccentric calf-lowers to my regimen. These are the opposite of calf raises; you start on tippy toes, then lower yourself down with your bad leg.

Training Log Week 111			
Day	Date	Notes	Mileage
Thurs.	3/17/11	Simple day, starting with a 5-mile elliptical. Later I ran 7 miles on the beach. The footing was challenging, but I kept the pace manageable. I felt no adverse effects from yesterday's heavy workload. According to his blog, Berra did an 8-mile tempo run at 6:10-6:15 pace, with a 1-mile warm-up and a 2-mile warm-down. He totaled 11 miles for the day. That said, I'm becoming less obsessed with Berra's activities. As my training schedule becomes clearer, I'm starting to focus on getting into the best shape I can.	12.0
Fri.	3/18/11	Strong day. Did a light speed workout: 2 x 200m, 2 x 400m, and 5 x 800m, all at 6 min pace. Total work was 8 miles, including warm-up and warm-down. Berra did "an easy 5" in "30-some min."	8.0
Sat.	3/19/11	Started my day with the Ocean Drive 5K. Cobi Morales, a good local runner, won in 16:14. I finished second in 16:25. Considering my last few days of work, I was happy. I felt fine after, so I opted to run at the Hurricane Invitational Track Meet. I ran 400m in 54.6 sec and the 400m hurdles in 62 sec. (See Race Report section.)	8.0
Sun.	3/20/11	Paying for yesterday's hurdles shenanigans. Sore all over. Hit the elliptical for an easy 30 min in the early afternoon. Later I returned to the gym for the rowing machine and did 5 x 1 min w/1 min rest.	5.7
Mon.	3/21/11	Stair workout; 18 reps (both up and back down). Averaged about 50 sec (up) per each 8-flr rep.	4.8
Tues.	3/22/11	As my shift in strategy takes shape, it's clear that I need to get closer to 100% healthy and change the way I approach workout intensity. Specifically, I need to train at less than race pace, which will allow me on the track more often (e.g., upward of 5 days per week). In this spirit, I only did 30 min on the elliptical.	4.3
Weds.	3/23/11	Busy workout day. Started with a light weight workout (mainly bench presses, backward lunges, and calf raises) at 1p. Later, I did a 30-min elliptical, and I upped the resistance one level. (Perhaps my strength training was starting to pay off!) After the elliptical, I jogged 1 mile to Alex's for a flexibility appointment, but we had a schedule mix-up. I walked home and did additional weights, including runners' curls and more backward lunges. I also did a 5 x 1 min rowing intervals (250m per min). This was my 777th straight day of training!	6.9
Total		Averaged 6:47 per mile for the week	**69.1**

---

100 www.achillestendon.com/PreventingInjuries.html

Training Log Week 112			
Day	Date	Notes	Mileage
Thurs.	3/24/11	Experimented with muscle activation therapy (MAT) – a massage-like technique in which trigger points supposedly activate muscles that are not firing properly. It felt like it worked; my only concern was that in my 6.3-mile run later, I could barely manage 7:00 pace. I may try again and will monitor the results.	6.3
Fri.	3/25/11	Light weights at noon; 30-min elliptical in the evening.	4.4
Sat.	3/26/11	On the track today: 2-mile warm-up and straight into 20 x 100m @ 5:00 pace w/60m active rest (2 miles total). Even with the active rest, I completed the 2 miles of speed work in 12:16. Thus, I combined a strong aerobic effort with 20 pickups at faster-than-5K pace – but the pickups were moderate enough that they should not wear me down.	4.0
Sun.	3/27/11	Back on the track today: similar to yesterday, 1-mile warm-up in 5:51, then 10 x 100m @ 4:40 pace w/60m active rest, then 2 min recovery; 10 x 100m @ 4:40 pace w/60m active rest, then 3 min recovery; 5 x 100m @ 4:40 pace w/60m active rest. Warm-down about 1.5 miles.	6.9
Mon.	3/28/11	Weight circuit at noon, mixing in one upper body, core, and lower body set into each phase of the circuit: (bench, leg lifts, quad extensions; lats, cross-over crunches, step ups; bicep curls, hyperextensions, hip adductions; triceps, sit-ups, calf raises; runners' curls, woodchops, stairs). Track work at 6p following the same format as the previous 2 days: 100m fast followed by 60m rest. I added drills to my warm-up and warm-down and totaled 6.5 miles at 6:35 pace for the workout. I feel no ill effects from being on the track in this fashion 3 days in a row.	12.0
Tues.	3/29/11	Bryan came over to try a weight circuit (similar to yesterday's) at noon. We adjusted all the machines beforehand so we would not interrupt the circuit, then we got into it: 45 sec per station (but if either of us felt the burn, we called 'time' and moved on. The idea is to build strength but be able to recover by the next day. On the track I adjusted the workout to be 8 x 200m @ 30 sec w/200m active rest. Despite being my fourth track workout in as many days, I felt great. Standard warm-up, warm-down and drills applied.	6.6
Weds.	3/30/11	Easy day; felt a *little* tired from four straight track sessions (but not too tired, really). Jogging, strides, drills, stretching, then a 30-min weight circuit and 30-min elliptical later.	4.4
Total		Averaged 6:51 per mile for the week	44.6

Dietary Research and Findings

The Pros and Cons of Magnesium: I learned of magnesium's lactate buffering properties early in my research, and some additional research I conducted indicated magnesium offered recuperative properties as well. An article by Dr. Krista Scott-Dixon, a researcher at York University, underscored magnesium's ability to alleviate cramping and aid the sleep cycle.[101] Dr. Mark Sircus, an expert on magnesium, was cited in multiple publications promoting the topical application of magnesium oil to reduce inflammation and stimulate faster regeneration of tissue.

But experimentation has its pitfalls. I experimented with magnesium supplementation by eating more magnesium rich foods, taking magnesium pills, and spraying my legs down with an Epson salt solution. I noticed a difference in muscular recovery. However, I think I found the limits of how much magnesium a person should absorb. I woke up one night with a stomach ache and diarrhea.

For 10 to 15 minutes I felt progressively worse and feared that I would have to go to the hospital. Suspecting magnesium was the culprit, I drank two bottles of water and ate several pieces of calcium-rich bread. Then I hopped into the shower to wash the Epson salt off my legs. In the shower, I flexed every muscle in my body trying to induce a lactic response. Basically, I was hoping that the calcium would inhibit any further absorption of magnesium, that the water would dilute any residual magnesium in my stomach, and that a lactic response would drive my pH level down (assuming that a high pH might be the cause of my condition).

I don't know what did the trick, but within a few minutes I felt better. Within 30 minutes, I was back in bed, thankful that it was just a close call. I cut my supplementation notably (but kept the Epson salt spray rubdowns).

---

101 Source: [Google: krista scott-dixon phd + magnesium + bodybuilding supplements]

Day	Date	Notes	Mileage
Training Log Week 113			
Thurs.	3/31/11	Morning stair workout: 20 min of continuous movement, up and down – 9 reps total; 90 sec rest, then 4 hard 'up' reps with easy downs. In the evening I ran the Nike Thursday Night Tempo; one of the good distance guys dragged me through a torture chamber (5:52 pace), but because of the effort I put in on the stairs, this didn't discourage me.	8.7
Fri.	4/1/11	Morning weight circuit with Matt; short on time, so we only did 23 min. Based on the specific demands of the 800m distance, I decided to increase the weight and decrease the time for each station from 45 sec to 30 sec. At the end of 23 min we felt like we had run a few miles, but we got the benefit of upper body, core, and lower body exercises. In the afternoon we did cardio: 20 min elliptical, followed by 5 x 1 min rows, followed by 10 min elliptical. Rowing is getting much easier with practice. Time for a Friday night cheat meal!	5.7
Sat.	4/2/11	Rested this morning, then ran to John Cormier's place in the evening for lower-body strength work (squats, hamstring lifts, box jumps, and kettle bells). Did 22 min elliptical and a jog home to warm down.	6.3
Sun.	4/3/11	A little sore from yesterday's weight workout, but not too bad. My glutes are the most sore, which pleases me. These are powerful muscles, yet I haven't done a good job exploiting them to their fullest. Morning session was 71-min elliptical (9.5 miles). In the evening I hit Flamingo Track for an extended warm-up and 2 sets of 10 x 100m with 60m active rest. I was a little slower than the last time I ran this workout, mostly due to yesterday's weights and the high heat/humidity. Calf is sore, but nothing traumatic.	16.3
Mon.	4/4/11	Calves feel fine, but everything else is fatigued. I hit the gym at noon hoping to do a weight circuit, but I knew that most the exercises would hurt more than help. So, I did the smart thing and just focused on areas that were not fatigued. It made no sense to do a hard workout in the afternoon, so I hit the elliptical for 40 min at up-tempo pace.	6.0
Tues.	4/5/11	I joined Track Club Miami for my first intermediate-distance intervals since the Indoor Nationals: 5 x 500m with "full rest" – exactly what I had in mind to get back into the swing of things. My hamstrings were a little sore from my recent workload but felt strong enough to handle 5 x 500m. I ran 60-64-sec 400m pace for the reps, then added a bonus rep at 66-sec pace. I wanted to compare this workout to one a I ran Dec. 15, 2009, but I don't know if we had more or less rest today. I skipped the warm-down to make a yoga class with John Cormier and his wife, Nawel. The class was full, but Nawel is an instructor and led us through the exercises. I want to incorporate more yoga as I did earlier in my comeback.	4.0
Weds.	4/6/11	Started the day with a mid-afternoon weight circuit (35 min). I was a bit tired from yesterday's workout, so I nixed the afternoon stair workout and went out for an easy 7-mile run, (mostly on the fairways at the Miami Beach Golf Club). It was troublesome; first my GPS battery died. Fortunately I had already established 7:00 pace, so I felt good about my exertion level and distance. Second, yesterday's workout caught up with me quickly. By Mile 5 I was spent.	7.0
Total		Averaged 6:45 per mile for the week	**54.1**

Race Reports, Records and Results

2011 Ocean Drive 5K/Hurricane Invitational: On March 19th I ran the Ocean Drive 5K. Cobi Morales, one of Miami's better local runners jumped out to an early lead and stayed strong to win in 16:14. I finished second in 16:25. Considering my previous days' workouts, I was quite happy with the time.

I felt fine afterward, so I opted to run at the Hurricane Invitational later in the day. This is where I clocked 1:57.5 in the 800 meters in 2010. That obviously wouldn't happen after a hard 5K, but I wanted to have some "fun" after a tough winter track season. I also wanted to face an old demon.

I competed in two races plus a field event (the triple jump). The racing was designed to remove a mental block dating back to high school. Back then, I routinely would experience excruciating pain for up to 20 minutes after a race – pain that did not justify racing. I never realized why this happened (in hindsight, probably the lactic acid cycle), but as a Master the pain had not been as intense. Nonetheless, the memories remained, and I avoided racing more than I probably should have. I set out to break that mindset.

I started with the 400 meters and ran a 54.6 seconds. Not bad considering my earlier 5K. I pushed hard and after the race I focused on how I felt. It hurt, but consistent with my Masters experiences, it was nothing like the old days: maybe five points on a 10-point scale. In the old days, I would consistently hit 10 on the scale.

I followed the 400 meters up by running the 400-meter hurdles. I can run over hurdles better than most, but that didn't mean I belonged in that race. I ran an amusing 62 seconds, which earned me second-to-last place in the field of Division I college athletes. But I didn't care; I was there to have fun and race hard enough to feel pain. The 400-meter hurdles was a race that would satisfy both criteria. The pain was a similar to what I experienced in the 400 meters – only five points on the 10-point scale. That was enough to ease my "race apprehension syndrome."

With more than enough racing out of the way, I tried my hand at the triple jump. Unfortunately, the qualifying board was 41 feet from the landing pit. I had pretty good leg strength, but I wasn't delusional. I made two attempts and fouled on both tries for not reaching the pit – coming up about a foot short. After that, I headed home.

2011 USATF Florida Championship: On May 15th my prerace routine included fending off my hard-partying Australian friend James "Cashy" Cashmore with all I had. Cashmore, his wife, two complete strangers he met at his bed & breakfast, and Jamie and I all went to Miami's Sugarcane restaurant for dinner. This presented several problems:

Problem #1: Sugarcane doesn't serve light pre-race meals. Sugarcane serves dates wrapped in bacon and glazed duck presented atop a Belgian waffle, draped in syrup.

		Training Log Week 114	
Day	Date	Notes	Mileage
Thurs.	4/7/11	Hectic day at work, so no morning session; flexibility session with Alex before the Thursday Nike run. First half of tonight's run was hard-packed sand, second half on pavement – 6:00 pace out; sub-5:30 pace back. Felt like a good hard run. Standard warm-up and recovery.	5.0
Fri.	4/8/11	Last hectic day at work for a while, thank God. Feel sluggish; haven't been sleeping much. Started with 30-min weights at noon; later I ran to a nearby grassy field and – after two warm-up miles – knocked off another 10 x 100m w/60m active rest workout. The reps were at 5:00 pace, and total set took 5:51 to complete.	5.7
Sat.	4/9/11	John Cormier introduced me to another strong Masters runner, Al Ray. Al, John, and I met in Fort Lauderdale for an interval workout. Being sprinters, Al and John proposed 2 x 300m and 1 x 200m at 90% effort with full rest. I wanted more volume and slower, so I compromised: I added some extra 300s during their rest periods to get 7 x 300m and 1 x 200m – but I ran my reps a little off their pace (for obvious reasons): 43.0, 43.4, 42.4, 42.2, 43.8, 27.2, 42.3, and 41.7 sec, respectively. The track facility had ice tubs, which we took advantage of after spending a fair amount of time in the heat. Later I hit the beach to relax, but I didn't last long. I was wiped. I napped and then felt good enough to hit the elliptical for 35 min.	8.1
Sun.	4/10/11	Well-needed sleep-in for recovery, followed by a walk on Lincoln Road with Jamie. Later John Cormier and I met Karl and John Mederos for some track work – of easier intensity than yesterday. John Mederos, who won the Miami Tropical 5K the year before my first win, chose 5 x 400m w/2-3 min rest, then 5 min break, then 4 x 200m w/2-3 min rest. I logged 71.0, 70.2, 69.7, 67.1, and 65.3 sec for the 400s, then 30.3, 29.7, 29.6, and 28.2 for the 200s. I kept my pace reasonable but still probably should have worn flats instead of spikes. I hopped on the infield and did 5 x 100m w/60m rest – for a non-stop 800m in 2:45. No warm-down because we were late for dinner, but after dinner I logged a 30 min elliptical with resistance at 12. I'm clearly getting stronger.	8.0
Mon.	4/11/11	Some days you just don't realize that you're working hard until you crash. Started with 30 min of circuit weights at 1p. I upped the weight on many of the machines and pushed hard the entire 30 min. I'm now better at quickly switching stations, and it's kicking my butt. At 5p I ran 6 miles. It was 82 degrees -- perfect acclimation weather, considering my big races take place in July. I ran at a fairly easy pace for the first mile (6:44). I felt a bit sluggish from the weekend's work and my earlier weights session. By the second mile I was cruising at sub-6:20 pace. I ran on grass as much as possible. The last 2 miles were especially hard. Mile 5 was 6:35 but felt like Mile 3 of a 5K. The last mile, I focused on form and got back under 6:20 to finish. Muscularly, I didn't tax myself too much but still induced complete exhaustion.	6.0
Tues.	4/12/11	After a full night's sleep and an afternoon nap, I was ready for the Tuesday track workout. I was still fatigued, but the workout wasn't going to be overly taxing: 4 x 800m w/3-4.5 min static rest. A youth team was on the track when we got there, so we did our first two reps in Lane 6. According to my GPS that was 900m, not 800m. My first rep was 2:17 for 800m, 2:35 total. My second rep was the same. The third and fourth reps were in the normal lane, and I clocked 2:25. After a recovery, I hopped on the field for 6 x 100m strides.	5.5
Weds.	4/13/11	Focused on recovery; 30-min circuit weights with Matt and Brian – still felt rough – then off to Alex for flexibility, then used a coupon for a hydromassage at Planet Beach Contempo Spa. Later I did a 1-hr elliptical.	8.6
Total		Averaged 6:35 per mile for the week	46.9

Day	Date	Notes	Mileage
Training Log Week 115			
Thurs.	4/14/11	Took the a.m. off to rest up for a tough evening session. Jogged 3 miles on roads and grass to Miami Beach Golf Club, then I eased back to 7:00 pace before launching into 10 x 100m w/60m active rest (6:15 for the full mile). After that, I plodded to the Thursday night temp run (3 miles, 7:09 pace). The tempo added 3.55 miles (6:06 pace, first 800m on sand) to the tally. Afterward, my legs were dead. I'm pretty sure it's impossible to develop sharp speed with legs as dead as mine. I believe my key focus has to be building aerobic capacity without falling behind in speed.	10.8
Fri.	4/15/11	In Newport RI for a wedding. Marked my 800th training day at the Newport YMCA with 20 min stretching/drills/strides, then a 30-min weight circuit, then a 50-min elliptical. I spent 10 min on their stretching bars until I banged my shin (but it was a good warm-down despite that incident.)	7.2
Sat.	4/16/11	Similar to yesterday. Hit the YMCA, where I loosened up before a stiff 30-min weight circuit. I stretched on the "monkey bars" for 10 min, followed by a 40-min elliptical. Wanted to save some strength for John Riley and Courtney Sullivan's wedding!	5.8
Sun.	4/17/11	Woke a little sore after an awesome party the night before. Not surprisingly, I took the morning off. Jamie, Rick Miller, John Burke, and I grabbed breakfast, where I ate like a pig. After, Jamie and I drove to my cousin's house in Massachusetts to visit for a few days. After a 1-hr nap, I was good to go for a 2-hr elliptical. I still felt good after that, so I stretched for 30 min then did 8 hard sprints (5-10 sec each), with enough rest to avoid hitting a lactic wall. I felt *fast*.	17.5
Mon.	4/18/11	Sore in the a.m.; 1-hr elliptical.	8.7
Tues.	4/19/11	Grabbed a great massage then joined my Eliot Track Club compatriots for a workout at Harvard -- first time back since the world record debacle a couple of months ago. (No bad feelings -- too many *good* memories to hold a grudge.) The workout: 4 x 800m at 2:25 w/400m rest, then 1 x 400m at 68 sec, then 3 x 50m sprints. The first rep felt hard, but the next two were fine, and the final was only kinda tough. All were on pace, and I suffered no lactic burn. Consequently I opened up a 63 sec 400m, which was fast but still fully aerobic. Warmed down with Joanie Bohlke, a blazing fast F35 middle distance runner. I finished with 3 x 50m sprints, and I can feel my speed coming back. The combination of my aerobic base, resurgent speed, and upcoming anaerobic phase promised to be a deadly combination. I was hoping everything would come together by summer. If so, I would have a very good shot of placing high at the world championships and winning a national title.	9.8
Weds.	4/20/11	Jamie and I spent much of the day in transit to Miami. Luckily, today was a planned easy day. Bryan and I hit the gym for 20 min of upper-body weights and 30 min on the elliptical.	4.3
Total		Averaged 6:48 per mile for the week	**64.1**

Problem #2: People really enjoy what Sugarcane serves. This makes it *very* difficult to be seated for your table for four when you show up with two additional strangers — making your total six.

Problem #3: Cashy doesn't eat quickly. This is mainly because Cashy drinks quickly… very quickly.

Despite resisting Cashy's pleadings to "rip it up" after dinner, my head didn't hit a pillow until nearly 1 a.m. Worse yet, my pre-bed weight was 159 pounds, way above my preferred race weight of 150 pounds. I woke up at 5 a.m. with a modest headache… but *no* pre-meet headache is modest at 5 a.m. After an hour, I fell back to sleep -- two hours before my alarm clock sounded. Not surprisingly, I awoke slowly and required an extra-long hot shower. Though none too confident about my chances of running a decent time, I was actually starting to feel half-normal… And then things got ugly.

I learned the meet started an hour late (perhaps due to the drizzle that was falling) and was nearly that far behind schedule. The first event of the day, the 5,000 meters, was still being contested. I decided to turn the negative into a positive, check in, hit the local supermarket to stock up some post-race bananas and yogurt, then relax.

Unbeknownst to me, the Florida chapter of USATF hadn't quite figured out how to convert South Florida's rabid population of 5K road racers into track addicts. The meet was thinly attended, and by the time I returned from the store 20 minutes later, the 800 meters was on track to start as scheduled. Instead of having more than an hour to warm up and relax, I had 30 minutes: just enough time to do two quick laps and three quick drills before changing into my uniform, lacing up the spikes, and running two quick strides. By then, the field was heading to the starting line; I hurried to the official to grab my hip-number and lane assignment... But they didn't have my name on the list.

This glitch was weeks in the making. The registration web site wouldn't allow me (a Master) to sign up for the open 800 meters, which is where I wanted to compete. I had contacted the meet director and thought the issue was solved... but clearly, it wasn't. They delayed the start of the race and bounced me from official to official until someone came up with the brilliant idea of simply writing me onto the list and sorting it out later.

So with a wet track, a body heading into cool-down mode, and a head/heart that was losing focus and interest, I responded to the gun. My strategy was to open with 58 seconds for the first 400 meters by getting a good break and vying for position behind the lead runner, but when I got to the breakpoint, no one else was there. I later learned that Florida's faster 800-meter runners attended a track meet in Jacksonville instead. I hit the 400-meter mark in 58 seconds as hoped, but my haphazard pre-race experience left me with little desire to push the pace. I got all the way to the final straightaway before I finally decided to throw in a modest surge. I crossed the line in 2:01-ish.

It was still a solid effort and gave me plenty of valuable information. On January 15, 2011, I ran a 2:02.6 to start my indoor track season, just seven weeks prior to Indoor Nationals. At this meet, I ran about a second faster with less effort and I still had over 10 weeks before Outdoor Nationals. Considering the circumstances, I was satisfied.

Training Log Week 116

Day	Date	Notes	Mileage
Thurs.	4/21/11	Logged some easy miles before the Nike Thursday Tempo Run. Started with 2 miles at 6:30 pace, which felt great from the start. I'm now tracking heart rate (HR), which was constant at 151-153 bpm until the last part of the warm-up. Next I slowed to 7:30 pace before kicking off 10 x 100m w/60m active rest (5:46 for the total mile, 162bpm). After 20 min rest, I ran the tempo run (sub-6:00 pace), taking note of my HR at different splits. My beginning rate was high (93bpm) because of the work I did prior, but the first two miles were at 168 bpm or lower and I finished 3.5 miles at 173bpm.	7.6
Fri.	4/22/11	Noon circuit weights (33:20; 101 bpm avg/134 bpm max), then 30 min stairs (133 bpm avg/152 bpm max). Coming down between sets, I hit each stair quickly to keep my heart rate above 130 bpm before reaching bottom. Later, I did 4 miles (7:14 pace, 150bpm). Heat and muscle fatigue cause a high bpm at slow pace.	8.2
Sat.	4/23/11	After a long night's sleep, I ran 10 miles at about noon – 80 degrees and humid. My goal was to keep my HR at about 150 bpm (aerobic). The first 3 miles were easy, and I maintained the zone at 6:30 pace – but it got harder, and by the last 3 miles I was at about 7:25 pace.	10.0
Sun.	4/24/11	4p weight circuit (15 min, 110bpm) with Bryan, followed by 30-min elliptical (110-140bpm). Next I headed to John's for another 30-min easy elliptical (110bpm), accompanying him as he warmed up. Next we did squats (3 x 10 @ 115, 205, and 205lbs), calves (3 x 10 @ 180lbs, 135lbs, and 135lbs), and box jumps (3 x 10, stacked 10 high). We capped the workout with 6 x 40m sprints with a full recovery.	8.3
Mon.	4/25/11	Sore from yesterday, clearly overtaxed my hamstrings. Hit the gym late for 30-min elliptical (135bpm) I reached 110 bpm pretty quickly but took about 10 min to reach to 135bpm. Every weight exercise except quads proved fruitless, so I went for a 6-mile recovery run. My HR hit 150 bpm at only 7:00 pace, but it held steady – indicating I might truly have been recovering.	10.3
Tues.	4/26/11	Pre-breakfast elliptical (30 min, HR 130-154bpm). At 5:30, hit the track with John Cormier. Workout was as many 200m reps as possible w/30 sec rest while maintaining aerobic HR zone (135-155bpm). We did 9 x 200m in 27-30 sec before John's calves cramped and we decided to stop.	10.3
Weds.	4/27/11	Started so late, my "a.m." workout began at 2:30p. Aiming for recovery, I started with a 30-min weight circuit, then 10-min elliptical. HR was under 93 bpm for 10 min, under 111 bpm for the next 20 min or so, and then under 130 bpm until the final 3 min of the workout (134bpm). I went outside for 5 miles and the HR jumped to 150BPM pretty quickly (7:00 avg pace).	6.5
Total		Averaged 6:58 per mile for the week	61.2

Miscellaneous Research and Notes

Heart Rate Training: When I got home from the Masters Indoor Nationals, two packages were waiting for me -- an under-desk bicycle and a heart rate monitor. The under-desk bike was something of a gimmick I decided to experiment with to increase my daily caloric burn. The heart rate monitor was a more well-thought purchase. I had been researching heart rate-based training and its kissing cousin lactate-threshold training for awhile. Rick Miller had sent some very detailed research on heart-rate training that he found on the Let's Run message boards that made a lot of sense to me. By Week 116 in my training log, you'll notice I started measuring most activities by heart rate beats per minute (BPM) as well as by time and distance.

The under-desk bike was not the most sophisticated piece of equipment. I tossed it under the desk and gave it a whirl. Within a few seconds my heart rate popped 20 percent, from 60 BPM to 72 BPM. It stabilized around that level as I pedaled intermittently while working on my computer.

I didn't break a sweat, but I got warm enough to switch from a long-sleeve shirt to a T-shirt. Nothing to write home about, but I figured if Paavo Nurmi got some benefit from walking a 10K every morning, I might get a little something out of that. When I checked the digital display at the end of the day it said that I had turned the crank over 6,000 times and done a total of 55 minutes of work. Granted, it was all very low intensity stuff. However, over the course of an entire day, that probably added up to a lot of calories. It may have provided some recovery benefit, as well because extra blood circulated through my body. It wasn't something I could credit knocking seconds off of my 800-meter time, but it made me feel a little bit better about my sedentary day job.

Unlike the under-desk bike, the heart rate monitor quickly became what I would describe as a mandatory weapon in my training arsenal. For most of March 2011, I simply wore it on runs to monitor what was going on with my body

Training Log Week 117

Day	Date	Notes	Mileage
Thurs.	4/28/11	Erratic sleep killed my a.m. workout. I was tired by evening as well, but I headed out. I felt surprisingly good, even at 80 degrees – and I averaged well below 7:00 pace for 7 miles w/out a huge spike in HR (about 151bpm, steady). This may indicate yesterday's recovery session worked, and I'm growing more confident in HR training as a principle.	7.2
Fri.	4/29/11	John and I ran hills. We started with 1 mile jogging/strides to warm up, then we ran 8 hills. The pace was variable – John erred toward fast; I erred toward slower – but we would stop when our HR reached 150bpm. The next rep would start when John's HR got back down to 135bpm. I kept my HR in a similar range by doing high-knees during our recovery jog-downs. I capped the workout with 3 x 8-sec hard strides up the steep side of the hill. After, I was fatigued and my right Achilles tendon hurt. I walked home (1.5 miles) at a strong pace to keep my HR in the 110-120 bpm range. Later, I did a 30-min elliptical at a solid intensity and some upper/lower/core weight work.	6.8
Sat.	4/30/11	Elliptical session (45 min); later I did 5 strides, the final 2 at near full speed.	6.5
Sun.	5/1/11	Hard elliptical (30 min), starting at high resistance and easing back to Level 12 (still higher than my norm). HR went from inactive 77 bpm to 146 bpm from 20-min mark until finish. Later I jogged to John Cormier's (1.5 miles, 6:18 pace, avg HR 132bpm) for squats, calves, and box jumps. Immediately after, we jogged to Flamingo Track for 8 x 60m strides with ample recovery. Felt fast and strong and jogged home.	7.9
Mon.	5/2/11	Hard elliptical (50 min, Level 12) because I've been doing a lot of high-impact work lately. Followed with 5 hard strides. I feel my body is adjusting well to the speed; I wonder if part of this is because I've started experimenting with Epson salt and magnesium oil.	7.5
Tues.	5/3/11	Morning elliptical (30 min, moderate pace). Evening track workout: a few 200m strides at 6-min pace to warm up, then 14 x 200m w/pace *and* rest determined by HR (155 bpm max, sub-145 bpm recovery). This forced longer rest periods, so my total time/pace was slower than when I run my 'X' x 100m workouts. I will try this workout again to compare data and determine if it is an optimal way to spend my track time.	9.0
Weds.	5/4/11	Easy pre-breakfast elliptical (30 min). Afternoon weight circuit with Bryan (avg HR 108bpm, max HR 140bpm), immediately followed by another 30-min elliptical (avg HR 125bpm, max HR 140bpm).	8.6
Total		Averaged 6:45 per mile for the week	**53.4**

during different training scenarios – but by mid-April, after some additional research, I was using it not just to monitor my body but to guide it through workouts and govern effort levels.

For the uninitiated, heart rate training seems daunting and confusing – and to make matters worse, everyone's optimal heart rate training zones are different... so there's no standardized chart you can consult when deciding how you should train each day. Entire books have been written on the science of heart rate training, and theories differ on the best ways to calculate your resting heart rate and your maximum heart rate.[102] But once you've done the ground work to calculate your zones, the concept is fairly simple.

Calculating your resting heart rate is relatively easy. Strap on your monitor or accurately take your pulse when you first wake up in the morning – or wear the monitor and chill out on the couch in a totally relaxed, near-napping state for 10-15 minutes. Calculating your max heart rate is a little trickier. The old formula, subtracting your age from the base number of 220, has been proven unreliable over years of testing. A newer formula, 205 BPM minus half your age, is said to be better for athletes – but this too can be wildly inaccurate. (My co-author's max rate has repeatedly tested between 196-200 BPM while the formulae say he should max out at 180-185 BPM.)

The only real way to calculate your maximum heart rate is to push yourself close to your max. Fortunately you don't need to run a half-marathon or some similar great distance to do so. A simple, short track workout should get you close to the accurate measure you need. *(I issue this advice with the normal caveat: Consult your physician before beginning training to be <u>certain</u> you're in sufficient health to be running hard.)* At the track, do your customary warm-up and stretching as you would before a race or hard workout, then run 1 x 800 meters all-out, followed by two minutes rest, followed by 1 x 400 meters all-out. The highest heart rate you record during or after the intervals should be your max – or very close to it.

With these baseline numbers, you can calculate your training zones, of which most coaches and physiologists say there are five:

➤ Recovery (50-60 percent)
➤ Aerobic (60-70 percent)
➤ Steady State (70-80 percent)
➤ Anaerobic (80-90 percent)
➤ Sprint or Red Line (90-100 percent)

Note: The percentages above represent the difference in BPM between your *resting heart rate* and your *maximum heart rate*, not the percentage of your maximum heart rate alone. (e.g., If your resting rate was 60 BPM and your max rate was 180 BPM, a 50 percent "recovery" run would *not* be 90 BPM, it would be 120 BPM.)

A number of Web sites will help you calculate your training zones, and depending on the formula the site uses, you might find the zones differ by a few BPM from site to site. I used famed British coach Brian Mackenzie's site (www.brianmac.co.uk/hrm1.htm) to calculate mine because he provides descriptions of the physiological effect each zone is designed to stimulate; however, based on the calculator he uses, some people may need to fudge their age to arrive at their true max heart rate.

How you apply heart rate training will vary according to the distance at which you intend to compete. As an 800-meter specialist, I intended to spend more days on the track working in the upper heart rate zones than perhaps a marathon specialist would. However, one principle holds true no matter how you leverage this style of training: recovery runs are essential, and recovery runs are *sloooow*. The biggest mistake athletes of all levels make is training too hard on recovery days. When Rick Miller adopted this method of training, he was certain the either the monitor or the math was wrong. His slow days were at nearly 9:00-mile pace. We later learned this is common.

---

102 *Heart Monitor Training for the Compleat Idiot*, by John L. Parker Jr. (yes, the same John L. Parker Jr. who wrote the great *Once a Runner*) is one such book. Lydiard's books and others also address the concept.

Mark Gomes' Heart Rate Measurements, Spring 2011		
Resting Heart Rate:	55 BPM	
Maximum Heart Rate:	180 BPM	
Zones	Min BPM	Max BPM
Recovery	118	130
Aerobic	130	143
Steady State	143	155
Anaerobic	155	168
Sprint/Maximum	168	180

Training Log Week 118

Day	Date	Notes	Mileage
Thurs.	5/5/11	No Cinco de Mayo party for me. Morning rest; afternoon strength work with John: a variety of drills and moderate-intensity strides, followed by 10-12 bounding drills... 45 min of solid work. We added 4 x 30-sec stair sprints. Later, I returned to the stairs for 30 min of aerobic work: 13 x 12flr reps, double-step up and quick single-step down. I stayed in my steady-state HR zone, averaging 150bpm. Total time = 30:12.	6.5
Fri.	5/6/11	*Very* sore from yesterday; 30-min recovery elliptical and rest.	4.2
Sat.	5/7/11	Not recovered enough to work hard today. Elected to rely on my slow-twitch muscles and do my slow distance run. Set my HR target at 155 bpm and settled in to 6:40-6:50 pace until Miles 6-7, when I had to back off to keep my HR constant. Oddly, in Mile 8 I was able to increase the pace again w/out a rise in HR.	8.0
Sun.	5/8/11	That evening, still sore, I went to John's for plyos and hills. We did box jumps (lower height, higher reps than last week, with a focus on greater jump speed), then proceeded to MacArthur Causeway Bridge for 4 downhill sprints (2 for quickness, 2 for speed) and 3 high-intensity uphill reps with walking rest. We finished back at the gym with squats. This week, we upped the weight and lowered the number of reps per set. We did this because the squats are to build power, just as the box jumps are for explosiveness, the uphills are for strength, and the downhills are for quickness. Later I logged a 30-min elliptical (Level 12) and 5 x 1 min rowing session. My strength is improving on both of those machines.	7.2
Mon.	5/9/11	Logged a 6-mile run similar to my 7-miler on April 28th – HR 152bpm, avg pace 6:45 – mostly on grass in warm conditions, which represents an improvement. After the run, I did upper-body work (bench, curls, pull-downs, and triceps) and core work (various crunches). I also did 2 sets of abductors and adductors. For the first set, I did 10 reps at my college weight. For the 2nd set, I kicked the weight up 10-15%, but I only did 5 reps.	6.0
Tues.	5/10/11	*Still* not fully recovered from May 5th's strides and plyo work. Glutes/hamstrings are very sore, borderline strained. Yet another lesson to ease into a new training phase. Been sleeping well though: 8 hrs per night plus naps. John and I hit the track but decided that recovery was prudent. I did a lot of stretching and drills, followed by a 1-mile warm-up in 6:27. I stayed on the infield wearing a new pair of Vibram Komodos. My feet need strengthening – as I suspect do most people's – but I will *ease* into these. We worked on start drills and fixed a problem with John's start by forcing him to run *on* the line instead of in the lane. This limited his wasted lateral movement. Later I logged a 30-min hard elliptical and reached a HR of 140 bpm by the 10-min mark. I held my pace, which gradually edged my heart rate deeper into my steady-state zone.	6.0
Weds.	5/11/11	Started the day with a hydro-massage, immediately followed by PT at Alex's office. He worked almost exclusively on my calves, Achilles, and feet. He could have worked my glutes/hamstrings, but they're not "problem areas"— just slow to recover from last week's plyo overload. In the afternoon I copied my May 5th stair workout: 13 x 12flrs, double-step up/single-step down. Total time was a little off from May 5th: 30:23, possibly because of heat. Avg HR was similar (144bpm). Next I did 20-30 min upper-body weights.	4.8
Total		Averaged 6:38 per mile for the week	**42.7**

Training Log Week 119

Day	Date	Notes	Mileage
Thurs.	5/12/11	Easy day: easy 30-min elliptical, easy 30-min run (golf course), easy drills, 4 x 50m strides. Feel healthy.	8.9
Fri.	5/13/11	Today's goal was to hit every muscle type, energy system, and training phase in 75 min or less. (I've concluded the quickest work should be done early to ensure optimal neuromuscular uptake. Thus, I've prioritized my activities from fast to slow.) That requires an extra good warm-up. I started 20 min of dynamic stretches and drills, then went right into 3 strong 50m strides. I moved to stairs: 8 x 6 flrs @ 95% effort w/walk down recovery. My HR progressed from 141 bpm to 160 bpm fairly linearly. Next was 5 x 1-min rows, w/1 min active rest (HR of 150 bpm each rep). Last, I hit the elliptical (Level 12) for 20 min, ramping my pace and ramping my HR from 140 bpm to 154bpm. Throughout the workout, my HR remained aerobic, but I still worked my ATP/creatine phosphate system (strides) and my anaerobic/lactic system (stairs, rows) – so each system got some work.	5.1
Sat.	5/14/11	Easy 30-min elliptical.	4.3
Sun.	5/15/11	Woke up on 6 hrs sleep after dinner with James Cashmore and friends. Won the Open 800m at the debacle that was the USATF Florida Championships (see Race Results section), then added some Masters jumping events and 1,500m Run (1st place) for additional work. Later, I hit the elliptical (45 min, avg 137bpm). The last 10 min were tough (fatigue was setting in), but I got through it with a little help from Ozzy Osborne.	9.0
Mon.	5/16/11	Scheduled easy day: 30-min circuit weights, then 30-min elliptical. Achilles is hurting a bit today.	4.2
Tues.	5/17/11	Track day. Warm-up of stretching, massage (especially on the Achilles), 1 x 400m @ 7:45 pace, more stretching, 1 x 400m at 5:24 pace, more stretching, 1 x 800m at 5:08 pace, then drills. Workout = 1 x 1 mile, 2 x 400m, 2 x 300m, and 2 x 200m. We got 10-min rest after the 1 mile, and 2 min static rest between all other reps. The track was packed, and Bryan Sharkey and I spent most laps running wide to avoid people. Adjusted times (based on Garmin) were 4:39 for 1 mile; 61.1 and 58.6 sec, respectively, for the 2 x 400m; 43.2 and 43.3 sec for the 2 x 300m, and 27.4 and 26.7 sec for the 2 x 200m. My max HR in the 1-mile rep was 175bpm, which surprised me because it felt easy. I didn't go above 170 bpm again until the final 200m rep. Easy 1-mile warm-down, and later I snuck in an easy 35-min elliptical session.	9.0
Weds.	5/18/11	Recovery day: 30-min elliptical and 4 x 150m strides. Achilles is still sore, but holding steady.	4.7
Total		Averaged 6:43 per mile for the week	**45.1**

Cross Training and Sprints: One strategic dilemma troubled me as I sought to integrate heart rate-based training and plan workout paces and recovery more logically: How could I prevent the mistakes of my winter season and improve my strength and raw speed while still training at paces that allowed adequate recovery? I decided to increase the emphasis on circuit-weight workouts and 100-meter sprints.

I used the heart rate monitor to reach my aerobic zone and remain there for as long as possible each day without deadening my legs – combining weight circuits, 100-meter sprints, and elliptical sessions into single, continuous workouts. I aimed to top off my aerobic capacity while developing my legs' fast-twitch muscle fibers. I wanted a smooth transition from my base phase to my anaerobic phase later in the season.

I investigated how Emil Zatopek incorporated sprints and strides into his training regimen. Remember, Zatopek won the 5,000 meters, 10,000 meters, and marathon at the 1952 Olympic Games. There is no debating that he was a distance runner. Despite this, he incorporated a disproportionate amount of 100s, 200s, and 400s into his training. He was widely criticized for this but was famously quoted as saying, "I already know how to run slow. I must learn to run fast by practicing to run fast." He once said, "If I run 100 meters 20 times, that is 2 kilometers and that is no longer a sprint." Zatopek's sprints were *not* all-out efforts; however, they were much faster than the other running he would do. This was very similar to my "nonstop 100s" workout (see Training Log).

Zatopek's training philosophy was inspired by Paavo Nurmi, a 5,000-meter and 10,000-meter specialist from the 1920s who ranks among the greatest Olympians of all time (12 medals). In the book *Lore of Running*, author Timothy Noakes noted that when Nurmi was in his early-20s, his training included long morning walks (at least 10,000 meters), cross country skiing, and 10,000 meters worth of sprints ranging from 80 meters to 800 meters. Nurmi would often run short sprints at the end of his walks and training runs and was rumored to occasionally grab onto the back of moving trains, which would pull him along faster than he could run on his own.

Nurmi's and Zatopek's dominance as distance runners during their respective eras suggests that incorporating sprints and strides into your aerobic training regimen is extremely effective. More circumstantial evidence supported this. Rick Miller had long suggested that athletes who played soccer exhibited a proclivity toward successful distance and middle distance running. Miller ran for a highly successful high school program in New York, with very experienced track coaches who fostered multiple state champions. Yet he was amazed each spring when two or three soccer players would come out for winter or spring track and make the team – with no cross country season under their belts or summer distance running. But soccer games and scrimmages are – at their core – a series of sprints and recoveries: sprint to the ball, engage, recover; sprint to the ball again.

Here is one *important* note: Mixing aerobic and sprint training differs greatly from mixing aerobic training with lactic threshold (anaerobic) training, which is widely considered to be suboptimal.

Training Log Week 120

Day	Date	Notes	Mileage
Thurs.	5/19/11	First workout with Moses Washington[103] at the Miami Gardens Athletic Complex. Long warm-up and Achilles massage, then did a full "Coach Ward" with drills. Workout was 10 x 400m @ 70 sec (cut to 7 x 400m when I screwed up the pace on the first 2); 1 min static rest between reps. I logged 62.6, 65.1, 66.3, 63.5, 62.0, 64.7, and 66.0 sec, respectively. My HR hit 171 bpm in Rep #3 and ended at 177 bpm on Rep #7 – 2 bpm higher than my previous hard workout. Maybe my central nervous system is giving my body more leeway for punishment. After dinner, Rick Miller and I hit the gym for some lower body work and 30 min on the elliptical.	8.2
Fri.	5/20/11	Recovery day. Miller, Bryan, and I did the now-standard 30-min weight circuit, immediately followed by 30 min on the elliptical. Later, I headed out to Ocean Drive for some stretching and strides. For a recovery day, it was pretty hard. I may have to rethink off-day workouts now that I'm hitting the track more aggressively.	4.3
Sat.	5/21/11	Long, easy day. After relaxing all day, I did 70 min on the elliptical. Hopefully, today's "break" gives my legs enough rest before my usual Sunday night workout at John's gym.	10.0
Sun.	5/22/11	Neither John nor I was fully recovered from our recent work, so we started with a lot of stretching and a quick warm-up on the elliptical. After a set of squats, we focused on upper body (bench presses, chin-ups, and power pushups). Assuming our legs couldn't handle anything explosive, we hit the stairs: 5 x 60 sec double-stepping, fast single-stepping down for recovery. It was walking pace, but it was tough. My HR jumped immediately to 150 bpm (although it never broke 155bpm). Either my heart is getting stronger, or my legs just couldn't muster real work. Warmed down with a 5-min elliptical, then much later I did another 30-min elliptical at a very easy pace.	7.0
Mon.	5/23/11	Woke up feeling much better, but took some PT at Synergy Wellness Clinic in downtown Miami. (I had a Groupon for massage, and learned they do ultrasound and e-stim – and they work with my health insurance! I won't replace Alex, but I may use Synergy for issues my insurance will cover.) Dr. Gus Marshall recognized my issues with no prompting, performed e-stim on my back, ultrasound on my calves, then finished with some manual work – a very productive session. After PT I met Bryan for 35 min on the elliptical. That evening I ran to Flamingo Track (1 mile, 5:22 pace), then I did 10 x 100m @ about 15 sec per, keeping my HR at 155 bpm or less – still in my steady state zone, allowing me to save anaerobic work for later in the week.	6.8
Tues.	5/24/11	Tues. night speed work at Booker T Track: 5 x 500m @ 70 sec (400m) pace. I hit each time as planned, but I left disappointed; I guess I expected a breakthrough after last week. I walked instead of ran a warm-down, to protect my Achilles, then hit the elliptical for 35 min. I added some light squats, lunges, reverse lunges, runners' curls, and chin-ups for good measure.	8.5
Weds.	5/25/11	Recovery day. Pre-breakfast elliptical (30 min), then 30 min more at noon, plus some light weights. I had an appointment with Alex at 4p, and he worked the calves and Achilles good. I walked 3+ miles around town doing errands, then around 9p I stretched and did 5 x 150m strides.	8.5
Total		Averaged 6:51 per mile for the week	53.2

---

103 Moses Washington was a U.S. Junior National Champion at Florida's' Carol City High School – where he now coaches. He won virtually every major high school 800-meter race and had a high school PR of 1:48.5 – which he lowered to 1:47.9 at the University of Oklahoma. In his 30s, he was still a sub-1:50 threat.

Chapter 14
Face the Electric Time Shock Now

Weeks 121-130

In November of 1984 (my freshman year of high school), like thousands of boys around New England, and probably the nation, I watched Boston College quarterback Doug Flutie complete a ridiculous Hail Mary pass to Gerard Phelan with just seconds remaining on the game clock to shock the University of Miami. Coming from a working-class family, I knew little about college – but I knew someday I wanted to go to BC.

By spring of my junior year of high school, my awareness of college had changed. I was excelling in math and doing well in other subjects – and my achievements on the track were garnering some attention. I received recruiting requests from prestigious schools like Harvard and Cornell, but the biggest excitement for me was coming home one day to find a letter from Boston College.

BC invited me for an overnight. I was out of control with excitement. On the first day, I was given a walking tour of the campus. The next day, I was taken to Alumni Stadium, where the BC football and track teams competed. The locker rooms were nice, but the school's record board was what really caught my eye. The times and distances were *insane*. I was overwhelmed.

I got to watch a BC track meet. There weren't many spectators, but that was fine with me. I sat high in the stands and silently rooted for the home team. The times were fast, but compared to the school's record board, it was a big relief. Some of the 800-meter and one-mile times were slower than mine, so I knew I could hang. Then came the biggest surprise of the trip – track coach Randy Thomas told me that he would be offering me a full scholarship!

There were no words to describe the feeling. Things like this only happened in movies. Not only was I going to college, but I was going to Boston College – on a full scholarship to run track! My home track was going to be at Alumni Stadium, the same stadium where Doug Flutie played out his college career. I wanted everyone to know about it, and soon that wish came true too. I was named "All-Scholastic" by *The Patriot Ledger*, the primary newspaper of suburban Boston. They ran a photograph and a detailed interview – an interview in which they asked where I would attend college. I was pretty happy to say "BC." A few days later, *The Patriot Ledger* spread the word across much of Massachusetts. Soon after that, the other college coaches stopped calling. I was spoken for and couldn't be happier. It was a huge relief going into my senior year.

My final season of outdoor track, I went on a tear – establishing new school records in the half-mile and mile. After winning the Massachusetts State Qualifier meet, Coach Dave sprung the news on me: The 1988 State Finals and 1988 New England Championships would be held at Boston College. I couldn't believe it. My high school career was going to end on the same track where my college career would soon begin.

At the State Finals, I looked for Coach Thomas. I was still waiting for my scholarship paperwork. Not seeing him before the meet, I turned my attention back to the competition. Once again I'd be racing my nemesis Jamalh Prince from Cambridge Rindge & Latin. Prince won this race the year before (the race in which Scott Cody out-leaned me), but I was a year stronger now and had run a faster time than Prince at the Eastern States meet indoors. Now, one last time, we'd see who was the state's fastest miler.

It was a dogfight from the start. Prince led and I followed. He pushed hard. I hung close, running with him stride for stride. As we completed our third lap, the bell signaled one to go. Prince sped up. I went with him. As we rounded the track, I could tell we were alone. With half a lap to go, I surged with everything I had left. Prince responded by unleashing his vaunted kick. It was too much. I couldn't hold on and finished second. I ran 4:17 – a school record – but it wasn't good enough.

Later that week, I called Coach Thomas at BC. I still hadn't received the scholarship paperwork and was getting concerned. I was relieved to finally hear his voice when he answered the phone, but that was about as good as the conversation got. When I asked where I could find my scholarship papers, Coach Thomas explained that he had given out too many scholarships but that he would help me get financial aid. I didn't understand what financial aid was, so I asked.

"It's a loan to pay for your tuition," he explained.

"A loan?" I replied. "So, at some point I'll have to pay it back?"

"Yes, but I'll take care of you next year," he replied.

I was only 17 and naïve to the college game, but I was pretty certain that I had been tricked. He had offered me the scholarship but never put the promise on paper. By that point in the year, scholarships had been awarded to everyone. Everyone but me. In an instant, a four-year dream evaporated. If I didn't understand what betrayal felt like before, I did then. A rush of blood went to my head. My body felt like it had been lit on fire. I was as angry as I had ever been, and I lashed out:

"Randy?" I asked.

"Yes," he replied.

"Fuck you!"

I slammed the phone down. I was in shock. The next week was a blur. I don't remember running. I don't remember talking to anyone. I only remember telling Coach Dave what had happened and asking him what I was going to do. I don't remember him having an answer.

The following week I ran a poor race and finished fifth at the New England Championships. I remember hating the medal they gave me, and I remember learning that Jamalh Prince would be going to BC on a full scholarship. I couldn't have been more humiliated. I sat by myself on the football field after the race, changing out of my racing shoes. I was too busy pouting to notice a lanky figure standing over me.

"Nice race," the figure said.

I disagreed, but thanked him anyway.

"I'm Mark Lech. I coach at Northeastern. I heard about you from Coach Day."

Jane Day was another coach at Stoughton High. Coach Dave must have told her what had happened.

"I can only offer you a half-scholarship, but if that works, I can have paperwork ready in a couple of days."

My head down, I mustered a few words in a low voice, "Can I ask you two questions?"

"Sure," he responded.

"Does Northeastern go against BC?"

"Yeah. We race them a lot."

I felt a familiar rush of blood in my head. A renewed wave of anger swept over me. I was still sitting quietly, but inside of me things were very loud.

"What's your other question?" Coach Lech inquired.

"Where do I sign?"

I thought about that day more than a few times in the weeks leading up to the 2011 Masters Nationals. In essence, it was the start of things. That day didn't mark my first step on a track or my first first-place finish, but it was the platform I needed to right perhaps the biggest wrong I'd been subjected to at that point in life. It set the stage for my early triumphs, and at the same time it set the stage for my later regrets. Less than two years after that disappointment, I would dominate BC, prove my point to Coach Thomas, and not long after that I would get more satisfaction throwing back beers with my BC friends than leading them around the oval... And 20 years after that, I was thinking about all the things I might have done.

Now I was two years deep into a mission that meant very little to anyone around me but myself. Only my closest runner friends could possibly understand (and half of *them* probably thought I was wasting my time – and far too much effort – on a race that few people had heard of and even fewer would see). But validation is a strange desire. It starts with a discrete topic – in my case a need to see if my unrealized college talent was real – and it expands... I wasn't just proving my talent anymore; I was proving that you can make up for lost time, that you can be forgiven for sins – that while Father Time is the one competitor who remains undefeated, you can add a lot of rounds to the fight. It was a comforting emotional transformation – empowering. Which prompted another recurring thought, a diametric opposite:

What if I lost?

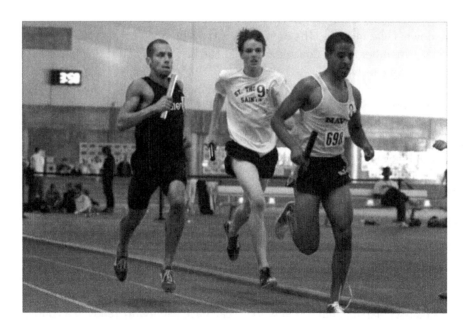

Mark Gomes (L) chases two collegians in the failed world record attempt at Harvard, February 2011.

Training Log Week 121			
Day	Date	Notes	Mileage
Thurs.	5/26/11	My kryptonite is speed. The workout was 6 x 300m @ 43 sec (sub-1:55 pace) w/3 min rest. This was my hardest workout in recent memory. I didn't make it to the final rep and was in *agony* for 20 min after. John clocked me at 42.3, 42.3, 43.0, 43.7, and 44.1 before I reached failure. I must improve here. My only solace was seeing another running laying on the track in agony. I've never seen him before, but he was running some *very* fast 200s earlier. He might make a good training partner for John… assuming he ever comes back! I didn't catch his name.	5.7
Fri.	5/27/11	Recovery day: easy 60-min elliptical at noon; drills and strides in the evening. I visited the Synergy Wellness Clinic for my Achilles and hamstring.	9.0
Sat.	5/28/11	Another recovery day. I've been reading Tim Noakes' *Lore of Running* – a 900-page beast of a book that is required reading for any runner. Today, I read a section on recovery and overtraining. After perusing the list of symptoms, I opted for lots of sleep, reading, and an easy 30-min elliptical. On a brighter note, my Achilles and hamstring feel great! Yesterday's PT got it back to 95%.	4.0
Sun.	5/29/11	Woke up around noon feeling great. Ran a pre-breakfast, dual-mode 7 miler. (Dual-mode meaning I kept the first 6 miles in my aerobic zone and then pushed hard the last mile.) It was 86 degrees when I started the run, but I'm heat acclimated now. I wanted sub-40:00 for the first 6 miles, but a quick open spiked my HR too soon, and I had to back off the pace to stay aerobic (40:34 through 6 miles). I ran the final mile in 5:53. Later I met John for weights/plyos and downhill strides. On the third stride, I felt a swelling in my hamstring and immediately shut things down. It was sore but didn't feel injured – but better not to take chances.	7.0
Mon.	5/30/11	Awoke fearing the worst; time to test the hamstring. Could've been better; could've been worse. Feels like I need a wk of rest and PT. With 6 wks until Worlds, I should be fine. I headed straight to Synergy Wellness Clinic for e-stim and ultrasound. Later I did 30 min on the elliptical very easy (just to keep my streak alive).	4.3
Tues.	5/31/11	The hamstring and Achilles felt better, but not close to 100%. I also felt a bit run down and residually sore from Sunday's workout. Despite this, the creature of habit in me thought to hit the track. Good sense prevailed when I called Coach Dave for a second opinion. Unsurprisingly, he advised me to take it easy for another couple days. He reinforced that a few days of rest can be worth more than a few days of hard work. I've done some hard work over the past few wks, so a rest is due. I logged an easy 45-min elliptical and light weights. I didn't feel a single twinge in my hamstring, so I knew I could at least lift weights if all else failed.	6.0
Weds.	6/1/11	Easy 30-min elliptical and a session with Alex for more PT. I felt ok – maybe a little bit sore from yesterday's weights – but I felt ready to get back to a hard-easy-hard schedule. For me it was more beneficial to go extra hard on hard days and extra easy on the easy ones, and I was trying to perfect the art of supercompensation – that optimal balance between hardwork and rest that leads to the greatest muscular development.	4.2
Total		Averaged 7:05 per mile for the week	40.2

Injury Reports and Medical Findings

At this point, I had found a solid balance between training hard and staying healthy. I had no way of eliminating the calf pains that would crop up after hard workouts, but I now had an effective physical therapy routine for eliminating them during my off days. For the most part, going into my biggest races ever, I was healthy!

Dietary Research and Findings

Coconut Water: When I started seeing coconut water drinks popping up at local road races, I had to check it out. After doing some research, I figured it was worth trying. The main benefits are post-workout hydration and potassium replenishment. A serving of coconut water provides the roughly the same amount of potassium as a banana (~450 milligrams) with 75-percent fewer calories and lower sugar levels (something I became increasingly sensitive about). To be honest though, I didn't like the taste. More importantly, between bananas, Muscle Milk, Vitamin Water, and other foods like salmon, I had plenty of tastier ways to replenish my potassium levels.

Note: If you plan to add coconut water to your training diet, read the label! Many varieties have added sugar that makes them just as caloric as sports drinks or soda. Additionally, what many consumers see as a positive might be a negative for endurance athletes: coconut water has far less sodium than Gatorade, and as we've discussed, sodium is essential to replenish – especially after long workouts.[104]

Training Log Week 122			
<u>Day</u>	<u>Date</u>	<u>Notes</u>	<u>Mileage</u>
Thurs.	6/2/11	Today, I set out to "destroy myself." I met John for a light workout at Miami Gardens: stretching, 1 lap easy jog, followed by full drills. Next, we did 12 x 100m @ 800m goal pace (1:56) w/90 sec rest. Hammy tightened on the final rep; nothing major, but I shut it down. After lunch, I walked 3 miles while running errands (and hit 120 bpm while doing so). Late afternoon, John and I did a repeat of the morning's 12 x 100m work – but w/only 45 sec rest. That was challenging. We followed it with bursts: 6 x 6-sec uphill bounds and 6 x 6-sec "fast feet" downstairs. I hadn't done a "real" cardio session yet, so I joined the Thursday Night Nike Run. I suffered through 6:05, 6:14, and 6:16 mile splits (18:35 total). Usually, that would be easy. This time it took 3 min for my HR to hit 160bpm; 4 min more to hit 170bpm, and 5 min later it hit a near-max 175 bpm and held steady until the end. I even hit 178 bpm for a burst – my highest HR yet recorded. I jogged home exhausted.	5.5
Fri.	6/3/11	Recovery day. Took a 3-mile walk in the morning before visiting Synergy Wellness Clinic for the usual battery of e-stim and ultrasound therapy. Synergy and Alex have been *critical* for my ongoing recovery. Remember, I strained a hamstring less than a wk ago, and I'm an old dog. Later, I logged an easy 30-min elliptical and did some light lifting.	4.0
Sat.	6/4/11	Bryan Huberty, Dan Potter, and I ran a track workout at Moore Park (a nice facility situated along the Route 195 causeway). I worked on an abbreviated, but still effective, warm-up routine: 50m skipping, easy 400m (2:00), dynamic stretching, moderate 400m (80 sec), full drills/stretching, 2 strides. The workout: 1 x 800m, 1 x 600m, and 2 x 400m, all @ 68-sec 400m pace, w/200m jogging rest. After a 10-min break, I ran a hard 300m. I logged 2:13, 1:41, 66 sec, 64 sec, and 40.7 sec, respectively. I felt strong, but I took some oxygen and a Muscle Milk Light to start the recovery process. Back home, I did some assorted weights, 10 min of elliptical, and some strides/light bounding.	5.0
Sun.	6/5/11	Didn't sleep well, and after some lunchtime errands I napped again until 3p. Then I hit the stairs for 30 min non-stop with no HR restriction – double-step up, single-step down "fast feet" style. Both my "up" times and "down" times were faster than a month ago, but last month I restricted my heart rate, so it's hard to compare my progress. I spent 5 more bpm going up and 11 more bpm coming down today. I did manage one additional rep this time, as well. It was great work and felt low-intensity.	4.8
Mon.	6/6/11	Met Northeastern University teammate Jayme "Fish" Fishman[105] for a ~7-mile "recovery" run while he was visiting Miami. The pace was a little faster than I expected. Fish is in good shape, and apparently he is contemplating some Masters racing like me. His wife Gretchen was a national-class race walker (tougher than you think), so their kids may have some legitimate talent. That afternoon I had a PT and massage session, and that evening I jogged to Flamingo Track to oversee Matt Kiss in an interval workout. Feel fully recovered.	8.7
Tues.	6/7/11	Slept in but still felt tired. Hit the track in Miramar at 1p and it was Africa hot. I started with my new, abbreviated warm-up routine and tried some Ice Cube on my iPod to wake me up. (No dice. Tried MuteMath. Better.) I ran the same workout as Saturday: 1 x 800m, 1 x 600m, and 2 x 400m, all @ 68-sec 400m pace, w/200m jogging rest – followed by a 10-min break and a hard 300m. I opened fast (31 sec) and reigned it in, but too much – 2:15 for the 800m. It felt *much* tougher than that. The 600m was 1:41, back to what I expected. Then 66 sec and 64 sec for the 400s. Pretty much on pace, but I felt wiped. I sucked down some oxygen and hit the locker room for some cold water. With 3 min rest left, I still felt bad. I paced off the starting spot and then I was off. I felt rough, but with 100m to go, I heard Moses Washington cheering me on. When I crossed the line, I missed the 'stop' button on my Garmin several times. I finally hit it at 42 sec. It took a while, but I recovered and did some 50m strides. When I checked my watch later, it said each lap I ran was long – which would explain why they felt so bad. According to Garmin, the adjusted times were 2:05, 1:35, 62 sec, 59 sec, and 37 sec, respectively. After dinner, Matt and Bryan came over for weights work.	9.5
Weds.	6/8/11	Pleasantly surprised. Sore, but not too sore. The Achilles was stiff, but not too stiff, and the hamstring felt 100%. I slept much of the day and did an easy 30-min elliptical.	4.1
Total		Averaged 6:26 per mile for the week	41.5

---

104 Source: Segterra [Google: "insidetracker" + coconut water]

105 Jayme Fishman was an accomplished Massachusetts high school runner who posted some respectable times at Northeastern University and captained the cross country team in 1993.

Training Log Week 123

Day	Date	Notes	Mileage
Thurs.	6/9/11	Potentially a break-out day! Started with a Moses Washington track workout at Miami Gardens: 6 x 200m w/2 min rest. I logged 26.4, 26.0, 28.1, 27.9, 27.9, and 27.8 sec, respectively. I hurt after the last one, but the times were fantastic. A few hours later I felt recovered enough to hit the Nike Run for a tempo – clocking 17:30 for 5K. Clearly, something is starting to click. I have to make sure I take care of myself and induce a peak when it matters most.	6.5
Fri.	6/10/11	Racing tomorrow. Easy 30-min elliptical and lots of rest today.	4.2
Sat.	6/11/11	Progressed through my now-somewhat-complex pre-race routine (see Race Results section) and turned in a 1:57.4 3rd-place finish in the Elite Open Invitational meet, behind Moses Washington and a guy named Terry Charles. It was the #1 Masters 800m time in the U.S. so far this year – and I did it after a monster workout just days before. I hit the elliptical later for a 30-min recovery session and did some core work. I could envision Nick Berra in my sights!	6.5
Sun.	6/12/11	I woke up paranoid that I somehow induced a premature peak. I spent hours searching for research, and I called Coach Dave. The prevailing sentiment is that my workload is still too great to have induced a peak. I spent the entire day recovering but decided on a long session of moderate-intensity work when I finally got after it at 10:30p: 45-min elliptical, then 2 hrs of upper/lower weights (heavy load, high rest). Then, I headed outside for a full set of drills and 5 x 150m accelerations. I continued with 4 x 3-step stair bounds, 2 x 3-stair jumps, and 2 x 4-stair jumps... all with eccentric calf drops to get back down the stairs. I figured it was bed time, but to be sure I tried one 12-flight stair climb; 6 flights in it, I knew I was done. It was close to 3a.	7.4
Mon.	6/13/11	Surprisingly wasn't a complete mess after yesterday. Fatigued, but not more than usual. Felt I made a major breakthrough in fitness. Did an easy 30-min elliptical before breakfast (1p, after the late night). In the evening, I took an easy jog with Matt Kiss to Flamingo Track and did assorted drills. After dinner, I hit the elliptical for another easy 30 min. Lots of activity, but nothing taxing.	10.4
Tues.	6/14/11	Workout was 8 x 500m with 2:30 rest. However, one of the run-clubbers pushed my competitive buttons. Robert Johnson had been improving greatly while I was largely absent from the Tuesday crew and took over as the "top gun." What came next was predictable. I hammered every rep from the start. At first, Robert held tight, only fading in the final 100m. As the reps wore on, I pushed to shake him earlier. By Rep 4, I was tired and posted my slowest time of the workout (still a quick 1:25), but Robert was spent and lagged far behind. We gathered for one more hard rep and battled for the first 200m, at which point my base training trumped his speed. I posted a 1:22, my fastest of the workout. Robert showed a lot of guts. My times compared to April 5th, but the rest was nearly 1 min shorter. After dinner, I felt good, so I decided to move forward with a 30-min non-stop stair workout. After the stairs, I headed outside for plyos: 4 x 3-step stair bounds, 2 x 3-stair jumps, and 2 x 4-stair jumps... all with eccentric calf drops to get back down the stairs.	8.0
Weds.	6/15/11	Was due for a super-easy day: easy 30-min elliptical, PT session at 2p, nap at 4p.	4.0
Total		Averaged 6:43 per mile for the week	**46.9**

Technical Tip – *Tapering, the period in the training cycle in which an athlete significantly reduces his workload in an effort to be rested and ready for his goal event, might be the only enjoyable period of a workout program. But like almost every training technique, even this happy time is not immune from controversy. Some sources suggest a gradual taper – where you reduce your maximal weekly workload from 100-percent effort down to about 50-percent effort over a four-to-six week span – is the best way to keep your body in equilibrium and not disrupt your diet or sleep patterns. Other sources suggest the benefit of a gradual taper is offset by the aerobic capacity you lose, and you can taper in as little as three weeks.*

I opted for a short taper in preparation for the 2011 Masters National Championships. I felt I knew my body's rhythms and recovery times well enough that rest was not a problem (via supercompensation), and my greater concern was avoiding injury. I started exercising extreme caution during hard workouts, but I didn't start backing my effort down until two to three weeks before my date in Cleveland.

Race Reports, Records and Results

2011 Elite Open Invitational: Miramar, June 11th – I ran this local meet to build race experience ahead of the monumental races to come. The seeding sheet told me I'd get my butt whipped. Moses Washington was the top seed, with a 1:51, and the next seed was a younger 1:55 guy. The only other competitor was older and out of shape – and he pulled out of the race at the last second. (Probably wise.)

Although only three of us made the start, I drew the sixth lane while Washington was assigned the fourth and Charles the fifth. When the gun went off, it didn't take me long to question the stagger – I got off to a fast start, but those guys went by me like I was standing still. They hit the break-point and quickly cut into the first lane. I knew better. The shortest distance between two points (in this case, the break-point and the far turn) is a straight line. I wasn't going to get close enough to those guys to draft off them, so I made my way to the first lane gradually.

As I passed the 200-meter mark, John Cormier called out the splits: 26, 27, 28...

Twenty-eight seconds was a little slower than I wanted, but not bad. I was comfortable. The second 200 meters was so quick and easy, I don't even remember it. All I remember is *not* getting a 400-meter split. That's right; they didn't even have a clock at the finish line. In any case, I sensed I had run a decent split and continued on. Around 500 meters it got harder to breathe. I started exhaling deeply and deliberately.

I could see that Terry Charles was no longer pulling away. I thought to myself, "Less than 300 meters to go. Relax down the back stretch and it's a 200-meter kick." I could hear John counting off 1:23, 1:24, 1:25 at 600 meters.

At that point, I knew I was going to put up a number: 1:25-high plus 32 seconds for the last 200 meters would make 1:57-high. Hearing 1:25 only made me feel stronger. I started my kick and closed the large gap between me and Terry Charles a little. I wasn't going to catch him, but he gave me something to chase. Predictably, I started to lock up down the final straight away. The next time I looked up, the finish line was just inches away, and I ran right through it. I doubled over in exhaustion but didn't feel too bad overall. The final reps of my workouts felt much worse. Clearly, the lactic acid buffers did a great job. More importantly, I got the time: 1:57.42 – a new Masters PR for me and the fastest time by an American Master at that point in 2011.

2011 USATF National Championships (Men's Masters 1,500-Meter Invitational): University of Oregon, June 26th – My silver-medal performance in Albuquerque, combined with my strong time at the Elite Open earned me a once-in-a-lifetime opportunity: The USATF invited me to compete in an exhibition race – the men's Masters 1,500 meters – at the USA National Championships. This is the Super Bowl of American Track & Field. In 2011, this was the qualifying meet to select the men and women who would represent the U.S. at the World Championships in Daegu, South Korea, the only way the stage would have been bigger was if it were an Olympic year. TV crews, a sold-out stadium, and more past, present and future U.S. Olympic icons than you could count... all congregated at the University of Oregon's historic Hayward Field, the house that Pre built. Even though I wasn't training to run a fast 1,500, there was no way I could say no!

Rick Miller and I met in the Portland airport late on the Thursday night before my Sunday race. We rented a car, stopped at the fantastic Le Bistro Montage for dinner,[106] then immediately headed south toward Eugene. We crashed in a hotel when we were both too tired to drive any further, and by noon the next day we reached TrackTown USA. I can't even describe how cool it was to be there, like a child's first visit to Fenway Park or Wrigley Field. The crowd within was just starting to build at Hayward, but it was already larger than I had ever seen at a track meet.

We took in some sights, snapped some photos, and ran into Jeff Caron from New Balance Boston – which sent a number of contenders to the meet. But with 48 hours until race time, I focused mostly on laying low and staying out of the sun. By Sunday I felt like a kid at Christmas; I couldn't wait to get on the track.

---

106 www.montageportland.com

Training Log Week 124			
Day	Date	Notes	Mileage
Thurs.	6/16/11	Still sore from Tuesday. Mental note: Speed work and tempo runs can happen on the same day, but speed work, stairs, and plyos cannot. Spent most of the day recovering and opted to join the Nike tempo run (17:37 through 5K, 177 bpm HR max), and add some core work and 10 x 90m strides (focused more on form) afterward. Later I did a 30-min easy elliptical and some lunges at an increasing weight.	8.0
Fri.	6/17/11	Rest day w/1-hr PT session. Easy 30-min elliptical and 30 min weights.	4.2
Sat.	6/18/11	Nearly recovered from Thursday but was a bit tired; spent most of the day resting (in bed and by the pool). Bryan joined me at the Moore Park track at 7p. Workout was 12-16 x 200m @ 29 sec w/200m jogging rest. (Bryan opted for slower reps.) It was drizzling, so my flats were sliding, but it didn't hold us back. We hit our splits, but by Rep 7, I knew 12 would be my limit. It was getting sequentially harder. I averaged 28.6 sec (1:54 pace for 800m) w/only 83 sec rest. A year ago I averaged 28.2 sec for 8 reps w/a full 2:00 rest. Progress!	4.0
Sun.	6/19/11	Slept well and napped well. Hit the gym with Bryan at 6:30 for 60 min elliptical, 30 min weights/core, then stretching and 5 x 60m strides. Felt great physically and mentally. Not concerned about overtraining again, after yesterday's 200s proved to be non-taxing.	8.5
Mon.	6/20/11	Read Nick Berra's blog post of his most recent workout: 4 x 400m (2 @ 67 sec and 2 @ 65 sec) w/3-min rest, immediately followed by 4 x 300 (2 @ 46 sec and 2 @ 45 sec) going off every 2 min. I decided to duplicate his effort and compare... After a standard warm-up, I got to work. It was 87 degrees and very humid, but after months of heat acclimation, I could power through a blazing sun. This was planned; my most important races would be in July. Despite an effort to start reasonably, I opened my first 400m rep w/a 29-sec 200m. (After months of running 14-sec 100s and 29-sec 200s, my body didn't know any other speed... awesome, but not practical.) I backed off and completed Rep 1 in 63.4 sec, a full 3 sec faster than Berra. It was time to settle down. I logged 65.1, 63.2, and 61.9 sec, respectively, for the next 3 reps (2.5 sec faster than Berra on average). For the 300s, I logged 43.9, 45.3, 45.6, and 43.8 sec, respectively, and bettered Berra by 1.3 sec on average. Over the course of 800m, that would equate to a 4.75 sec gap – but I knew it wouldn't be that easy. Still... more progress.	5.6
Tues.	6/21/11	Easy day. Bryan and I hit the elliptical and some weights. Later, I visited Alex for flexibility and some PT.	4.3
Weds.	6/22/11	Hitting the track every other day as part of my "mesocycle" (multi-wk plan) to work progressively harder for 3 wks then take it easy in the 4th wk. However, my body told me the time for an easy wk came early. I was still sore from Monday's workout, so I hit the roads for an aerobic 6-miler. I hadn't run roads in awhile. I played it safe and wore my heavier, but supportive New Balance 1226 trainers with orthotics. I ran by heart rate, not pace, so I didn't care about weight. I headed out at 6p, but it was still 87 degrees (and humid, of course). This matched my last aerobic road run, with the only difference being the heavier shoes. I ran 41:34 with an avg heart rate of 152bpm. A month prior I ran 40:34 with an avg HR of 156bpm. I believe those are similar efforts, and given that I had entered my speed phase, I was happy to see I was holding my aerobic capabilities.	6.0
Total		Averaged 6:47 per mile for the week	40.6

Just before starting my warm-up, I ran into Ryan Hall – one of America's elite distance runners. We exchanged pleasantries and a meet volunteer snapped a photo. As I completed my warm-up, the meet officials called for all Masters 1500-meter competitors to gather in the waiting area. There I saw Dan O'Brien, whom I had met earlier in the meet. As he was prepping a segment while broadcasting for NBC, he looked over at me and said "Good luck".

"See you on the podium in a few minutes," I answered.

"Yeah?" he asked.

"Yeah. I'm feeling it," I answered. And I was. I was nervous, but physically and mentally I felt ready. I was confident in my training and perfectly warmed up. Even though the competitors list was a veritable who's who of Masters runners, including my nemesis Nick Berra, I felt ready to do battle. The officials lined us up, and adrenaline did its job: it felt like every other race I had run. I took a quick knee (my pre-race ritual); the starter gave the command; we approached the line, and the gun went off.

Nick Berra and Christian Cushing-Murray were in the outside lanes and got out quickly to gain position, as I expected. I lined myself up to tuck in behind Berra, who took the lead. Lance Elliot and Mike Blackmore trailed close behind me. For the next three minutes and 30 seconds, that's how it remained. It couldn't have looked like much to the people watching, but to me it was a 3.5-minute tour of the Nick Berra Torture Chamber.

Berra set a strong pace. He was clearly gunning for a sub-4:00 finish and had taken us through the quarter mile in 63 seconds, then the half mile in 2:08. As a 1:57 half-miler, the pace was comfortable enough for me, but I felt a little stiff considering there was still 700 meters to go. The third lap was very challenging. I knew I'd be okay if I could make it to the 1,200-meter mark intact, but that was no sure thing at that point. Berra remained intent and plowed though the 1,100 meters in three minutes flat. The bell rang; the crowd roared, and more adrenaline flowed. I needed that. I expected things to pick up, and I had no problem staying stride for stride with Berra as he gradually accelerated. At the 1,200-meter mark, I thought, "Made it. I might have this now." But I knew not to kick yet, not against Berra.

With 150 meters left, I couldn't take it anymore. I went and went decisively. I passed Berra high on the turn and quickly dropped into Lane 1. I intentionally positioned myself in the center of the lane to force any challengers as wide as possible, but I was careful not to leave enough room for anyone to sneak by me on the inside. By the end of the final turn, I would be fairly close to the rail, but not so close as to risk tripping over it. The tactic was sound. I had used it dozens of times before. Only once had it failed after I made a decisive pass to take the lead. That one time? In Albuquerque against Nick Berra.

Berra must have seen the daylight between me and the rail and thought he had enough time to hit it with one last surge before I closed the door. He's a fierce competitor. That said, he's also among the greatest gentlemen you'll ever meet. If he thought he saw daylight, I'm sure it looked like fair game. He came close up my inside; our feet tangled, and the disruption caused me to slow for a split-second and caused him to run right up my left shoulder.

In real time, I didn't know it was him. All I knew was I was being forced outside, and I instinctively recoiled to avoid being knocked over. Then, I reacted like I always have in those situations… I took off. My old kick was back and I was cruising.

With 60 meters to go, as usual, I went into full rigor mortis. With about 30 meters to go, my body hit a new level of tightening up. I scrambled to find any remaining muscles to call on. My glutes, obliques, and calves were the only things not on fire, so I called upon them… and they did yeoman's work for five agonizing, exhilarating seconds. Then I was across the line. No one in front of me. On the most storied track in America, I had won. I honestly couldn't believe it until I heard the commentator call my name.[107]

I collapsed onto the track, debilitated by oxygen debt and lactic acid. It was agony, but worth every moment. Next I was rushed to the podium, where I was greeted by 10,000 cheering fans and a gold medal. Ryan Hall, seated nearby, congratulated me. It was the greatest athletic moment of my life. Soon, I was on the practice field gathering my things with Mark Cleary, Chairman of the USATF's Masters Invitational Program Committee. My phone, now in hand, was buzzing like crazy. Innumerable emails, texts, and calls from friends and family watching online were fighting to get through. That's when it really hit me. A wave of accomplishment and joy swept over me. I lurched, weeping uncontrollably. But the next text changed everything. This time it was on Cleary's phone. It said I was DQ'd.

Considering what happened in the winter, I didn't think his joke was funny, but I could appreciate the dark humor. But as a couple of seconds passed, Cleary's face remained stone cold. He wasn't kidding. He accompanied me to the Protest Area, where although still slightly delirious with fatigue, I requested access to the official results. The results did not reference which USATF Rule I had allegedly broken. Any violation was supposed to be referenced there but none was. I was verbally informed that the disqualification was in reference to Rule 163.3 of the 2011 USATF Competition Rules (obstructing the progress of a fellow competitor by not running in a straight line down the straightaway).

The only thing about the race I remembered that could have prompted such a ruling was on the final turn, when Berra and I tangled. But he came up on me, and I was still accelerating at the time – it wasn't obstruction. And when I took off, I won by nearly a full second – quite a margin over the final 100 meters.

---

107 Race video/audio: [Google: Mens Masters 1500 - USA Outdoor Track 2011]

Training Log Week 125			
<u>Day</u>	<u>Date</u>	<u>Notes</u>	<u>Mileage</u>
Thurs.	6/23/11	Recovery + travel day: 30-min elliptical and I snuck in a 35-min massage at Synergy Wellness Center. The therapist, Maria Sosa, is quickly becoming a valuable addition to my regimen. After that, I headed to Oregon to meet up with Rick Miller and get to Eugene for the USATF Championships. Hard to believe I'll be racing at Hayward Field!	4.3
Fri.	6/24/11	Miller and I met in Portland last night, as planned. We stopped at the fantastic Le Bistro Montage for dinner. After a great meal, we drove halfway to Eugene and crashed at a hotel. We reached TrackTown, USA around noon today. My race was scheduled for 1:15 on Sunday, so I wanted my last two workouts to take place at that time. I hit Hayward's practice field for a full warm-up, followed by 8 x 75m accelerations. I threw in some bounding exercises for good measure but shut it down early. After a 20-min elliptical, I was ready for dinner.	4.0
Sat.	6/25/11	Big rest day. I slept late and stayed in bed as much as possible. Miller and I hit the gym at 1:15, exactly 24 hrs before race time – an easy 30-min elliptical. After, we headed to Hayward to check out the main events. I met up with Bernard Lagat and Galen Rupp again. I also met Chris Solinsky, the largest distance runner I've ever seen (listed at 6'1"/165lbs). He made me wonder if more muscle is the future of distance running. Solinsky is a *great* guy. Lagat makes graciousness an art form, but Chris is right there with him. We talked the 8-10 mph wind, which hits directly on the back stretch. His advice solidified my strategy: hang and kick. I went back to bed for a nap, then grabbed a light dinner with a *little* bit of everything (red meat, veggies, bread, pasta), then back to bed again.	4.3
Sun.	6/26/11	Race day. Unfortunately not a good one, two great performances ruined in a split sec. (The Race Results section has all the details.) Aside from being at Hayward Field in front of 10,000 cheering fans, it was a normal, text-book warm-up and race. We opened with a 2:08 for the first 800m, and I closed the 1,500m in 1st place with a 4:01.7 – but it would not stand...	2.2
Mon.	6/27/11	After 16 hrs of travel, I reached Miami around noon. Depressed and trying to figure out how to shake the awful feeling after yesterday's disqualification. I mustered a 30-min elliptical in the evening.	4.6
Tues.	6/28/11	Still depressed about Eugene. Walked to Alex's for rehab, then did 8 x 200m (avg. 28 sec each w/2-min rest) that evening. Full upper- and lower-body weights.	4.0
Weds.	6/29/11	Haven't slept well in days. Sunday's disaster still occupied my mind during any quiet moment. Recovery day of 30-min elliptical at quick pace (~4.5 miles).	4.5
Total		Averaged 6:43 per mile for the week	**27.9**

I quickly filed (and paid $100) for a written protest of the officials' ruling. Minutes later, I was informed that my protest had been reviewed but would not result in any amendment of the initial decision. Although video of the race was available, I was told that it had not been reviewed, nor would it be. I requested further edification regarding the protest ruling and an audience with the ruling reference. Both requests were denied.

By pure happenstance, Rick Miller was at the final turn where the infraction supposedly occurred. He said to me, in the midst of my protest, "I saw the whole thing. As a friend, I'd be honest with you to save you the time and trouble if I thought you were wrong, but if this holds up it's one of the worst DQs in the history of the sport."

I wandered aimlessly for awhile. Eventually, we hopped in the rental car and departed TrackTown for the airport. The ride to Portland was not as fun as the ride to Eugene had been.

At the airport, Miller and I grabbed a bite to eat. I wasn't very hungry, so I had a few Sprites and a soup. Then I just moped for awhile. Miller provided good company, as he always had in my darkest hours. It had been a long time since those services had been required, but he wasn't rusty.

After a while, he asked, "When does your flight take off?"

"10:25. Why?"

"It's 10:05."

"Oh, shit!"

I grabbed my bag, dropped $15 on the counter, thanked Miller, and rushed off.

Predictably, the security line was slow. It took 10 minutes to reach the metal detector. When I got there, my day of bad luck continued. I was chosen for a random search.

The TSA officer did a thorough job, which I fully understood, but I couldn't help but think, "Why me…"

When the inspection was done, I gathered my stuff tossed on my sneakers (untied), and made a break for the gate. I sprinted non-stop, dodging people and suitcases along the way. I made a sharp turn into the gate area and simultaneous stepped on the brakes and handed my ticket to the lady at the desk.

"Am I too late?"

"Almost… hurry up!"

Again, I sprinted. This time, down the jet way. As I boarded the plane, I sighed in relief and dropped to tie my shoes. Witnessing the ridiculous spectacle, a flight attendant handed me a water. I thanked her and looked up to see how many first-class passengers I had embarrassed myself in front of. And there he was…

Sitting in his pilot's uniform was none other than Captain Nick Berra, justifiably chuckling. I was still on a knee with my laces untied, belt and other possessions cradled in my hands. My humiliation was complete and total. Once again, I was not good enough. I mustered a guffaw and shook his hand. It was then I realized that his goal of breaking 4:00 in the 1,500 meters evaporated when we collided on Bowerman Curve. Despite my bitterness, I could empathize with him. I shamefully walked down the aisle, slumped in my seat, and festered in my latest failure.

But at 40 years old, I still believed… That which does not kill me will make me stronger. It was time to knuckle down.

2011 World Masters Athletics Championships: On Thursday, July 8th Jamie and I reached Sacramento for the Worlds. It's an oddity of Masters racing that sometimes the world championship meet is held before the national championships. Finding venues large enough to host must be challenging, and the events are produced by completely separate athletic governing bodies… and because Masters qualifying is based solely on time and not on a top-three finish in a meet (like the Olympic Trials, for example), the race organizers can schedule as it suits them.

Nonetheless, although I was pretty amped up to race against the world's best, I felt a little strange coming into the meet three weeks before my scheduled peak. Presumably this would be the toughest Masters competition I would face, but my sole point of focus was winning a national championship. In theory that should have take most of the pressure off. However, after the disaster in Eugene, seeing the world's elite challenged my self-confidence.

For Jamie and me, the marveling commenced as soon as we hit Hornet Field at Sacramento State, when two *ripped* 70-something guys jogged by. I don't mean ripped for 70 years old. I mean ripped. Sure, Father Time had delivered some shots to their outer bodies, but the engines were clearly intact and firing on all cylinders.

On the field, another male athlete approached the pole vault pit in full stride, pole in hand. He only got a few feet of air, but when we saw the 'M-90' on the back of his singlet, our jaws nearly hit the pavement. This guy was pole vaulting at 90 years old!

After picking up my competitors packet, we headed to the stands. We found seats next to a lone spectator wearing an athlete's badge. He looked about 40, so I couldn't help but take a peek at his name: Neil Fitzgerald. I knew this name from the seeding sheets. He was registered to compete in the 800 meters. I introduced myself. He cordially reciprocated.

Training Log Week 126			
Day	Date	Notes	Mileage
Thurs.	6/30/11	Nike Run Club (tempo day). 1.25-mile warm-up @ about 6:30 per mile. 2-mile tempo run (10:48). HR was 170-175 bpm for first 3.5 min, then above 175 for 5.5 min, with a max HR of 178 bpm (tying my personal record). Good hard work -- an effective remedy for my post-Oregon depression. I'm starting to feel better.	7.8
Fri.	7/1/11	Recovery day. Brisk 30-min elliptical.	4.5
Sat.	7/2/11	Started with a 2-mile warm-up to the golf course (12:56), w/a HR goal of 140-165bpm. At 2 miles, I did 10 x 100m at race pace on the fairways w/enough rest to allow the HR to ease a bit. After the 10th rep, I headed home but added a couple of miles for good measure.	6.0
Sun.	7/3/11	Early evening: brisk 30-min elliptical. Late evening: full warm-up and 5 x 150m on Ocean Drive with slow walking recovery. Ended the day with 30-min easy weight/core work, followed by light stretching.	5.9
Mon.	7/4/11	Finally let go of Eugene enough for a long night's sleep. Aside from grabbing some supplements in the early a.m., I slept from midnight until 2p. I was a bit groggy until my workout @ 5:30p. I felt a little off until I kicked on some gangsta rap and launched into the session: 4 x 200m @ 27 sec w/45-50 sec rest – basically a 1:48 800m in just over 4 min. Logged 24.7, 26.3, 24.6, and 27.8 sec, respectively, w/50 sec rest. Later, I did some light stretching, and 5 x 60m strides. (I ran right past Lebron James, who was cruising Ocean Drive in a red Range Rover.) I hit the gym for a full upper- and lower-body weight workout and a brisk 30-min elliptical.	6.5
Tues.	7/5/11	Today was all recovery. After an easy 30-min elliptical, I relaxed, got some PT at Synergy, and hung out at the Booker T track meet-up, just to be social.	4.4
Weds.	7/6/11	Starting Friday I expected to race 3 times in 4 days at the World Masters Championships in Sacramento. I was not 100% recovered from Monday's monster session, so I visited Alex around mid-day. In the late afternoon, I did 30 min on the elliptical, grabbed a little protein and my racing flats, and headed outside for a warm-up and 4 x 60m strides plus 3 quick sets of stair-bounds (3 x 24 stairs, 2-3 stairs at a time). Then, a little more protein, some ice, and dinner (lamb, to top off my iron stores). I'm ready for Worlds; after racing the country's best Masters 1,500m runners at Hayward Field, I'm not sure that much would intimidate me anymore.	5.0
Total		Averaged 6:40 per mile for the week	40.1

"So…" Neil continued, "You're the guy who ran 4:01 in Oregon a couple weeks ago, right?"

"Yeah," I said and promptly changed the subject. "How's your season been?" I asked.

"It's going well," he replied. "I ran 1:56 last weekend."

Fitzgerald's time was a full second faster than my best for the year… which *had been* the fastest time in the United States. I also learned he coached youth track and, before attending Brown University, had gone to high school in California – where he ranked among the state's best all-time 800-meter runners with a 1:50 flat. Jamie and I wished him good luck and excused ourselves, and I got back to the task at hand: preparation.

For most meets, I had a fixed regimen that involved a lot of rest, specific foods/supplements, and specific activities… all carefully timed and coordinated to get me to the starting line prepared for a perfect performance. Despite this, for most meets, I continued to be myself. Jamie was largely unaffected. We'd talk, laugh, eat, watch TV, etc. This was not "most" meets. This was rarified air. Poor Jamie. I don't know how many eBooks, HBO Go episodes, and Netflix movies she perused while we were in Sacramento, but like an FBI agent on a protective custody case, she dutifully sat silently in our hotel room for five days. As for me, I did little more than lie in bed, nap, eat, and do warm-up exercises.

In the World Championships, a competitor had to advance through a quarter-final race and a semi-final in back-to-back days. The final was held just under 48 hours after the semis. I approached every race with an equal level of intensity and precision. Within four hours of each race, everything was according to my standard pre-race script. Mentally, things were a lot more intense though.

There were 12 runners per race and only eight lanes, so some runners had to share a lane for the first 100 meters. The officials had an elaborate set of rules to determine who got what lane and with whom. I couldn't figure it out; all I knew is that I'd be placed somewhere on the track among 12 of the best Masters 800-meter runners on the planet.

I had read the seeding sheet before the race because I wanted a sense of how fast I'd have to run to make it past the first round. The number I came up with was pretty close to 2:00 on the dot. I thought it incredible that two dozen 40-year-olds were still running two-flat for 800 meters. As luck would have it, Neil Fitzgerald and I would tangle in the quarterfinals.

With 20 minutes until the quarterfinals race, the meet officials gathered us combatants under a tarp located just outside the track at the beginning of the final straightaway. Soon enough, it was coliseum time. An official herded us onto the track in time to run a wind sprint or two, then they walked us down the length of the straightaway to the start. This was clearly for show...

As it turned out, Fitzgerald and I didn't have to tangle at all. In the first three heats we witnessed many competitors succumbed to the rigors of travel, the Sacramento heat (mid-80s), or simply the pressure. The times were awful. I determined that a 2:06 or 2:07 would advance me to the semifinals. I told Neil as much, hoping he'd take the hint and not take the race out too fast.

Sure enough, when the gun went off, Neil and I held back. Pascual Morcillo of Spain took the early lead, but he wasn't exactly scorching up the track. Morcillo led us through 400 meters in a pedestrian 63 seconds. The next 300 meters were uneventful, but down the final straightaway a few guys got spunky. I kicked into third gear and cruised in for third place and an automatic trip to the semis in 2:07.2. Fitzgerald finished just ahead of me in 2:06.8.

The semi-final heat and lane assignments were released on the Internet while I rested in my hotel room. There would be two heats with 12 competitors in each heat. Half would move on to the finals and half would go home.

The race sheet provided good news and bad news. The bad news was that I was placed in the first heat (no benefit of seeing the competition run before me, as was the case in the quarterfinals). The good news was I was assigned to have Lane 5 all to myself. According to the rules, the top two finishers in each heat would automatically advance. The final eight spots would be awarded based on time. Following my strategy from the quarters, I looked down the list and figured out what it would take to *not* be one of the 12 people to go home. I determined that I would be best served by finishing third or fourth with a time of 2:02 or so. By finishing third or fourth, I would have beaten most of the 12 people in my heat and would likely have a faster time than at least four or five guys in the second heat.

Just before the race, I learned of a change to the lane assignments. Instead of getting Lane 5 to myself, I would share Lane 4 with none other than Neil Fitzgerald. It seemed like fate demanded we clash. As we awaited the start, I decided I wasn't going to waste energy fighting him for the lane lead. I figured he might be thinking the same way, so I asked him. He wanted to start fast, and I wanted him to do so. Seconds later, the starter called us to our marks, fired the gun, and we were off.

Jamie Heilpern, an American, made it clear what position he wanted: the lead. He sprinted ahead, while Patrick Robinson, another American followed close behind. After that, there was a nice juicy gap, so I slid right in. Heilpern took us through the 200 in 27 seconds. "Fast," I thought, "but fine. I'm down with it."

As we rounded the turn, Heilpern decided that 54 seconds would be a little fast for the first 400 meters and eased off. We still cruised through in about 56 seconds. I felt a little lactic heaviness in my legs, but my lungs were fine. At the 450-meter mark I starting breathing a little heavier. As usual, I embraced it. The next 200 meters were a blur. I usually spent the third 200 meters of an 800-meter race trying to hold it together and get ready for the final kick, but in this race there was nothing to hold together. I was moving fast, but it didn't feel all that fast. We passed 600 meters in just under 1:28, and I knew I was good to go. I felt ready to kick, but if I eased in I'd finish around 2:00, well under my 2:02 goal time. By the time we hit the home straightaway, I had pulled even with Heilpern and was happy with that position. There was no need to turn on the jets. Fitzgerald had other plans. With about 70 meters to go, he flew by me and Heilpern in what looked to be high gear and easily took the race as we coasted the final meters.

On the big board that loomed over the track, Fitzgerald's finishing time was already on display. 1:58.3. Shortly after, Heilpern's name popped up (1:58.6), immediately followed by mine (1:58.8). There was not a bead of sweat on my body! A thin mist, yes. But no beads. I couldn't believe it; I just basically coasted a 1:58! I strutted off the track and made eye contact with Nick Berra.

"You guys weren't messing around out there," he said. My confidence soared.

I stuck around for a look at the second heat. Mathematically, I could still be eliminated, but 10 of the 12 runners would have to go faster than my 1:58.8 for that to happen. They opened slowly in 58 seconds, which likely meant a fifth-gear sprint for the finish. They didn't disappoint. Down the final straightaway the mad rush ensued. Three guys finished within three one-hundredths of a second of each other: Nick Berra, Brian Sax (another American), and Rich Tremain from Canada, respectively. Berra's 1:58.8 led the group, which meant that I had the third-fastest time of the semis. It also meant that I'd get Lane 3 to myself in the finals.

Based on how the semis had gone down, I figured most of the field was tired. I wasn't. As such, I wanted the finals to be fast-paced. I didn't like the idea of leading most of the race, but I would have if I had to. That being said, I felt *someone* would take it out.

In the 36 hours leading to the finals, I prepared *exactly* as I had for the semis. Jamie and I slept at the same time, for the same number of hours, and ate the same foods at the same places.

Despite this, by race time, I felt a little different. My warm-up went well, but my two warm-up 400 meters were fast. My first, which I used simply to loosen up before stretching, was in 71 seconds. My second, which was meant to get my engine revving before doing my drills, was a comfortable 63 seconds. But I was uncharacteristically uncoordinated during my drills. One last time, the officials ushered us onto the track, paraded us past the spectators, and set us in our lanes. I felt a little out of sorts, but couldn't put my finger on how or why.

The gun went off, and I rounded the turn quickly and comfortably. I wanted to be among the first to reach the breakpoint so I could pick my spot among the leaders. As I suspected, a few guys started fast. I think Heilpern was among them, but I wasn't really paying attention to who was who. I was laser-focused on running a perfect race.

We reached 200 meters in 27 seconds, and I was happy with my position – hanging in fourth off of Nick Berra's shoulder. The pace was fast, and that was what mattered. As we rounded the turn, my happiness dissipated. The leaders weren't as enthusiastic about the 27-second open as I was. Things slowed noticeably and I was faced with my first dilemma of the race. A decent gust had developed on the home straight. If I took the lead, I would also have to take the wind. But if I stayed there, the first quarter would surely be slower than I wanted.

I decided to save my strength for the third 200 meters and held my position. We went through the 400 in 57.3 seconds, reflecting a marked slowdown. By the time we rounded the corner, Berra had taken the lead and I knew exactly what I would do.

We hit the back straight and I moved outside. The wind was at our backs, and it was time for me to take a shot. I pulled even with Berra, then shifted into fourth gear. I was careful to exert just enough energy to pull ahead and grab Lane 1 before the final turn. For the first time in the entire competition, I had the lead.

There was no time to enjoy it though. I focused on executing a flawless final kick. Having learned a lesson in Eugene, I clung tight to the rail so nobody would think to pass inside. Then, with 150 meters to go, I turned on the afterburners.

With 100 meters to go, I was clearly in front. I just had to hold on, and I could achieve something I never thought possible when my comeback began: a world championship. In a space the length of an over-sized parking spot, time seemed to stop. With 70 meters to go, a lactic acid tsunami crashed upon me. My legs slowed and my face tensed.

"Come on, come on," I thought. "You can win this. Just. Keep. Moving."

And moving I was. But out of the corner of my right eye, I a tall figure came into view. Then another… and another… It was Fitzgerald, and he had two guys hot on his heels: Rich Tremain and Brian Sax. I reached deep to hold my lead, but it was no use. These guys were going by and there was nothing I could do to stop them. Just like that, my long-shot at a World Championship was gone. I crossed the line fourth, just fractions ahead of Berra, and clapped my hands in futility. I looked toward Jamie and my mom and shrugged my shoulders like, "I did all I could."

And I had. I looked up at the big board and saw I had run 1:56.2, my fastest time since my days at Northeastern University. Two years prior, I was just another 38-year old guy. That day, I was the #4 Masters 800-meter runner on the planet. And I had 18 days to reach my true goal: a national championship.

Training Log Week 127			
Day	Date	Notes	Mileage
Thurs.	7/7/11	Nice easy 30-min elliptical. Racing at Worlds tomorrow!	5.0
Fri.	7/8/11	World Championships! Getting through the quarter-finals was easy (2:07). Warmed-down with 30 min on the stationary bike at the hotel.	4.2
Sat.	7/9/11	Stationary bike warm-up, plus strides in the a.m. World Championship semi-finals in the p.m. Ran a comfortable 1:58.75. Felt great!	4.5
Sun.	7/10/11	30 min on the stationary bike, plus pre-race drills and strides. Timed the workout to correspond with tomorrow's race time. Keeping the body in synch...	4.3
Mon.	7/11/11	15 min on the stationary bike, plus strides in the a.m. World Championship finals in the p.m. (4th place in a Masters PR of 1:56.20!). Light warm down jog afterwards.	5.0
Tues.	7/12/11	30 min on the stationary bike. So long Sacramento!	4.3
Weds.	7/13/11	Quasi-recovery day. Around 3p, I went to Synergy Wellness for physical therapy. At 9:30p, I hit the gym with Bryan. We did an extended session (45 min) on the elliptical, followed by a full, but moderate weight workout. I also did some dynamic stretches to shake the legs out. Still feeling the effects of racing at Worlds, but recovering quickly.	6.5
Total		Averaged 6:33 per mile for the week	33.8

2011 USATF Masters National Outdoor Championships: Jamie and I made the trek to Baldwin Wallace College in Berea, OH. Here I would achieve my ultimate victory or suffer a final defeat. We arrived a couple of days early for the July 30th race, partly to get acclimated and partly because we were told by the USATF to expect a potential qualifying round – even though Nick Berra had mentioned to me that the USATF often plants that expectation and then realizes they have a small enough field to cancel the preliminaries.

Berra's words proved true, and thus began the waiting game again: a couple more days in a cookie-cutter hotel room for Jamie, more downtime for me to visualize the upcoming race, scrutinize my pre-race routine down to the microsecond, and stew in a thick glaze of stress. On Thursday afternoon, after we arrived and checked in, I took advantage of Baldwin Wallace's top-rate athletic facilities and snuck in a 30-minute elliptical session, followed by a few strides. Then it was back to the hotel.

On Friday I fulfilled my pledge to train every day until the 2011 Masters Outdoor Nationals. I did the easiest possible 30-minute elliptical session and that was it. Before I left the gym, I stared blankly at the machine for a few moments. For more than two years, I spent countless hours on machines just like that one. Books and entertainment gadgets made the experience more enjoyable while the machines saved me from injury – and I was sure that similar machines would serve a large role in my fitness going forward – but it wouldn't be the same. The sessions before that day served a purpose toward an emotional goal; after this, I questioned if my motives would ever be as strong. And the difference between looking back on those two years with a sense of redemption, or a sense of futility and regret, would come down to two minutes on the Baldwin Wallace track.

I awoke the next morning, the day of the 2011 US Masters Nationals 800-meter run, with a palpable sense of dread. The race had driven my every decision for the past two and a half years.

Training Log Week 128			
Day	Date	Notes	Mileage
Thurs.	7/14/11	Tough day. I was sore from yesterday's weight work and perhaps underestimated my level of recovery from the Worlds. I headed to Nike Run Club around 7p. It was 88 degrees, but I couldn't resist wearing my World Championships T-shirt (silly). I did a full set of dynamic stretches and a 3-min 800m to warm up, plus about 400m of skipping with full arm motion (something I may need down the final straightaway at Nationals). A guy named Kerry Sullivan came along for the ride.[108] I decided run briskly, but not too hard – a good decision. A couple miles in, I felt tired. My HR was over 170 bpm and closing in on my max. Apparently, the heat, dehydration, and last night's workout were taking a toll. Plus, my T-shirt was soaked and weighing me down. My main goal on Thursday nights is to get my HR near its max for 5-10 min, so mission accomplished. I matched my HR best of 178 bpm. After, Kerry and I chugged some water and did 4 x 90m strides.	4.2
Fri.	7/15/11	Recovery day: 30-min elliptical, but I completed the greatest number of "miles" I've done in a 30-min session. After, I hit the weights for easy upper, lower, and core. Capped the day with strides, to keep my speed honest.	4.8
Sat.	7/16/11	Good sharpening day. Started w/a recovery massage at 1p. I did 10 x 100m strides and light jogging on the artificial turf at Curtis Park. Next, I hit the track intending to run 4 x 200m w/short rest. After my second rep the officials shut the park down for the evening... 15 min early. Too bad. I was running fast (25.8 and 26.5 sec). Booker T. Washington was still open, so I met John Cormier there for more 200s. Very fast (including a 25.1) but took ample rest.	5.0
Sun.	7/17/11	Recovery day. Sore from yesterday's intervals, so I got plenty of bed-rest and took it easy on the elliptical.	4.3
Mon.	7/18/11	Still stiff from Saturday's workout. Was considering racing a local meet tomorrow (400m, to sharpen up for Nationals), so I took it easy again. Started w/a 1-hr PT session at Synergy in the afternoon. Later, I did 4 x 90m strides followed by a moderate 30-min elliptical. After, I did very easy weights (again, just to stay sharp).	4.6
Tues.	7/19/11	The track meet was a bust. Nobody came, and the track was asphalt, with a bit of sand, gravel and standing water. Racing 400m would have been ill-advised and slow at best. Back in South Beach, the 2 hrs of driving sapped our will to work, so we kept things to a standard warm-up and 8 x 90m strides (30m acceleration, 30m hold, 30m coast/decelerate). I hit the elliptical for 30 min when I got home.	6.0
Weds.	7/20/11	Back was still sore and stiff. I visited Alex, which helped a lot. Next, I headed straight for some EMS and ultrasound at Synergy. It also helped, but I was still stiff in the evening. A 30-min elliptical loosened it back up a bit, but I was growing concerned this would be an issue. I underestimated my recovery time from the recent sharpening sprints. And I had only 10 days until the big dance.	4.5
Total		Averaged 6:36 per mile for the week	33.4

I knew I was ready. The two weeks prior had gone very well. I focused on three things: speed, speed, and speed. I performed short, sharp sprints on a near-daily basis. At the end of my final session, I clocked a 24-second 200-meters, my fastest since college. There was no telling what I was ready to run. I was clearly at my absolute peak.

So why the dread? Simple. Regardless of my conditioning, my indoor and outdoor track seasons had been cursed.

The February world record attempts ended in failure and disqualification. In March, I was 50 meters from winning the USATF Indoor National Championship but was chased down by Nick Berra. In June I was the first across the finish line at the prestigious Masters Invitational 1,500 Meters at the USA Outdoor Track & Field Championships and was awarded the gold medal... but 30 minutes later I was disqualified and the medal was gone (along with what turned out to be one of the fastest Masters 1,500-meter times in the world in 2011). Lastly, just a few weeks prior, I led a field of the planet's fastest Masters runners down the home stretch at the World Championships. But that chance at glory evaporated just seconds from the finish as I was passed by three well-pedigreed members of the sport's royalty. I travelled home with nothing.

As the setbacks mounted, I always forced myself to redouble my resolve. Always get off the mat and fight on. However, the punches were piling up. Fighting harder made each subsequent failure tougher to accept, and in the dark corner of my mind I wondered: Maybe some greater force would simply not allow me to win. Maybe it was karma for squandering my talents at a younger age. Maybe, despite all my work, I just didn't deserve it.

---

108 Kerry Sullivan is a top-notch sponsored triathlete. He's one of two athletes behind the Rock Star Triathlete Training Academy. To top it all off, he's a Massachusetts boy (Carlisle High School).

		Training Log Week 129	
Day	Date	Notes	Mileage
Thurs.	7/21/11	Back was stiff again this morning, but noticeably better than yesterday. I visited Synergy Wellness for a recovery massage with Maria Sosa. Later, I headed to a hot (90 degrees/65% humidity) Nike Run Club. I'd recently been shortening the tempo distance and upping the intensity, so I decided to start easy and slowly accelerate for the entire run. When we started, I ran the first mile with the 6-min group. Bryan and I accelerated into Mile 2. I was glad he came along because I nearly missed a key turn. With a mile to go, Bryan went his own way and I picked up the pace. I hammered the next half mile and then really hammered the last one (especially the last quarter). Unfortunately, I accidentally stopped my watch at 1.67 miles. But I was cruising and felt good. My heart rate reached 185 bpm toward the end, destroying my old record of 178. I think the trick was the gradual acceleration, which left me with enough strength to go super-lactic in the final min. I certainly felt the burn.	3.8
Fri.	7/22/11	Recovery day: 30-min elliptical.	4.9
Sat.	7/23/11	*Still* feeling the effects of overdoing it this week, so I started with a lot of skipping and dynamic stretches. Eventually, I loosened up and did a 4-mile run with 10 x 100m non-stop strides mixed in. My pace was solid. The strides were full and strong. I completed the 4-miles in 26:32 (6:38 pace).	4.5
Sun.	7/24/11	Today was my 900th straight day of training! I remember the day, 2 years ago, when I decided that I would train every day until the 2011 USATF Masters Outdoor Championships. I was running with Terry Pricher and had racked up about 50 straight days. Terry didn't like the idea because recovery days are important. But neither of us understood the power of cross-training… Today was a recovery day, starting with a 4-mile walk around South Beach. Later, I did 30 min on the elliptical at a moderate pace, plus some light weights. It was likely my last weight workout of this incredible 2-year-plus mid-life crisis. Now every time I do something, I wonder if it's the last time.	4.8
Mon.	7/25/11	Easy day: 30-min elliptical. Tomorrow will likely be my last real workout.	4.8
Tues.	7/26/11	After consulting Erik Nedeau and Moses Washington, we decided on a race simulation for the final workout. Scheduling resulted in an 11a, 92+-degree start time. I ran 1 x 400m, then 2 x 200m at race pace (or faster), w/only 45 sec rest. After a 52-sec opening 400m and a 28-sec 200m, I gutted out a 26.8-sec final 200m – easily one of the toughest workouts I've ever run. I was in pain for hours. I hoped it was a sign I was ready…	1.5
Weds.	7/27/11	Super easy 30-min elliptical. In fact, I did the workout shortly after midnight to maximize the rest time between the next session.	4.0
Total		Averaged 6:24 per mile for the week	28.2

Psychologically, I felt if anything went wrong in Ohio, there would be no getting off the mat. There would be no redoubled resolve. There would be no tomorrow. Thus, the pressure on the morning of that race was the greatest I ever felt. Physically, I was ready for anything. Mentally I was fighting a multi-nation army: the losses, disqualifications, chances for redemption. All the work. All the miles. All the people that had given so generously of themselves on my behalf. It was all I could do to hold it together.

Everything else was business as usual – maybe better than business as usual. As I expected, a lot of the big guns from Worlds elected to pass on the meet. They had peaked in mid-July, ran their best races, and were likely off enjoying barbeques and family vacations and the other things normal folk do with their summers. No Neil Fitzgerald; no Brian Sax nor Jamie Heilpern on the seed sheet. It would be me and one familiar foe: Nick Berra. I had edged Berra at Worlds, with my fourth place to his fifth place, but by the narrowest of margins – and given our track record, I knew I could not underestimate him. But I was due one more surprising challenge.

"Mark Gomes?" a lanky guy inquired, approaching me as I was taking the field to begin my warm-ups.

I had not met this runner before, but I recognized him from my pre-meet research. His name was Blair DeSio. The day before, I had watched him challenge for Nationals gold in the 400 meters against Eric Prince, arguably the most dominant Masters sprinter in the game that year. (Prince was crowned Masters 400-meter champion at Worlds and went on to win triple gold at Nationals.) DeSio showed no shortage of speed for a one-lapper, and I was about to find out what he could do for two.

"Blair DeSio," I replied. "Nice to meet you." DeSio was extremely friendly and had no idea that his mere presence was threatening my fragile psyche. I did my best to be cordial before getting back to my warm-up, but the voices from the dark corner of my mind were starting to whisper again. I shut them out and got back to my jogging, stretching, and drills.

Before I knew it, I was headed to the check-in tent, joining the six men that stood between me and my Masters dream: Dave Brown, Gary Rossen, Kenny Walker, John Zuehlke, Blair DeSio, and of course, Nicolas Berra. The officials gave us our instructions and race numbers. They escorted us to the track and up to the starting line.

It was go-time.

I was seeded second in Lane 2. As the top seed, Berra stood behind me in Lane 1. DeSio was just ahead in Lane 3. I took a knee for a moment, then stood and thought, "This is it. Run a clean race. This is it."

Without another moment to spare, the starter commanded us to our marks. He raised the gun, and fired.

With intimate knowledge of Berra's racing tactics, I expected him to start conservatively. There was a bit of a breeze, so he was unlikely to lead early. Conversely, I figured that DeSio's natural speed would take him out quickly, whether he meant it to or not. Sure enough, as we reached the 100-meter cut-in point, Berra was nowhere in sight, but DeSio and I were almost even. I eased up just enough to give him the lead. He took it and led the pack down the back straight.

It was a hot, humid 90 degrees out there. My breathing elevated a little sooner than usual, but I was ready for that because of all the heat training in Miami. We went through the first lap in 58 or 59 seconds, and it felt like a brisk jog – but that didn't necessarily leave me calm and collected; I needed to push DeSio out of his comfort zone before the final turn because I *definitely* didn't want him around for a 100-meter sprint. However, the headwind on the back straightaway had become fairly stiff. I let the tall DeSio lead for awhile longer but stayed glued to his tail. It was like running behind an 18-wheeler. Being short hadn't always been good in life, but it was good for that.

Halfway down the back stretch, I felt I'd let it go long enough. I pulled into the second lane, picked up the pace, and took the lead. I continued to push the pace until we hit the final turn. There, I eased up just a bit, saving some strength and waiting to see if anyone would challenge me wide. Nobody bit. As the final straightaway approached, I thought to myself, "Explode at the corner. Fourth gear, fifth gear, and the afterburners. Everything… Leave nothing in the tank."

The second I hit the straightaway, I took off like I was coming out of blocks. As I took that first explosive step, I caught a blur of blue in my periphery. It was Berra. As predictable as the change of seasons, he was right there with 100 meters to go.

I had a flashback to the Indoor Nationals. I called on every muscle in my body, swung my arms hard, and focused on the form that I had practiced every day since Albuquerque. In an instant, I accelerated to full speed and knew that there would be no lactic acid wall this day. The blur of blue disappeared from the corner of my eye and I was alone. Still I pressed. DeSio may still have been back there. Berra seemed to always find another gear. "Go!" I urged myself.

The finish line loomed closer.

"Go!" I commanded. Then closer… "Go, go, go!"

A step from the finish, I couldn't stand the suspense. I broke a golden rule and glanced over my right shoulder. Sure enough, Berra was close behind…but not close enough.

Still in full stride, I raised an arm to the sky. Rick Miller erupted at the edge of the track. I looked at him and waved an umpire's "safe" signal with a quizzical look. No yellow flags. No disqualification. John Cormier ran onto the track and gave me a bear hug that nearly crushed my ribs. Jamie was waiting at the exit gate near the finish. She threw her arms around my neck and burst into tears. I held her close and whispered in her ear, "It's over, baby…"

It was over. I had done it. I was a national champion.

Training Log Week 130			
Day	Date	Notes	Mileage
Thurs.	7/28/11	Jamie and I arrived at Baldwin Wallace College in Berea, OH – the proving ground for a 2 1/2-year dream. I did an easy 30-min elliptical, followed by a few strides to stay sharp. All that mattered from that point forward was rest.	
Fri.	7/29/11	Fulfilled my pledge to train every day until the 2011 Masters Outdoor Nationals: easiest possible 30-min elliptical.	
Sat.	7/30/11	2011 USATF Masters National Championships: standard warm-up plus 800 meters. First place!!!	
Sun.	7/31/11	Yesterday marked 906 days in a row of training and/or racing. Today I did nothing!	
Total		Averaged 6:24 per mile for the week	28.2

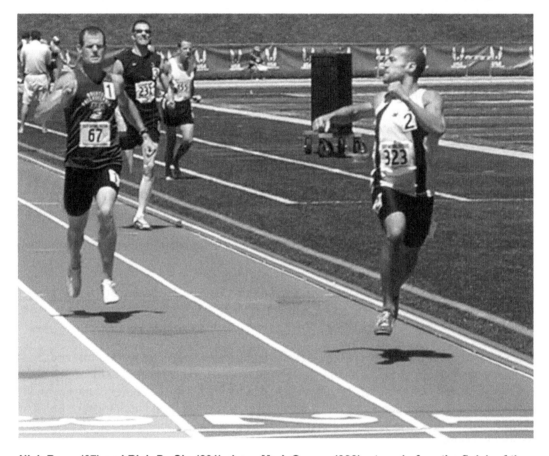

Nick Berra (67) and Blair De Sio (231) chase Mark Gomes (323), steps before the finish of the 2011 USATF Masters National Championships 800-meter run, at Baldwin Wallace College.

Chapter 15
One Year Later

The year following my championship was a good one. Jamie and I spent three months travelling Europe. (After everything I put her through, she deserved nothing less.) Thanks to modern technology, I was able to work on trains, planes, and automobiles, making the trip possible while still running my business.

We spent a week in Budapest with a new friend, Gabor Pasztor,[109] and his family. Pasztor is the mystery sprinter that appeared in my log on May 26, 2011. John Cormier befriended him and introduced me. As it turns out, Pasztor was a professional soccer player in Europe before switching to track and field. He ran 20.88 for 200 meters in March and looked poised to qualify for the Olympics before injuring his foot, just three weeks before the cutoff date.

As for my running career, after two and half years without a day off, I was ready for a long respite. The transition from hardcore training to "normal life" seemed easy. For a month it was. Then, for some reason, I stepped on the scale (probably because my clothes were all feeling tight). I was shocked to find I gained *18* pounds. It dawned on me: I had transformed my body to be as fast as I was at 16 years old, but my body wasn't 16 anymore. Being faster than forty was returning to being fatter than forty.

I estimated that I was eating about 2,000 more calories per day than I was burning. In training, my daily regimen burned 1,000 calories per day or more. Now I was burning zero. Plus, I had traded in my celery for burritos. One steak burrito with all the fixins is about 1,000 calories… 1,000 extra calories eaten, plus 1,000 fewer calories burned, equaled a 2,000-calorie difference in my lifestyle.

So much for my new culinary habits. I cut back on the fast food and took up flag football. I hadn't played in a couple of years and missed it. I found a Sunday game, and in addition to the Sunday games, I would hit the beach to play catch a couple times a week. Going deep for an hour was like running a speed workout… Pretty soon, I trimmed down, sped up, and shook off the rust.

The only problem with football was recovering from the games. I played hard and couldn't walk for days afterward. I also was getting banged up from diving, cutting, and the inevitable collisions that took place. For a non-contact sport, flag football was doing quite a number on me. After enough time away from the track, I decided to balance out the football with some running.

It was then that I remembered something: I don't like running that much. Plus, I knew if I started running on a daily basis again, I would likely reinjure myself. And I certainly didn't feel like resuming ice baths and visiting physical therapists. Then I came to a new conclusion: I didn't need running… I needed *"No Running."* I needed a daily exercise regimen that would be fun and low-impact. This would allow me to fully recover in between the football and high-intensity workouts I loved to do.

Considering my final year of training, it should have been obvious. Most of my off-days were spent on elliptical machines, just as Nick Berra spends many of his in a Hydroworx pool. A few more Internet searches validated my idea. I found out that Olympians like Galen Rupp were spending more and more time using low-impact aerobic

---

109 Pasztor returned to Miami and started a career as a personal trainer and speed coach for professional athletes. He plans to focus on the 400-meter distance going forward. Keep an eye out for him in the Diamond League meets.

techniques like underwater jogging. In fact, many of the world's top athletes are learning that aerobic conditioning is best done using low- or no-impact methods, saving their bodies for the important aspects of their training that require high levels of impact (like speed work).

I started cycling, went back to weight lifting, and eventually stumbled upon a relatively new machine called the ElliptiGO. As the name implies, the ElliptiGO is just like an elliptical machine with one critical difference... it's not stationary. The elliptical propulsion mechanism has been integrated into a bicycle frame allowing the user to simulate running without being trapped in the gym. On their Web site, I discovered a laundry list of elite athletes that use the ElliptiGO for aerobic conditioning, including numerous 800-meter and 1,500-meter runners. Distance phenom Adam Goucher was on the list. I was sold.

The No Running program has worked out great for me. Excluding the occasional 5K tempo run, I haven't gone for a jog since the 2011 Masters Nationals. Despite that, I clocked a 2:00.4 800-meters at an indoor meet in early 2012 — just two-tenths slower than I ran at the Indoor Masters Nationals the year before! I was so shocked that I was compelled to share my findings with friends, family, and anyone else that cared to read my ramblings. I launched the NO RUNNING group on Facebook: www.facebook.com/groups/NoRunning/.

Final Thoughts

Looking back on it all, it's amazing to think how much one e-mail can change a life. A few years ago, I was a weekend warrior with nagging regrets about my athletic past. A few years before that, I was a troubled substance-abusing divorcee rushing headlong toward 200 pounds (and maybe a date with an early death). Now I've never felt more comfortable in my own skin. And surrealistically, I find myself sitting in front of a computer screen putting the final touches on a book about how I became a national track and field champion.

In the end, the biggest change was mental. I was suffering from issues stemming from my youth, and eventually I sought counseling. There, I came to realize that I was the victim of psychological abuse and neglect as a child. A lack of paternal guidance my fear of making even the smallest missteps took a heavy toll. I'll be working to reverse those effects for years to come.

As a result, I now have a greater appreciation for the protection my mother tried to provide. As for my father, he was the clear source of many miseries, but he also had his own crosses to bear. Seeing or speaking with him is still uncomfortable. Thankfully, he now demonstrates some understanding of what happened on his watch and seems to accept the consequences. He respects my need for space. I'm sure he hopes that time will heal some wounds, but for now, it's far too soon to tell. There's a long road ahead, but this one's neither paved nor measurable in miles.

I hope this story inspires you to chase your dreams and put to rest any demons that may haunt your past. I will testify that the reward is well worth the countless days of effort. I no longer ponder my past. That life sentence has been commuted. Instead, I have pictures and medals and new friends... and I get to spend the rest of my life playing the memories back in my head.

What's next? I've learned not to ask, but maybe it's time to start a family. In the meantime, my teammates and I are still chasing that 4 x 800-meter world record.

All the more reason to remain faster than forty...

Epilogue

A few thoughts from Jamie...

When a person in a relationship sets about to chase a dream, it's not just that person who is tested – it is the relationship itself... even more so when the second person in the relationship has no interest in the dream at hand. I didn't grow up around runners – in high school I regarded them like choir geeks – and it was a sport I couldn't care less about. Sure, when I found myself watching a track meet once every many years I can say I thought the 200-meter or 400-meter dashes were cool to see. I mean, those guys are fast! But the rest of it, and everything that went into training for it? Not on my radar... and it still isn't.

When Mark sparked the idea of making a comeback on the track, I really didn't think much of it: neither in a good way nor bad one. What did I care if he wanted to work out really hard and eat strange combinations of foods? Although I considered it some sort of mid-life crisis, I was okay. He wasn't blowing money at strip clubs, and he didn't purchase some obnoxious car. Other women have had it worse. And when it comes to relationships, I firmly believe that each person should pursue individual goals.

But I definitely was not prepared for what Mark's goal meant when it came to our life together *and* my life on its own! I first noticed the time commitment. When he was training multiple times a day, he was gone half the time. Next came the diet. (Pause here for an eye roll and a scowl!) When Mark's training started, I was just teaching myself to cook. I am miserable at cooking and don't much enjoy it, but I was excited by the idea of creating something new, sitting down as a couple once a week, and critiquing my concoction like the hosts on Food Network. But how the hell do you make dinner for someone who was constantly changing and scrutinizing everything they ate!? Then came the talk: talk of training techniques; talk of supplements; talk of recovery; talk of workout times; talk of nutrition. All. Running. Talk. And last but not least were the physical changes. I think I now understand how men feel as they watch their pregnant wives or girlfriends grow bigger. For Mark to run at an optimal level, it meant he had to lose a *lot* of weight, but I liked some meat on him. A waistline skinnier than my own was not sexy to me.

But the physical changes Mark put himself through opened my eyes to a different point. I supported him because I knew what he was doing, but sometimes the comments we would get from friends or acquaintances were rude or ignorant. People who hadn't seen him for a while would jokingly ask if he was sick or accuse him of not eating enough in ways that just weren't funny. It didn't make sense to me. Is it appropriate in our culture to approach an overweight person in this way? Why is it okay to do this to a skinny person? We both saw a new perspective on weight and society during this period in our lives.

It's a strange thing to support someone else's dream. You lose any plans during the time frame; you lose much of your spontaneity; you lose a part of you; you lose a part of him or her. If there hadn't been an end goal in sight, I don't know that I would have made it. I tried my hardest to be supportive at meets I attended although they were *beyond* not fun for me. Anyone who has spent time with an athlete knows that before a big event, the athlete goes into a zone where everything and everyone becomes non-existent. But I was nervous and proud during each race that I watched.

The U.S. Masters National Championship, the race that prompted it all, was overwhelming. I kept thinking, "What if he doesn't win...what then?" I think our friends and family feared the same thing, but for *my* sanity as much as his! When he crossed the finish line in first place, my tears definitely fell. Tears because he reached his goal – because he won for himself but also because he won for us. We had both sacrificed for that moment. And going onto the track to hug him as he cried his own tears of joy was a moment that made it all worth it. Despite my lack of interest in the sport of track and field, I love Mark and was in his corner every step of the way.

During his two-plus years of training, I became deeply thankful for Mark's track buddies because as he began to realize how much I hated everything running-related, he talked to me about it less and talked to them more. But apparently I will never escape all the talk of diet, supplements and training. (Hell, I know so much about it now, I could probably tell you what you are doing wrong in your own training.) People call our house on a regular basis for Mark's advice on how to train better. They come over to use his recovery equipment, to join him in workouts, and to use our gym. Helping others in the track world actually brings Mark a lot of happiness. And I have come to learn that runners are almost incapable of talking about anything besides running.

I tried running for a spell. I gave it a true and honest go; Mark even writes about it in this book. I did a few speed workouts and even some drills. In the end, it wasn't my thing. I believe in being physically strong, and I have embraced other healthy habits I absorbed by witnessing Mark's training routine, but – and he will second this notion – I believe to succeed you have to find a fitness program that works for you, and running wasn't it for me.

Mark was not blind to my sacrifices. He supports my interests now in a different way than perhaps he would have before this journey began. And I will remind him of this journey on the occasions when he wants to kill me for bringing home yet another pet or – should we decide to have children – when my belly expands at the same rate at which his shrunk. (And I will remind him that that too shall pass.)

Lastly, I have mastered the art of tuning out. So if you ever see me at a meet or a running club meet-up and I appear to be involved in a running/training/diet/supplement conversation, you might catch on that my mind is somewhere far, far away. Don't take it personally.

Credits

Photo Editor: Seth Kane

Cover Design & Illustrations: Joyce Hansen

Interior Design: Rick Miller

CPSIA information can be obtained at www.ICGtesting.com
Printed in the USA
LVOW02*0401271014

410601LV00013B/61/P